Applied Home Hemodialysis

Ankur Shah • Anjay Rastogi
Edgar V. Lerma
Editors

Applied Home Hemodialysis

A Clinical Guide

Springer

Editors
Ankur Shah
Warren Alpert Medical School
Brown University
Providence, RI, USA

Anjay Rastogi
UCLA Medical Center
Los Angeles, CA, USA

Edgar V. Lerma
Section of Nephrology
University of Illinois at Chicago/Advocate
Christ Medical Center
Oak Lawn, IL, USA

ISBN 978-3-031-77243-6 ISBN 978-3-031-77244-3 (eBook)
https://doi.org/10.1007/978-3-031-77244-3

This Springer imprint is published by the registered company Springer Nature Switzerland AG
The registered company address is: Gewerbestrasse 11, 6330 Cham, Switzerland

To my many mentors at Temple University Hospital, the Hospital of the University of Pennsylvania, and the Warren Alpert Medical School at Brown University who have molded me into the physician I am today, who have challenged me to think critically, encouraged me to pursue excellence, and inspired me to make a difference.

To my wife Courtney, my soulmate and guiding light. Your unwavering support has been the foundation of my success; your love has been my greatest inspiration. This book is dedicated to you, my love, for always believing in me and encouraging me to reach new heights.

Ankur Shah, MD

To all my mentors and friends at the University of Santo Tomas, Faculty of Medicine and Surgery in Manila, Philippines, and Northwestern University Feinberg School of Medicine in Chicago, IL, who have, in one way or another, influenced and guided me to become the physician that I am today.

To all the medical students, interns, and residents at Advocate Christ Medical Center, whom I have taught or learned from, especially those who eventually decided to pursue nephrology as a career.

To my parents and my brothers, without whose unwavering love and support through the good and bad times, I would not have persevered and reached my goals in life. Most especially to my two lovely and precious daughters, Anastasia Zofia and Isabella Ann, whose smiles and laughter constantly provide me unparalleled joy and happiness, and my very loving and understanding wife, Michelle, who has always been supportive of my endeavors both personally and professionally and who sacrificed a lot of time and exhibited unwavering patience as I devoted a significant amount of time and effort to this project. Truly, they provide me with motivation and inspiration.

Edgar V. Lerma, MD

Preface

In the evolving landscape of kidney replacement therapy, home hemodialysis (HHD) stands out as a modality that offers patients unprecedented control over their treatment and quality of life, yet remains underutilized. This comprehensive guide aims to illuminate the multifaceted world of home hemodialysis, providing health-care professionals, patients, and caregivers with the knowledge and tools necessary to navigate this empowering treatment option.

The journey of home hemodialysis is marked by both challenges and remarkable opportunities. As we explore its history, clinical outcomes, and practical implementation, we unveil a treatment modality that has the potential to revolutionize the way we approach kidney failure management. From improved cardiovascular outcomes to enhanced fertility options, the benefits of home hemodialysis extend far beyond the mere filtration of blood.

Applied home hemodialysis delves into the core aspects of HHD, beginning with the crucial decision-making process of dialysis modality selection and progressing through the intricacies of patient training, home preparation, and program development. We examine the many benefits of the modality and then delve into unique considerations and benefits for different populations, including pediatric patients, pregnant persons, and elderly patients, as well as the international applications and barriers to widespread adoption. As we face global challenges such as pandemics and environmental concerns, the relevance of home-based therapies has never been more apparent. This volume addresses these timely issues, offering insights into disaster management strategies and the concept of "green nephrology" within the context of home hemodialysis.

The authors contributing to this work represent a diverse array of experts in the field, bringing together decades of clinical experience, research, and patient-centered care. Their collective wisdom provides a balanced view of the promise of home hemodialysis, ensuring that readers are well-equipped to make informed decisions and provide optimal care. This book would not have been possible without the guidance and help of an amazing team at Springer Nature, including Hannah Campeanu, Janakiraman Ganesan, Margaret Moore, Ameena Qotbray, Jananee Ravichandran, and Anila Vijayan.

This book is intended for a diverse array of audiences, including both novice and experienced nephrologists who specialize in home hemodialysis, as well as internists, fellows, residents, and medical students. We also hope that people living with kidney disease and their advocates will find empowerment in our text. It is our hope that this comprehensive resource will serve as a catalyst for the continued growth and improvement of home hemodialysis programs worldwide, ultimately leading to better outcomes and enhanced quality of life for individuals living with kidney disease.

Providence, RI, USA — Ankur Shah
Los Angeles, CA, USA — Anjay Rastogi
Berwyn, IL, USA — Edgar V. Lerma

Contents

Contributors

Graham Edwin Abra Division of Nephrology, Department of Medicine, Stanford University School of Medicine, Stanford, CA, USA

Rebecca S. Ahdoot Division of Nephrology, Department of Medicine, University of California Irvine Medical Center, Orange, CA, USA

Maroun Azar Division of Kidney Disease and Hypertension, Brown Medicine, Warren Alpert Medical School of Brown University, Providence, RI, USA

Stephanie Braunthal Division of Obstetric Medicine, Department of Medicine, Warren Alpert Medical School of Brown University, Providence, RI, USA

Christopher T. Chan Division of Nephrology, University Health Network, Toronto and the University of Toronto, Toronto, ON, Canada

Kenneth K. Chen Division of Obstetric Medicine, Department of Medicine, Warren Alpert Medical School of Brown University, Providence, RI, USA

Justin Cheng Division of Nephrology, University Health Network, Toronto and the University of Toronto, Toronto, ON, Canada

David Clark Department of Medicine, Dalhousie University and Nova Scotia Health, Halifax, NS, Canada

Division of Nephrology, Nova Scotia Health, Halifax, NS, Canada

Gates B. Colbert Texas A&M College of Medicine, Dallas, TX, USA

Joel D. Glickman Perelman School of Medicine, University of Pennsylvania, Philadelphia, PA, USA

Gopa Green US Renal Care, Plano, TX, USA

Nupur Gupta Division of Nephrology, Indiana University School of Medicine, Indianapolis, IN, USA

Heedeok Han Division of Nephrology, Columbia University Medical Center, New York, NY, USA

Ramy M. Hanna Division of Nephrology, Department of Medicine, University of California Irvine Medical Center, Orange, CA, USA

Daljit K. Hothi Department of Pediatric Nephrology, Great Ormond Street Hospital, London, UK

Wael F. Hussein Department of Medicine, Division of Nephrology, Stanford University School of Medicine, Stanford, CA, USA

Shivam Joshi Division of Nephrology, Department of Medicine, Orlando VA Medical Center, Orlando, FL, USA

Kamyar Kalantar-Zadeh The Lundquist Institute at Harbor-UCLA Medical Center, Torrance, CA, USA

Tibor Rubin VA Healthcare System, Long Beach, CA, USA

Sean Kalloo Division of Nephrology, Department of Medicine, Columbia University Medical Center, New York, NY, USA

Department of Radiology, Columbia University Irving Medical Center, College of Physicians and Surgeons, New York, NY, USA

Edgar V. Lerma Section of Nephrology, University of Illinois at Chicago/Advocate Christ Medical Center, Oak Lawn, IL, USA

Matthew R. Lynch Department of Medicine, Warren Alpert Medical School of Brown University, Providence, RI, USA

Division of Nephrology, Brown Medicine, Providence, RI, USA

Iona Madden Department of Pediatric Nephrology, Great Ormond Street Hospital, London, UK

Brent Miller Division of Nephrology, Indiana University School of Medicine, Indianapolis, IN, USA

John Moran Department of Medicine, Division of Nephrology, Stanford University School of Medicine, Stanford, CA, USA

Elaine Phua Department of Renal Medicine, Royal North Shore Hospital, St Leonards, NSW, Australia

Carol Pollock Department of Renal Medicine, Royal North Shore Hospital, St Leonards, NSW, Australia

University of Sydney, Camperdown, NSW, Australia

Kolling Institute of Medical Research, St Leonards, NSW, Australia

Sindhuri Prakash-Polet Department of Medicine, Division of Nephrology, Columbia University Irving Medical Center, College of Physicians and Surgeons, New York, NY, USA

Anjay Rastogi UCLA Medical Center, Los Angeles, CA, USA

Ankur Shah Warren Alpert Medical School, Brown University, Providence, RI, USA

Yvonne Shen Department of Renal Medicine, Royal North Shore Hospital, St Leonards, NSW, Australia

University of Sydney, Camperdown, NSW, Australia

Sydney Dialysis Centre, St Leonards, NSW, Australia

Rachel Shi University of Central Florida, College of Medicine, Orlando, FL, USA

Karthik Tennankore Department of Medicine, Dalhousie University and Nova Scotia Health, Halifax, NS, Canada

Division of Nephrology, Nova Scotia Health, Halifax, NS, Canada

Jordan Thorne Department of Medicine, Dalhousie University and Nova Scotia Health, Halifax, NS, Canada

Bradley A. Warady Children's Mercy Kansas City, Kansas City, MO, USA

Hannah Webb Division of Nephrology, Indiana University School of Medicine, Indianapolis, IN, USA

Tanuja Yalamarti Division of Critical Care, Department of Medicine, Stanford University School of Medicine, Stanford, CA, USA

Samiya Yasin Division of Nephrology, Baylor University Medical Center, Dallas, TX, USA

Shahrzad Zonoozi Virginia Nephrology Group, Arlington, VA, USA

Home Dialysis: Dialysis Modality Selection

1

Samiya Yasin and Gates B. Colbert

Introduction

For many patients, the progression of kidney disease will be inevitable. As eGFR begins to fall below 15 ml/min/1.73, chronic kidney disease (CKD) progresses to stage G5, and dialysis or kidney replacement therapy (KRT) will need to be discussed. Once below an eGFR of 15 ml/min/1.73, the kidneys are unable to adequately clear uremic toxins and fluid to balance euvolemia [1]. Timing of when KRT will need to begin is highly variable and can range from weeks to possibly 1–2 years [2]. Ideally, these patients are already in an established nephrology CKD clinic where these vital discussions and planning can occur. The guidance of the nephrologist and nephrology team can help a patient avoid KRT as long as possible, while simultaneously planning for what will likely result in the future. This is a scenario where the best laid plans can truly optimize a patient and their families' expectations and improve outcomes.

Dialysis modality selection is critical for a patient and their caregivers to determine the need for the beginning of KRT and is a best practice for improving the experience while also optimizing cost [3]. Patients who begin to need KRT can choose from in-center hemodialysis (iHD), the most common modality in the United States, or home dialysis therapy. Home therapy comes in two varieties of peritoneal dialysis (PD) or home hemodialysis (HHD) (see Fig. 1.1). The selection of which therapy the patient should begin with is unique to each individual patient. Lifestyle expectations and realities are important to explain and educate prior to treatment selection. Surgical procedures will need to be planned: on the abdomen in

S. Yasin
Division of Nephrology, Baylor University Medical Center, Dallas, TX, USA
e-mail: Samiya.Yasin@BSWHealth.org

G. B. Colbert (✉)
Texas A&M College of Medicine, Dallas, TX, USA
e-mail: Gates.Colbert@BSWHealth.org

A. Shah et al. (eds.), *Applied Home Hemodialysis*,
https://doi.org/10.1007/978-3-031-77244-3_1

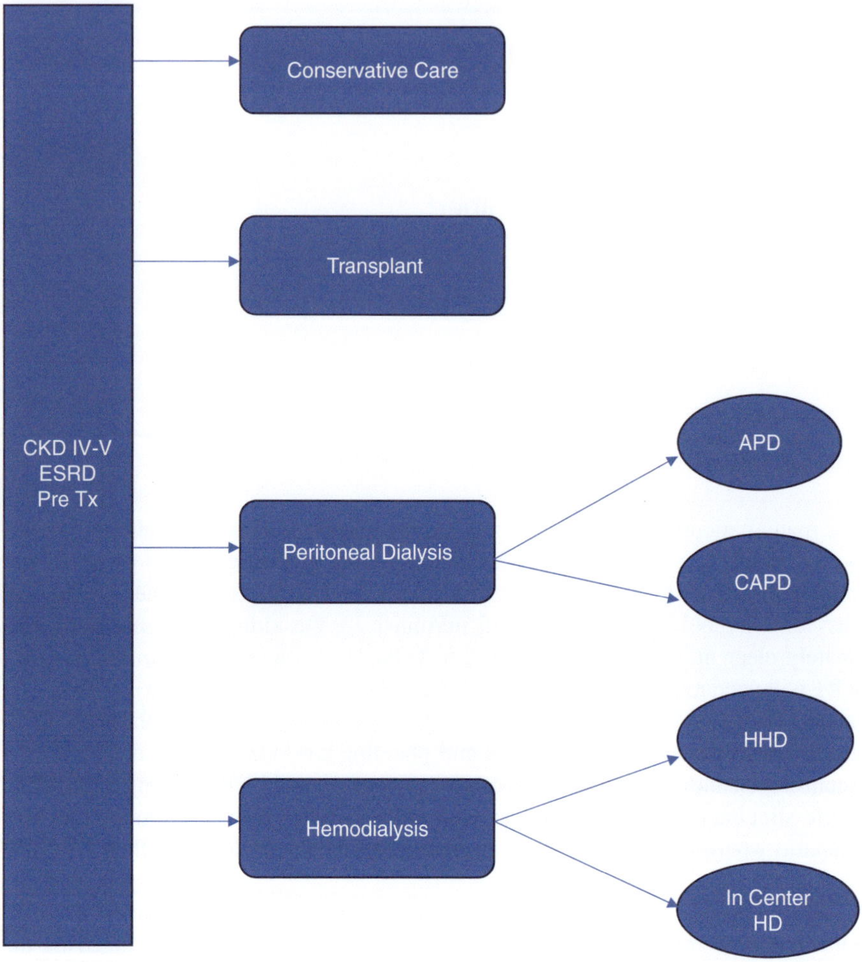

Fig. 1.1 Types of renal replacement therapy. *APD* automated peritoneal dialysis, *CAPD* continuous ambulatory peritoneal dialysis, *HHD* home hemodialysis

PD or on the arm if choosing hemodialysis for the placement of an arteriovenous graft (AVG) or arteriovenous fistula (AVF). As well, patients should have real-time education to not only raise awareness of their options, but also clear up misconceptions that may be based on previous family or friend experiences.

Dialysis Modalities

We will start with the treatment choice that most patients in the United States are currently receiving iHD [4]. Unfortunately, many patients do not have adequately planned dialysis education and selection and end up on this treatment modality as it is the most universally available and requires the least amount of preparation. iHD is a treatment modality that uses a semipermanent catheter in the chest or groin, or an AVG or AVF in the arm for dialysis access. Blood is removed from the patient using one of these options and is processed through a hemodialysis machine and returned to the patient. The blood is cleaned of uremic toxins, electrolytes, and drugs/medications while simultaneously removing excess fluid from the patient. The process lasts between 3.5 and 4 h per treatment and is usually performed 3 times per week at the hemodialysis center. This modality takes the least amount of patient time for treatment and is performed in a highly regulated and clean facility.

Patients enjoy a number of benefits from choosing iHD as their modality choice. First, it is the most hands-off healthcare treatment with the ability to receive dialysis treatments, vital medications, mineral replacements such as iron or vitamin D, and education from staff in real time. This is the most face-to-face time with medical professionals that a patient will have among the treatment options. Patients will be seen by a nurse and a patient care technician who perform their treatments and assure that all steps necessary to make the dialysis treatment safe and effective are taken. As well, they will have face-to-face contact with their nephrologist or provider between 2 and 4 times per month. Comradery among other patients receiving the exact same treatments cannot be understated as a community feeling can be achieved in many units. Downsides exist to this frequent treatment in a facility that should be considered. Frequency of exposure to other patients with chronic medical illnesses can pose a health risk to the treating patient. Patients may have to miss work, school, or family activities while they are away receiving treatment. It should be addressed as well that patients must adhere to the schedule they are assigned, with the expectation that moving their assigned time slot should be rare. Furthermore, the medical benefits of other dialysis schedules are not afforded to patients receiving thrice-weekly hemodialysis. Even still, the majority of patients in the United States receive iHD because of the comprehensive care it provides with the least amount of patient and caregiver support required.

Next, we will move to PD, which is a home therapy and the second most common modality in the United States and performed in approximately 11% of end-stage kidney disease (ESKD) patients [5]. Yet, PD is the most common modality choice in many countries around the world. PD is performed completely differently than the HD treatments. A catheter is placed in the abdomen in the peritoneal catheter that extends outside the abdominal wall. A patient will inflow a dialysate solution that will instill in their abdomen for 2–4 h before it is completely drained into a waste bag. This dwelling state occurs for multiple treatments, and it can be done with a manual exchange process or completed using a cycling (cycler) machine. Most patients at home use a cycler machine that performs these exchanges for the patient over a 10- to 12-h process. Many patients choose their treatment time to be overnight while they are sleeping as it is a very comfortable and perfunctory process. The dialysate fluid removes almost the exact same toxins and minerals as iHD, and can be titrated to remove excess fluid from the body through concentration gradient removal [5].

Many benefits exist with choosing PD as the modality choice for KRT. First, the patient may do all of their treatments in their own home at the daily schedule of their choosing. Patients usually only need to see their nephrologist and dialysis treatment team once a month, as compared to iHD which requires 3x per week visit to the dialysis center. Travel freedom is a commonly heralded positive as the patient can take their PD supplies and perform treatment while on vacation or visiting family in another state or possibly country. Patients also describe their empowerment they feel with performing their treatments and being an integral team member of their own health which allows for improved self-actualization with their condition. Drawbacks do occur, with the most unfortunate reality that the vast majority of patients on PD will not be able to stay on treatment, and will move to HD modality within a few years as their peritoneal membrane becomes insufficient. Patients also have to perform as their own nurse and technician, as the treatments are performed at home without physical healthcare worker help [6]. Additionally, patients may have a higher risk of infection if sterile technique performing the procedure or storing supplies [7, 8]. The patient and their family will also be responsible for maintaining and housing the equipment and medical supplies which may disrupt balance or use of their spaces.

A hybrid between the two modalities above, and one that is growing rapidly in the United States, is HHD. The name exactly describes what occurs with treatment and is currently being encouraged by Centers for Medicare [9] as a modality that should be considered on a greater scale. HHD is very similar to the hemodialysis procedure that is performed in-center, but is entirely completed by the patient and their caregiver at home. Most patients use an AVG/AVF for cannulation and are educated on successful and safe technique. Treatment can be the same amount of time or more, but usually is performed more frequently than 3 days per week. Patients can do more treatments per week to optimize fluid removal, and potentially mimic the kidneys which never take off days in normal function. In fact, one of the benefits of home dialysis is the avoidance of the unphysiology of thrice-weekly hemodialysis. Some patients also will choose to perform nocturnal hemodialysis where they use low flows on the machine for extended times of 8–10 h nightly.

There are many benefits to choosing this option for patients which will be elaborated in this text [10]. Performing treatments in your own home environment provides the same lifestyle benefits of doing PD modality. Patients limit office or clinic visits with the nephrology team to once a month, which is very helpful for those with limited mobility or transportation difficulties. Patients are doing dialysis more frequently than iHD which allows for a more physiologic removal of fluid and uremic toxins. Outcomes are better for patients on HHD [11], but this should be recognized as a possible result of bias given that "healthier" and motivated patients are usually preferred for this treatment modality. There is also an ability to limit contact with other patients in center who may have chronic or contagious illness, which can be a benefit for those that are immunocompromised. Downsides also exist as with every treatment modality choice. Treatments must be performed and monitored by the patient themselves or a caregiver, and family support can be critical to perform the treatment safely [12]. Cannulating with large bore needles and bleeding-prone

AVG/AVF can present dangers and risks if vigilance is not performed with every treatment. Storage of supplies and medical equipment is also required, similar to PD, which can disrupt home space usage and does require a monitored threshold of cleanliness and sterility. Additionally, as of this writing not all insurance options are available for this treatment and can vary by state within the United States or country.

Kidney Transplantation

The ultimate goal for most patients with advanced CKD is to avoid dialysis therapies altogether and receive a kidney transplant. Most patients will need to start on a dialysis modality, as the waitlist for a deceased donor kidney is several years in most states. Living donor kidney transplant organs that come from family or friends can allow patients to have a short wait time and also have better long-term outcomes. In short, a kidney transplant comes from a human donor, for now, and this "spare" kidney is surgically placed in the lower abdomen attaching to one of the great vessels [13]. The native kidneys are left in place to avoid complications of removal, and the new kidney performs the function of both together. Patients will need to take medications orally or by IV for the life of the kidney to prevent rejection, and most kidneys can last between 10 and 25 years. Patients with high-quality matched kidneys and who are excellent at maintaining their medications and follow-up surveillance have the highest chance of their new organ last a decade or longer. As medication regimens narrow and become more precise, we are seeing organ transplant have better life spans and fewer infectious complications of the transplant recipients.

The positive impact of receiving a kidney transplant and stopping dialysis completely cannot be understated. Many kidney transplant recipients preach that they feel they have "new life" and a freedom restored that they enjoyed prior to needing KRT. The patients are better able to maintain their electrolyte and fluid balance, require potentially fewer medications, and improve bone and mineral health after a kidney transplant. As well, daily or every other day treatments of dialysis are no longer required. Additionally, cardiac benefits exist with improved mortality rates [14]. The negative side of a transplant still exists, particularly when contrasted to the general population, despite a patient no longer requiring dialysis. Maintenance immunosuppressive medications will be required multiple times per day for the life of the kidney [15]. Patients are at higher risk for infection and cancer given the current medication regimen required. As well, any previous cardiovascular or bone comorbidities that may have occurred during advanced CKD or dialysis therapy cannot be reversed. Despite these drawbacks, receiving a kidney transplant is the highest level of improvement that a CKD patient can undergo to restore kidney function to normal.

Many patients choose not to undergo dialysis therapy completely, and instead choose conservative care [16]. This means the patient will accept medication and lifestyle management, but ultimately will not undergo machine therapy for prolonged life. This can be a higher quality experience for many patients who accept their mortality and ultimately choose the way that they will pass on [17]. Hospice and palliative programs are readily available to care for patients over the weeks to years that this process can progress. Additionally, many patients are not surgical candidates for a kidney transplant and thus must choose between ongoing dialysis therapy and moving to conservative management. This topic is beyond the full scope of this chapter, but is a subject that should be offered and encouraged in the right settings for patients or when they are ready to make a modality shift to conservative care.

Patient Goals and Priorities Assessment

SONG-PD, Patient Goals

Unfortunately, there is a lack of PD trials on person-centered outcomes based on patient preferences including ability to work, travel, and other dimensions of quality of life and this literature gap extends to HHD. The available trials have significant heterogeneity in measured and reported outcomes, as well as reporting bias which diminishes their reliability and validity. To address these concerns, one of the global initiatives, the Standardized Outcomes in Nephrology (SONG) initiative, aims to establish core outcome domains and outcome measures across the full spectrum of CKD [18]. We extrapolate those findings to HHD as they are the strongest evidence of patient priorities in the home.

The specific aims of Standardized Outcomes in Nephrology-Peritoneal Dialysis (SONG-PD) are to:

1. Describe the scope, quality, and consistency of outcomes used in PD trials
2. Identify outcomes that are important to patients and caregivers
3. Ascertain health professional attitudes, values, and beliefs regarding outcomes for PD trials
4. Generate a consensus-based prioritized list of core outcome domains
5. Establish a set of core outcome domains for trials conducted in people on PD [18]

SONG-PD uses a validated, robust, and systematic approach to develop a consensus-based prioritized set of core outcome domains to be reported in all trials in patients on PD. Once the SONG-PD core outcome domains have been established, the Outcome Measures Rheumatoid Arthritis Clinical Trials (OMERACT) filter will be used to identify or develop core outcome measures to ensure that measures are truthful, discriminative, and feasible [19]. Additionally, guidelines developed jointly by the Core Outcome Measures in Effectiveness Trials (COMET) and Consensus-based Standards for the Selection of Health Measurement Instruments (COSMIN) initiatives on methods for selecting outcome measures for core outcome domains will also be utilized [20]. To facilitate the translation of the core outcomes into trials and research, national and international stakeholders will be consulted and dissemination strategies will be developed. The impact of SONG-PD on improving the consistency of reporting directly meaningful outcomes across trials will be assessed. Ultimately, the implementation of a consensus-based set of high-priority outcome domains will enable patients and their clinicians to make informed decisions about treatment.

Medical Considerations (e.g., Patient's Health Status, Comorbidities)

As advances have been made in KRT, the patient population initiating treatment has become older and often has several comorbid conditions that become the major determinants of survival. Improvements in outcomes for patients with ESKD will depend in part on improvements in KRT itself, but also on the better understanding and management of those conditions which coexist that become the primary determinants of outcomes. The most important cardiovascular abnormalities in ESKD are ischemic heart disease, left ventricular hypertrophy (LVH), congestive heart failure, hypertension, and peripheral vascular disease. Chronic inflammation, insulin resistance, elevated calcium, phosphate products, and oxidative stress all constitute additional risk factors which are brought on by the condition of uremia. As is true in the non-uremic population, LVH is a risk factor for mortality in the dialysis population. Hypertension can be both a cause of kidney failure and a frequent com plication of CKD. However, several studies have demonstrated that low blood pressure is an important risk factor for higher mortality in dialysis patients [21, 22]. In all registries, the coexistence of diabetes is noted to have a negative impact on survival at all ages [23, 24]. The most commonly seen indicators of having a poor outcome in ESKD are increasing age, cardiovascular disease, diabetes, and poor nutrition as reflected by hypoalbuminemia.

Ever since the United States Congress approved Medicare coverage for ESKD treatment in 1972, dialysis gradually evolved toward a first-line treatment option for patients with ESKD, including elderly persons and individuals with debilitating comorbidity. This led to a fourfold increase in ESKD incidence over the last 3 decades, including a 13-fold increase among patients aged >75 years [25]. The ESKD care, which is mainly disease-centered and (dialysis) process-driven, may not be beneficial and may be potentially harmful or impractical for certain subpopulations [26]. Dialysis patients are frequently hospitalized, on average 11.8 days per year [27]. Chronic pain, fatigue, cognitive impairment, and depression are present in up to half of patients with ESKD [28, 29]. Twenty-five percent of 70-year-old patients starting dialysis in the United States survive <9 months, whereas 25% survive for >4 years. The survival benefit of dialysis treatment may be limited for patients with advanced comorbidities or ischemic heart disease [30, 31].

The best attainable goal is the deferment of morbidity and mortality and an improvement or maintenance of quality of life [32, 33]. Although the risks and burdens of many healthcare interventions are immediate, the benefits may be delayed or may not even materialize for patients with a poor prognosis [33–35]. Consequently, life expectancy is an important element of the risk/benefit profile of most dialysis-related interventions [23]. Moreover, the most appropriate care for patients with complex multimorbidities, as is the case for many dialysis patients, may differ substantially from the sum of the most appropriate care strategies of each discrete condition [24]. The underlying comorbid conditions may also influence the dialysis modality of choice. Patients with cognitive impairment or coagulopathies may not be a candidate for home-based therapies. Some medical comorbidities may further restrict the choice of PD including inflammatory abdominal disease, unrepaired/irreparable hernia, and ostomies or feeding tubes.

Lifestyle Considerations (e.g., Work, Family Commitments, Travel)

According to the EPOCH-RRT study, the inclusion of patients' priorities in the choice of dialysis treatment improves outcomes [36]. Home-based treatments (HHD and PD) merge flexibility, deliver a higher weekly dialysis dose, and require and value patient participation, and what is now called "patient activation," which is associated with a higher quality of life and better survival with a lower burden for society [37, 38]. Patients who are working may choose home-based therapies like automated peritoneal dialysis (APD) which will provide minimal interference with their work during the day. Some patients may continue to work from home while on HHD. Home-based therapies give flexibility to patients to plan changes in the dialysis schedules and make up dialysis sessions for upcoming travel. Patients can continue their PD while traveling as well. The dialysis solution and the supplies can be delivered to the destination or can be taken by the patient themselves. Similarly, some home HD machines are portable and can travel. Home dialysis involves family members and/or caregivers who became valuable allies in providing adequate patient care. Involvement in patient care can be rewarding, but this workload can overburden caregivers and patients, inducing depression, frustration, and, in some cases, even financial burdens [39, 40]. Hence, it is important to jointly make decisions regarding schedules to improve adherence and prevent dropouts.

Psychosocial Factors

Stressors in the life of a dialysis patient can include dietary and time constraints, functional limitations, loss of employment, changes in self-perception, alterations in sexual function, and fear of death. The demands of ESKD treated with hemodialysis include potential changes in a patient's status in marital, familial, occupational, and societal contexts; the expenses and worries associated with the treatment and the illness, and the uncertainty, anxiety, and costs entailed while waiting for a kidney transplant. In addition, treatment within a unit implies a complex relationship with dialysis personnel: physicians, nurses, technicians, and other staff. Adaptive coping can produce desired outcomes—full employment and successful function within a dyad and family. In the absence of such coping, disability and marital and family dysfunction can occur, as well as depression, anxiety, loss of one's role and identity, and development or worsening of alcohol and substance abuse.

"Psychosocial parameters" include the vast number of psychological variables and aspects of the social environment that affect all of us and are central to the patient's perception of quality of life. These parameters include individual demographic data (age, ethnicity, gender), physiologic measures (body mass index; cardiovascular, immunologic, and conditioning status), psychological and behavioral parameters (distress, personality factors, health-promoting or health-damaging habits), and social or environmental factors (e.g., occupational imperatives, level of social support, access to health care, residential characteristics, and socioeconomic status). Patient-level psychosocial parameters include personality factors, affect, and perceptions of distress, well-being, or illness; patient/spouse indices include marital satisfaction; and patient/physician/dialysis staff measures include satisfaction with health care, compliance with the dialysis regimen, and level, number, and quality of interactions with personnel and staff. Psychosocial factors might affect mortality outcomes through at least four mechanisms: access to health care, compliance with the dialysis prescription or medication regimen, nutritional status, and neuroendocrine or immunologic function [41–43].

Economic and Logistical Considerations

Dialysis therapy consumes up to 5–7% of total healthcare budgets, despite the fact that kidney failure affects only 0.1–0.2% of the general population in most regions [44]. Kidney transplantation is the most cost-effective choice of KRT. Although societal costs for out-of-center dialysis (e.g., home or self-care hemodialysis, or PD) are in general lower than those for iHD, these options are often underutilized [45] adding to the rising costs of dialysis. The economic impacts of ESKD and dialysis are significant. A large proportion of the impact is due to incurred healthcare costs for managing clinical complexity, comorbidities, loss of productivity, and associated premature mortality. From a societal perspective, ESKD affects the patient, caregiver, employer, and healthcare system. Patients with ESKD must manage direct costs of medical procedures, diagnostics, laboratory tests, medications, vaccinations, healthcare provider visits, hospitalizations, dialysis, transportation to and from appointments, and absenteeism from work due to these factors. With varying modalities for dialysis, including the option for more frequent home-based dialysis, the complexity of patient and caregiver burdens is high; especially as in varying instances, those caregivers may be unpaid family compared to paid caregivers in other instances.

Patients on dialysis are often unemployed, but not by their own choice. In the United States, >75% of patients are unemployed at the start of dialysis, compared with <20% in the general population [46]. Unemployment affects not only purchasing power but also lifestyle, self-image, and mental health. Moreover, loss of productivity owing to unemployment and/or the premature death of workers with kidney failure also has economic consequences for society [47]. Notably, patients receiving home dialysis are more often able to work, likely related to the flexibility afforded by their dialysis modality and reductions in time spent in dialysis units and with post-dialysis fatigue [4].

Managing Work and Social Life

An individual's social network, social integration, and social support are important determinants of health-related outcomes [48]. Dialysis and transplant patients are encouraged to return to work once their condition stabilizes. Support and encouragement at home and from the healthcare team are important. iHD patients should request a dialysis schedule that fits best with their work schedule. Many people who work prefer dialyzing at night because they sleep after dialysis and wake up feeling refreshed. Most dialysis units will make it a priority to schedule employed patients on a convenient shift.

Family Planning and Pregnancy

The pregnancy rate of women on dialysis is still very low when compared to that of the remaining population. According to the literature, there has been an increase in the success rate of these pregnancies, from 25% in the 1980s to more than 90% recently [49]. Most patients on dialysis have sexual dysfunction, amenorrhea, anovulatory cycles, decreased libido, polypharmacy, and depression [50, 51]. However, improvement in the adequacy of dialysis techniques and pharmacological and nutritional approaches for pregnant women on dialysis has provided a significant increase in quality of life and an increase in pregnancy success rates [51]. It was noted in various analysis that the pregnancy rate is lower among patients on PD compared to those on hemodialysis [52, 53]. Pregnancies that begin before the dialysis period or in the first year of it have more chances of reaching a favorable term, when compared to those from women who become pregnant after a considerable period on dialysis [51]. Some authors suggest that this fact can be explained by the greater fertility in women with previous residual kidney function [50].

Both hemodialysis and PD can be substituting therapy options in pregnancy. There are studies with similar outcomes with both techniques [52, 53]. The treatment modality should not be changed with the onset of pregnancy; however, if urgent start is necessary, it may be easier to start with hemodialysis, since the insertion of a Tenckhoff PD catheter in any period of pregnancy increases the risk of miscarriage [53]. The advantages of hemodialysis in pregnancy include less dietary and water restriction and less fluid overload; however, the cons include worse metabolic control with intermittent hemodialysis, need for anticoagulation, more hemodynamic instability, and less autonomy. The advantages of PD include better metabolic control, no need for anticoagulation, lower risk of hemodynamically instability, and preservation of residual function. The cons with PD include increased risk of infectious complications, intrauterine growth restriction, difficulty managing volume, and increased frequency of exchanges.

Despite all the progress made in this field, most newborns are premature, and maternal-fetal complications, such as gestational hypertension, anemia, infections, polyhydramnios, and fetal growth restrictions, are frequent [53]. Safe and effective contraception should be made available to women who wish to delay or avoid pregnancy and those who take teratogenic medications. It is of paramount importance that pregnancies in this high-risk population are planned, allowing the opportunity to counsel women about the impact of pregnancy on kidney disease and the impact of kidney disease on maternal and fetal outcomes.

The decision to proceed with or delay conception is highly individualized and is affected by the baseline health of the woman, the woman's age and comorbid conditions, and the anticipated wait time for a donor kidney, if applicable. Contraceptive decision-making therefore needs to balance patient acceptability and safety. Estrogen-containing methods, including oral pills, the transdermal patch, and vaginal rings, are less preferred in patients with ESKD because of the markedly increased cardiovascular risk in patients with ESKD and their association with increased blood pressure and thrombotic and vascular events. For women receiving dialysis, progesterone-only methods have a better safety profile, including the progesterone-only pill (desogestrel preparations), the levonorgestrel-releasing intrauterine devices, and the etonogestrel implant.

Travel Considerations

For many people who are on dialysis or have had a kidney transplant, the ability to travel is important to their self-esteem and lifestyle. This may include travel for business meetings, conferences or travel for leisure, or a family event such as a wedding. Most people who receive dialysis or have had a kidney transplant can travel safely and continue their treatment while away from home. Many dialysis centers have a staff member who is experienced in arranging dialysis treatments away from home (transient dialysis). Planning and arrangements should start 6–8 weeks prior. Resources are available to find dialysis centers around the world that are willing to accept transient dialysis patients.

Most HHD patients arrange for in-center treatments while traveling; however, those who wish to continue doing their own treatment should get approval from their dialysis care team to do home dialysis away from. Patients may choose to travel with their machines, supplies, and portable water treatment equipment. For example, some people use specially equipped travel trailers and do hemodialysis in campsites that have hook-ups for water and electricity.

Traveling is often easier for PD patients because they are not dependent on the availability of a dialysis center. Continuous ambulatory peritoneal dialysis (CAPD) patients carry supplies for the length of the trip or may also arrange for supplies to be delivered to a hotel or home at destination. Airlines make special rooms available for patients to perform CAPD exchange between flight connections. Cycler PD patients can arrange for supplies to be delivered to their destination. Smaller cycler machines are now available, which are easy to take on airplanes and to use in hotel rooms, campers, etc. Some cycler PD patients learn how to do CAPD on trips, rather than carry their cycler with them.

Long-Term Health Planning

Advance care planning involves planning for future healthcare decisions and preferences of the patient in advance while comprehension is intact. It is an essential part of good palliative care that likely improves the lives and deaths of hemodialysis patients. Despite evidence of substantial need, there has been less emphasis on palliative and other supportive interventions to address symptom burden, rehabilitation, and end-of-life care in patients with end-stage renal disease (ESRD). This care intends to neither hasten nor postpone death and should be offered simultaneously with all other medical treatments.

Dialysis Life Plan

Options for Changing Modalities

A single therapy option might not be adequate across a patient's entire life span, and many patients will require a switch in their treatment modality to adapt the treatment to their clinical and psychosocial needs [54–57]. Dialysis modality transition is not only to allow for technical optimization or improved patient survival, but the patient's experience associated with the transition should also be considered. Transition should not be considered as a treatment failure, but rather as an expected progression in the patient's treatment needs (see Fig. 1.2).

There are several reasons why a patient might change their treatment modality including: (a) previous modality failure such as PD or kidney graft failure; (b) unplanned dialysis start where there was no pre-dialysis education and patients were not informed of dialysis choices who may now wish to consider a different therapy option that better fits their lifestyle; (c) patients who have a change in lifestyle or circumstances or who wish to reconsider their initial modality choice; (d) medical situations that require a change in dialysis modality, such as peritonitis, vascular access problems, or hemodynamic intolerance, or that require more frequent treatment prescriptions; and (e) cessation of dialysis treatment to be replaced by kidney transplantation [58–61]. Short-term and long-term benefits and risks should be considered before transitioning from one modality to another.

Transitioning from iHD requires a significantly different mindset, which is a change from a "passive" to a "proactive" attitude, for both the patient and the healthcare team. Transitioning from PD to HHD would seem easier, as the patient is already performing self-dialysis care. However, the patient is required to learn new skills which are significantly more complex than those needed for PD. The main

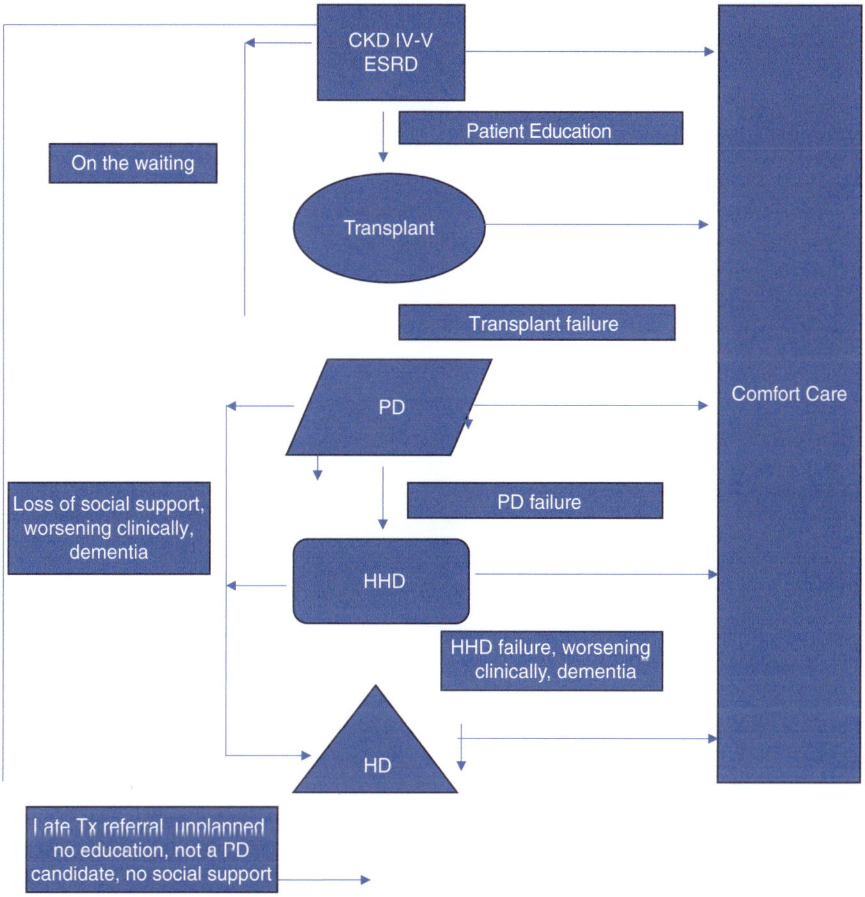

Fig. 1.2 Different pathways of renal replacement therapy

challenge for the healthcare team in this situation is to encourage the patient to continue home dialysis despite the increased complexity of the technique. Finally, managing transition from kidney transplantation back to dialysis poses a different set of challenges, especially as this transition is often psychologically difficult for the patient, so healthcare team needs to provide patient support for this change while promoting patient self-care and education on HHD.

Evidence has shown that among patients undergoing KRT, those who start on PD and then transition to HHD have some of the best outcomes by maximizing the benefits from home-based dialysis therapy while still capitalizing on the putative early advantages of PD and the potential survival advantages afforded by HHD [62, 63]. Therefore, HHD should be strongly considered for most PD patients in need of a new dialysis modality after PD, with the integrated home dialysis model as an expected progression in the patient's treatment options, a gradual move from one therapy option to another. This model should also be considered as an ideal dialysis strategy, especially if a kidney transplant is unavailable or there is a long waiting time on the kidney transplant list.

Transplant Candidacy

The 2020 Kidney Disease: Improving Global Outcomes (KDIGO) Clinical Practice Guideline on the Evaluation and Management of Candidates for Kidney Transplantation is intended to assist healthcare professionals worldwide who evaluate and manage potential candidates for deceased or living donor kidney transplantation.

Shared Decision-Making

Discussing all Choices Fully with Care Team

The most favorable approach in deciding the most appropriate course of action for an individual is shared decision-making, which provides evidence-based information to patients and families about all available therapeutic options in the context of the local situation. Providing accurate and unbiased information to support such decision-making is especially relevant for conservative care, to avoid the perception that this approach is being recommended to save resources rather than to pursue optimal patient comfort. Properly done, shared decision-making should avoid coercion, manipulation, conflicts of interest, and the provision of "futile dialysis" to a patient for whom the harm outweighs the benefits, life expectancy is low, or the financial burden is high. However, the views of care providers do not always necessarily align with those of patients and their families, especially in multicultural environments. Medical professionals are often not well prepared for shared decision-making, and thus, proper training is essential. Policy action is also required to create the proper ethical consensus and evidence-based frameworks at institutional and government levels to guide decision-making in the context of dialysis care that can be adapted to meet local needs [64–68].

Potential Need for Modality Changes Over Time

Transition is an intrinsic process in the life of a patient with kidney disease and should be planned and anticipated when possible. Before commencing the transition process, we need to address several aspects of patient care and ensure the patient is appropriately educated and prepared to transition to or start. We need to discuss with the patient the advantages and disadvantages of the dialysis modalities, as applicable to the patient's circumstances, explore the patient's apprehensions and misconceptions to address these concerns and fears, and ensure a timely transition in order to avoid complications associated with prolonged periods of graft failure, the pre-dialysis stage, or inadequate dialysis dose. It is important that the logistics of the transition are addressed, including vascular access preparation, in addition to ensuring all necessary home adaptations are in place for this treatment (including adequate space and specific HHD equipment) and explaining when and how patient training will be delivered. The patient and the care giver if applicable should be involved at every stage for better patient satisfaction, adherence, and quality of life.

Continuous Reassessment as Life Situation Evolves

It is important to realize that most of the ESKD patients with different accompanying comorbidities may have different rates of progression of their disease processes, for example, pulmonary fibrosis, pulmonary hypertension, or advanced heart failure. Although many patients in these circumstances will choose dialysis to increase longevity, some patients may prefer active medical management without dialysis. Patients who do choose dialysis in this situation, the appropriate intensity of dialysis, and other medical therapies will depend on the burden of the treatment and whether the intervention is for treatment versus prevention. Some patients may wish to receive interventions with modest or uncertain survival benefit because this may give them hope and the impression of control. Other patients in these circumstances may feel the gain in quality and quantity of life with the former treatment approach is small and may desire minimizing treatment burden as an equally important goal. Hence, it is important to reassess treatment options as life situation evolves to make sure patient preferences are honored at all times and the treatment option chosen does not cause more harm than benefit.

Conclusion

Patients who progress to needing dialysis therapy face a lot of decisions. The first should be to make sure they are safe and receive dialysis therapy expeditiously to secure their health and survival. Once this is obtained, education and shared decision-making should be performed with the patient about their many dialysis and transplant options going forward. Ideally, this scenario would happen before an emergent dialysis start has even occurred so that a patient may make an informed decision that matches their goals and aspirations for their life. Patients today have never had more options than in the past to perform dialysis in a facility, at home, while traveling, or even while working. Nephrologists and the nephrology team should take an active role in education and communication with patients about every step in this complex process. The best healthcare outcomes and patient actualization are achieved when knowledge is shared and patients feel secure in their healthcare process.

Key Points

1. Patients need adequate nephrology care and education prior to moving into chronic kidney disease (CKD) stage G5 for adequate dialysis planning.
2. Home dialysis prevalence in the United States is growing, which is being supported and pushed by national kidney initiatives and government payers.
3. All patients should be given options of dialysis modalities that are available which include education about switching modality if needed, but also with the ultimate goal of kidney transplant if possible.
4. Conservative care is a treatment plan for many patients with short life span expected or those with high comorbidities who would benefit more by medication management.

References

1. Australian Institute of Health and Welfare. Projections of the prevalence of treated end-stage kidney disease in Australia 2012–2020. Canberra: Australian Institute of Health and Welfare; 2014.
2. Liyanage T, Ninomiya T, Jha V, et al. Worldwide access to treatment for end-stage kidney disease: a systematic review. Lancet. 2015;385(9981):1975–82.
3. Himmelfarb J, Vanholder R, Mehrotra R, Tonelli M. The current and future landscape of dialysis. Nat Rev Nephrol. 2020;16(10):573–85. https://doi.org/10.1038/s41581-020-0315-4. Epub 2020 Jul 30
4. United States Renal Data System. 2023 USRDS annual data report: epidemiology of kidney disease in the United States. https://www.niddk.nih.gov/about-niddk/strategic-plans-reports/usrds/news/2023/usrds-releases-2023-interactive-annual-data-report. Published 2023. Accessed 2 Jan 2024.
5. Teitelbaum I. Peritoneal dialysis. N Engl J Med. 2021;385(19):1786–95. https://doi.org/10.1056/NEJMra2100152.
6. Jacquet S, Trinh E. The potential burden of home dialysis on patients and caregivers: a narrative review. Can J Kidney Health Dis. 2019;6:2054358119893335. https://doi.org/10.1177/2054358119893335.
7. Chui BK, Manns B, Pannu N, et al. Health care costs of peritoneal dialysis technique failure and dialysis modality switching. Am J Kidney Dis. 2013;61(1):104–11.
8. Evans LM. Peritoneal dialysis: one unit's response to improving outcome and technique survival. Ren Soc Australas J. 2012;8(3):114–9.
9. Morton R, Sellars M. From patient-centered to person-centered care for kidney diseases. Clin J Am Soc Nephrol. 2019;14:623–5.
10. Walker RC, Howard K, Morton RL. Home hemodialysis: a comprehensive review of patient-centered and economic considerations. Clinicoecon Outcomes Res. 2017;9:149–61. https://doi.org/10.2147/CEOR.S69340.
11. Rocco MV, Lockridge RS, Beck GJ, et al. The effects of frequent nocturnal home hemodialysis: the Frequent Hemodialysis Network Nocturnal Trial. Kidney Int. 2011;80(10):1080–91.
12. Tong A, Palmer S, Manns B, et al. The beliefs and expectations of patients and caregivers about home haemodialysis: an interview study. BMJ Open. 2013;3(1):pii: e002148.
13. Voora S, Adey DB. Management of kidney transplant recipients by general nephrologists: core curriculum 2019. Am J Kidney Dis. 2019;73(6):866–79. https://doi.org/10.1053/j.ajkd.2019.01.031. Epub 2019 Apr 11.

14. Augustine J. Kidney transplant: new opportunities and challenges. Cleve Clin J Med. 2018;85(2):138–44. https://doi.org/10.3949/ccjm.85gr.18001.
15. Davis S, Cooper JE. Acute antibody-mediated rejection in kidney transplant recipients. Transplant Rev (Orlando). 2017;31(1):47–54. https://doi.org/10.1016/j.trre.2016.10.004. Epub 2016 Oct 10.
16. Lanini I, Samoni S, Husain-Syed F, Fabbri S, Canzani F, Messeri A, Mediati RD, Ricci Z, Romagnoli S, Villa G. Palliative care for patients with kidney disease. J Clin Med. 2022;11(13):3923. https://doi.org/10.3390/jcm11133923.
17. Chiu HH, Murphy-Burke DM, Thomas SA, Melnyk Y, Kruthaup-Harper AL, Dong JJ, Djurdjev O, Saunders S, Levin A, Karim M, Hargrove GM. BC Renal palliative care committee. Advancing palliative care in patients with CKD: from ideas to practice. Am J Kidney Dis. 2021;77(3):420–6. https://doi.org/10.1053/j.ajkd.2020.09.012.
18. Standardised Outcomes in Nephrology—Peritoneal Dialysis (SONG-PD): study protocol for establishing a core outcome set in peritoneal dialysis. Karine E. Manera, Allison Tong, Jonathan C. Craig, Edwina A. Brown, Gillian Brunier, Jie Dong, Tony Dunning, Rajnish Mehrotra, Sarala Naicker, Roberto Pecoits-Filho, Jeffrey Perl, Angela Y. Wang, Martin Wilkie, Martin Howell, Benedicte Sautenet, Nicole Evangelidis, Jenny I. Shen, and David W. Johnson, on behalf of the SONG-PD Investigators. Peritoneal Dialysis International Volume 37, Issue 6, November/December 2017, p. 639–647.
19. Boers M, Kirwan JR, Wells G, et al. Developing core outcome measurement sets for clinical trials: OMERACT filter 2.0. J Clin Epidemiol. 2014;67(7):745–53. [PubMed] [Google Scholar].
20. Prinsen CAC, Vohra S, Rose MR, et al. How to select outcome measurement instruments for outcomes included in a "Core Outcome Set"—a practical guideline. Trials. 2016;17(1):449.
21. Iseki K, Miyasato F, Tokuyama K, Nishime K, Uehara H, Hira Y, Sunagawa H, Yoshiihara K, Yoshi S, Tomas S, Kowatari T, Wake T, Oura T, Fukiyama K. Low diastolic blood pressure hypoalbuminemia, and risk of death in a cohort of chronic hemodialysis patients. Kidney Int. 1997;51:1212–7.
22. Zager PG, Nikolic J, Brown RH, Campbell MA, Hunt WC, Peterson D, Van Stone J, Levey A, Meyer KB, Klag MJ, Johnson HK, Clark E, Sadler JH, Teredesai P. "U" curve association of blood pressure and mortality in hemodialysis patients. Kidney Int. 1998;54:561–9.
23. U.S. Renal Data System: USRDS 1997 Annual data report. Bethesda: National Institutes of Health, National Institute of Diabetes and Digestive and Kidney Diseases; 1997.
24. Canadian Organ Replacement Register: Annual Report 1998, Volume 1: dialysis and renal transplantation. Ottawa: Canadian Institute for Health Information; 1998.
25. US Renal Data System: USRDS 2011 annual data report: atlas of chronic kidney disease and end-stage renal disease in the United States. Bethesda: National Institutes of Health, National Institute of Diabetes and Digestive and Kidney Diseases; 2011.
26. American Geriatrics Society Expert Panel on the Care of Older Adults with Multimorbidity guiding principles for the care of older adults with multimorbidity: an approach for clinicians. J Am Geriatr Soc. 2012;60:E1–E25.
27. Davison SN. The ethics of end-of-life care for patients with ESRD. Clin J Am Soc Nephrol. 2012;7:2049–57.
28. McAdams-DeMarco MA, Law A, Salter ML, Boyarsky B, Gimenez L, Jaar BG, Walston JD, Segev DL. Frailty as a novel predictor of mortality and hospitalization in individuals of all ages undergoing hemodialysis. J Am Geriatr Soc. 2013;61:896–901.
29. Murtagh FE, Marsh JE, Donohoe P, Ekbal NJ, Sheerin NS, Harris FE. Dialysis or not? A comparative survival study of patients over 75 years with chronic kidney disease stage 5. Nephrol Dial Transplant. 2007;22:1955–62.
30. Chandna SM, Da Silva-Gane M, Marshall C, Warwicker P, Greenwood RN, Farrington K. Survival of elderly patients with stage 5 CKD: comparison of conservative management and renal replacement therapy. Nephrol Dial Transplant. 2011;26:1608–14.
31. Renal Physicians Association: shared decision-making in the appropriate initiation of and withdrawal from dialysis, 2nd ed. Rockville: Renal Physicians Association; 2010.

32. Bowling CB, O'Hare AM. Managing older adults with CKD: individualized versus disease-based approaches. Am J Kidney Dis. 2012;59:293–302.
33. Tamura MK, Tan JC, O'Hare AM. Optimizing renal replacement therapy in older adults: a framework for making individualized decisions. Kidney Int. 2012;82:261–9.
34. Smith AK, Williams BA, Lo B. Discussing overall prognosis with the very elderly. N Engl J Med. 2011;365:2149–51.
35. Reuben DB, Tinetti ME. Goal-oriented patient care—an alternative health outcomes paradigm. N Engl J Med. 2012;366:777–9.
36. Dahlerus C, Quinn M, Messersmith E, Lachance L, Subramanian L, Perry E, Cole J, Zhao J, Lee C, McCall M, et al. Patient perspectives on the choice of dialysis modality: results from the Empowering Patients on Choices for Renal Replacement Therapy (EPOCH-RRT) study. Am J Kidney Dis. 2016;68:901–10. https://doi.org/10.1053/j.ajkd.2016.05.010.
37. Baumgart A, Manera KE, Johnson DW, Craig JC, Shen JI, Ruiz L, Wang AY, Yip T, Fung SKS, Tong M, et al. Meaning of empowerment in peritoneal dialysis: focus groups with patients and caregivers. Nephrol Dial Transplant. 2020;35:1949–58. https://doi.org/10.1093/ndt/gfaa127.
38. Lightfoot CJ, Nair D, Bennett PN, Smith AC, Griffin AD, Warren M, Wilkinson TJ. Patient activation: the cornerstone of effective self-management in chronic kidney disease? Kidney Dial. 2022;2:91–105. https://doi.org/10.3390/kidneydial2010012.
39. Hoang VL, Green T, Bonner A. Informal caregivers' experiences of caring for people receiving dialysis: a mixed-methods systematic review. J Ren Care. 2018;44:82–95. https://doi.org/10.1111/jorc.12235.
40. DePasquale N, Cabacungan A, Ephraim PL, Lewis-Boyer L, Powe NR, Boulware LE. Family members' experiences with dialysis and kidney transplantation. Kidney Med. 2019;1:171–9. https://doi.org/10.1016/j.xkme.2019.06.001.
41. Kaveh K, Kimmel PL. Compliance in hemodialysis patients: multidimensional measures in search of a gold standard. Am J Kidney Dis. 2001;36:244–66.
42. Kimmel PL, Weihs KL, Peterson RA. Survival in hemodialysis patients: the role of depression. J Am Soc Nephrol. 1993;4:12–27.
43. Kimmel PL. Psychosocial factors in adult end-stage renal disease patients treated with hemodialysis: correlates and outcomes. Am J Kidney Dis. 2000;35:S132–40.
44. Vanholder R, et al. Reducing the cost of chronic kidney disease while delivering quality health care: a call to action. Nat Rev Nephrol. 2017;13:393–409.
45. Klarenbach S, Manns B. Economic evaluation of dialysis therapies. Semin Nephrol. 2009;29:524–32.
46. Erickson KF, Zhao B, Ho V, Winkelmayer WC. Employment among patients starting dialysis in the United States. Clin J Am Soc Nephrol. 2018;13:265–73.
47. Wang V, Vilme H, Maciejewski ML, Boulware LE. The economic burden of chronic kidney disease and end-stage renal disease. Semin Nephrol. 2016;36:319–30.
48. Sarason BR, Sarason IG, Pierce GR. Social support: an interactional view. New York: Wiley; 1990.
49. Reddy S, Holley L. Management of the pregnant chronic dialysis patient. Adv Chronic Kidney Disease. 2007;14(2):146–55.
50. Manisco G, Poti M, Maggiulli G, Di Tullio M, Losappio V, Vernaglione L. Pregnancy in end stage renal disease patients on dialysis: how to achieve a successful deliver. Clin Kidney J. 2015;8(3):293–9.
51. Jungers P, Chauveau D. Pregnancy in renal disease. Kidney Int. 1997;52(4):871–85.
52. Shilpanjali J, Blair G, McDonald SP. Pregnancy outcomes according to dialysis commencing before or after conception in women with ESRD. Clin J Am Soc Nephrol. 2014;9(1):143–9.
53. Chou Y, Ting W, Lin H, Lee N. Pregnancy in patients on chronic dialysis: a single center experience and combined analysis of reported results. Eur J Obstet Gynecol Reprod Biol. 2008;136:165–70.
54. Covic A, Bammens B, Lobbedez T, et al. Educating end-stage renal disease patients on dialysis modality selection: clinical advice from the European Renal Best Practice (ERBP) Advisory Board. Nephrol Dial Transplant. 2010;25:1757–9.

55. Moist LM, Lok CE. Incident dialysis access in patients with end-stage kidney disease: what needs to be improved. Semin Nephrol. 2017;37:151–8.
56. Chan CT, Blankestijn PJ, Dember LM, et al. Dialysis initiation, modality choice, access, and prescription: conclusions from a Kidney Disease: Improving Global Outcomes (KDIGO) controversies conference. Kidney Int. 2019;96:37–47.
57. Lambie M, Davies SJ. Transition between home dialysis modalities: another piece in the jigsaw of the integrated care pathway. Nephrol Dial Transplant. 2015;30:1781–3.
58. Lockridge R, Cornelis T, Van Eps C. Prescriptions for home hemodialysis. Hemodial Int. 2015;19(Suppl 1):S112–27.
59. Molnar MZ, Ichii H, Lineen J, et al. Timing of return to dialysis in patients with failing kidney transplants. Semin Dial. 2013;26:667–74.
60. Walker RC, Blagg CR, Mendelssohn DC. Systems to cultivate suitable patients for home dialysis. Hemodial Int. 2015;19(Suppl 1):S52–8.
61. McCormick BB, Chan CT, Group OHDR. Striving to achieve an integrated home dialysis system: a report from the Ontario Renal Network Home Dialysis Attrition Task Force. Clin J Am Soc Nephrol. 2018;13:468–70.
62. Nadeau-Fredette AC, Bargman JM, Chan CT. Clinical outcome of home hemodialysis in patients with previous peritoneal dialysis exposure: evaluation of the integrated home dialysis model. Perit Dial Int. 2015;35:316–23.
63. Nadeau-Fredette AC, Chan CT, Cho Y, et al. Outcomes of integrated home dialysis care: a multi-centre, multi-national registry study. Nephrol Dial Transplant. 2015;30:1897–904.
64. Moss AH. Revised dialysis clinical practice guideline promotes more informed decision-making. Clin J Am Soc Nephrol. 2010;5:2380–3.
65. Williams AW, et al. Critical and honest conversations: the evidence behind the "Choosing Wisely" campaign recommendations by the American Society of Nephrology. Clin J Am Soc Nephrol. 2012;7:1664–72.
66. Rinehart A. Beyond the futility argument: the fair process approach and time-limited trials for managing dialysis conflict. Clin J Am Soc Nephrol. 2013;8:2000–6.
67. Ladin K, et al. Characterizing approaches to dialysis decision making with older adults: a qualitative study of nephrologists. Clin J Am Soc Nephrol. 2018;13:1188–96.
68. Luyckx VA, et al. Developing the ethical framework of end-stage kidney disease care: from practice to policy. Kidney Int Suppl. 2020;10:e72–7.

History of Home Hemodialysis

2

Wael F. Hussein and John Moran

Introduction

In 1964, the first use of home hemodialysis (HHD) resulted from a need to dialyze a 15-year-old girl for severe kidney disease who, because of her age, would not be accepted by the "Admissions Advisory Committee" to receive in-hospital hemodialysis—the only available form of dialysis available at the time. Improvements were made to the dialysis machine, enabling her to receive dialysis at home with assistance from her mother, without the presence of nursing staff. It soon became obvious that given the limited funds, HHD was the best option to support the growing number of patients needing dialysis. Through the late 1960s and early 1970s, processes and equipment were further developed, and 40% of patients were maintained on HHD. This changed with the Medicare End-Stage Renal Disease (ESRD) program in 1973, which provided Medicare funding for dialysis, making access almost universal for all patients in need of the therapy.

What followed was an almost complete shift to facility-based HD driven by the development of industry-scale efficiencies that led to financial incentives favoring this modality. The ability to dialyze frail people and those with multiple comorbidities, and those with challenging home conditions, further contributed to the growth of facility-based dialysis. In parallel, peritoneal dialysis (PD) emerged as a safe and relatively easy modality, making it the preferred modality for home dialysis. All of these factors resulted in a rapid decline in the proportion of patients on HHD.

During the 1990s onward, HHD regained interest, driven by technological advances and observed benefits of HHD. More recently, the Advancing American Kidney Health Initiative encouraging more utilization of home dialysis, the expected advantages to the healthcare system (cost and staffing), together with the fact that

W. F. Hussein (✉) · J. Moran
Department of Medicine, Division of Nephrology, Stanford University School of Medicine, Stanford, CA, USA

A. Shah et al. (eds.), *Applied Home Hemodialysis*,
https://doi.org/10.1007/978-3-031-77244-3_2

PD is not suitable for everyone and not for an extended number of years, all contributed to a resurgence of interest in HHD.

In this chapter, we review the intertwining events, policies, and medical and technological advances that contributed to changes in interest in HHD and its uptake by the dialysis community (Fig. 2.1).

The Birth of Hemodialysis

The first attempt at treating kidney failure with hemodialysis was carried out by Wilhelm Kolff during World War II in the then Nazi-occupied Netherlands in 1943 in a patient with chronic kidney disease (CKD). The treatment was unsuccessful but revealed many issues that needed to be dealt with in establishing routine dialysis [1]. Kolff continued to treat patients with acute kidney injury (AKI), gathering more experience with patient management, dialysate formulation, and device design, but was only successful in saving the life of the 17th patient in 1945 [2]. After World War II, in 1947, Kolff sent four of his rotating drum artificial kidneys to England (Hammersmith Hospital, London) [3], the United States (Mt Sinai Hospital, New York) [4], and Canada (Royal Victoria Hospital, Montreal) [5]. In 1947, Kolff visited the United States, and as a result, Merrill and colleagues at the Peter Bent Brigham Hospital developed a modified version of Kolff's machine. The Kolff-Brigham device was used to treat AKI during the Korean War in the early 1950s [6].

Independent of Kolff and of each other, Alwall in Norway [7] and Murray in Canada [8] developed artificial kidneys of similar designs that had the added advantage of allowing controlled ultrafiltration. Murray soon abandoned this initiative to continue his work in heart surgery, but Alwall went on using his machine to treat both acute and chronic kidney failure, the latter with limited success, due to the intractable and universal difficulty in maintaining vascular access [9].

Despite the success of hemodialysis in treating AKI, it was not until Quinton and Scribner developed the arteriovenous shunt at the University of Washington, Seattle, in 1960, that it was possible to provide maintenance treatment without running out of suitable vascular access [10, 11].

The first patient to receive Scribner's shunt and maintenance dialysis for CKD was Clyde Shields, a 39-year-old man. The chronic program in Seattle at first used continuous HD [11, 12] with the Skeggs-Leonards "dialyzer," initially dialyzing patients for 12–24 h every 4–21 days [12]. The first dialysis of Clyde Shields in fact lasted 76 h [11]. Experience showed that more frequent HD was required to prevent or reverse complications of ESRD, in particular peripheral neuropathy, and the Seattle group eventually settled on dialysis thrice weekly as a compromise between providing adequate dialysis to individual patients and the need to provide treatment to as many patients as possible in a time of restricted resources.

Another innovation in Seattle was the development by Albert (Les) Babb, professor of engineering at the University of Washington of a central proportioning unit which could supply dialysate to four patients [13].

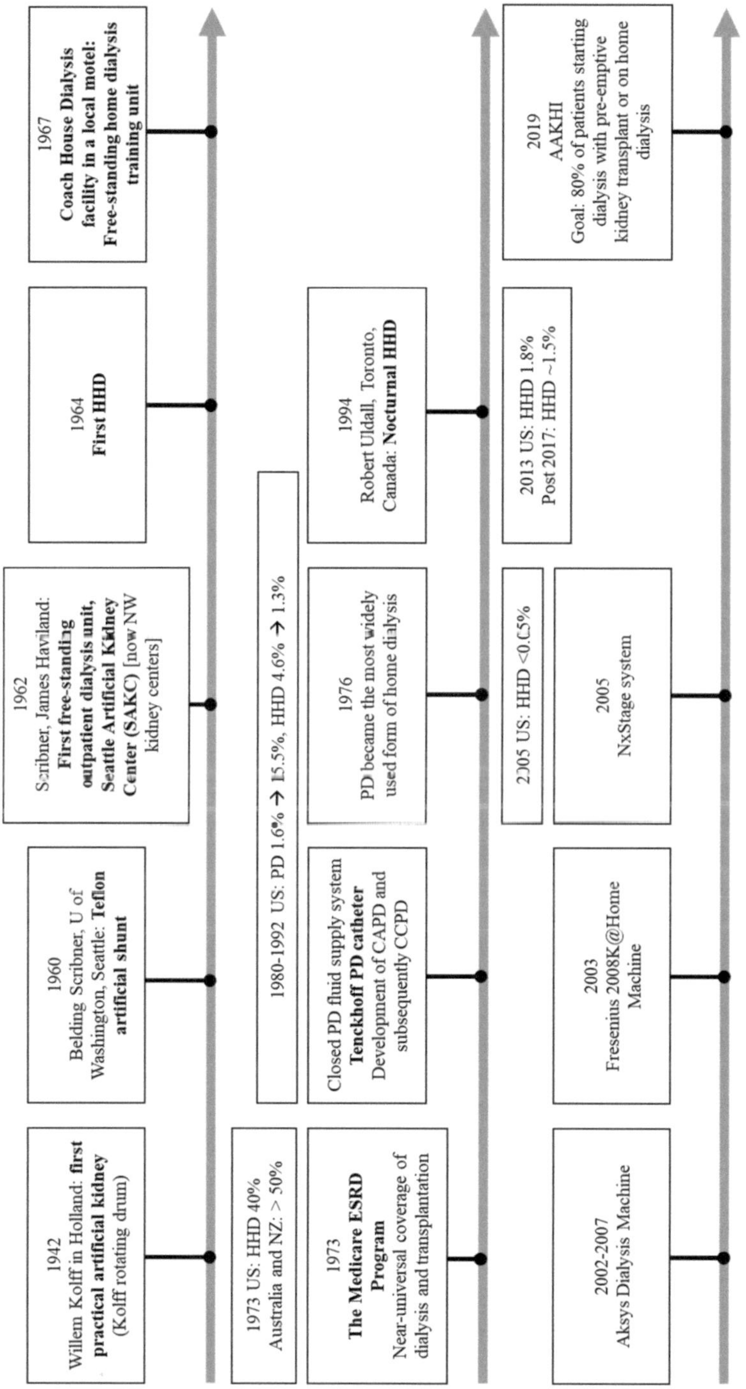

Fig. 2.1 Timeline

Kolff moved to the United States in 1950 and in Cleveland built a new device which became the first industrially produced artificial kidney, the twin-coil device marketed by Baxter Laboratories, Morton Grove, IL [14]. However, adoption of this new potentially life-saving device was slow; Kolff estimated in 1965 that there were about 500 devices in the United States, "but my guess is about half of them are gathering dust." [2] In 1962, Scribner and James Haviland established the world's first outpatient dialysis unit, the Seattle Artificial Kidney Center (SAKC), which has evolved to what is currently Northwest Kidney Centers.

Tight Funding for Dialysis

In the early years, the establishment of chronic hemodialysis was hampered by the lack of available funding, necessitating a process of patient selection. These issues were best documented by the Seattle group, who established a medical committee to establish medical suitability for the therapy with very stringent medical criteria, and a so-called "Admissions and Policy Committee" to review the patients who had been deemed medically suitable to select those few patients who could be offered the therapy. The excruciating decisions faced by this committee were presented to the general public in a dramatic and well-written article in *Life* magazine in 1962 [15]. Together with a 1965 NBC television documentary entitled "Who Shall Live?", this article led to widespread discussion in the medical and general community of the ethical issues involved in such patient selection [16].

The Birth of Home Hemodialysis

In 1964, all three groups most active in developing maintenance dialysis, Seattle [17], London [18], and Boston [19], turned to HHD to alleviate the problems of high cost and limited facilities for the management of increasing referrals of patients with ESRD. In 1964, *Caroline Helm,* the 15-year-old daughter of a friend of Babb, developed end-stage kidney disease (ESKD). Her age excluded her from consideration for the in-center HD program. At the request of Scribner, Babb assembled a team to develop a smaller HD machine, simpler for the patient to use at home [20]. This young lady was able to perform home dialysis with the support of her mother while continuing as an honors student in high school.

Concurrently, in Boston, HHD was developed by John Merrill using a twin-coil dialyzer, enabling HD to be provided at home [19]. Shaldon in London developed the concept of self-care HD, an important step toward HHD [21]. The first nocturnal HHD regimen was established by Shaldon, based on the development of fail-safe monitoring together with low-resistance Kiil dialyzers which eliminated the need for a blood pump (Baillod 1965, 1966) [22, 23]. Patients dialyzed twice weekly "overnight" for 13–14 h. This regimen improved the patient's quality of life by allowing more dialysis-free time for employment and family. In 1966, Shaldon set up the first dedicated independent HHD training center, the National Kidney Center, but this facility, despite great success in training patients from the UK and other countries, closed in 1968 due to insufficient funds [24].

Early Growth of HHD: Expansion of HHD as a Cost-Efficient Model

With tight resources, it did not take long for the dialysis community to recognize the need to increase utilization of HHD for its lower costs, since it did not require the presence of nursing staff. This encouraged Scribner and Shaldon to develop processes and equipment to simplify home dialysis and improve fail-safe monitoring of the procedure [17, 25]. In 1967, the Seattle group repurposed a local motel to establish "Coach House Dialysis" to provide HHD training [17, 20]. By 1970, more than 90% of their dialysis patients were on HHD [20].

DePalma in Southern California independently developed a simple machine suitable for HHD and trained patients to use it 6 days per week, the first use of short daily HD [26]. The clinical results were excellent, but the program eventually closed because of lack of funding.

The challenge of providing dialysis in the face of scarcity of resources provided a moral and ethical dilemma for public health and legislators. In 1962, James Shannon, Director of NIH, wrote to the Surgeon General describing the difficulties "created by Scribner's success: lives could be saved, but at a high cost to individuals and the country." Several initiatives attempted to address these financial and moral issues, including the Community Health Services and Faculties Act, Public Health Service making plans in 1963 for 14 demonstration chronic units in hospitals, and the VA planning to build 30 dialysis centers across the country [27]. In 1967, the Bureau of the Budget, prompted by the White House Office of Science and Technology Policy, formed an expert committee chaired by Carl Gottschalk. The committee recommended a national program supporting transplant, followed by home dialysis, then in-center dialysis [27–29]. All of these initiatives unfortunately were put on hold as attention and resources were diverted to the Vietnam War [27].

A Pivotal Point: The Medicare ESRD Program

Public funding through Medicare was enacted in 1965 to support the elderly. In November 1971, a patient received a truncated dialysis treatment on the floor of Congress at a hearing of the House Ways and Means Committee. It enabled legislators to see that he was a family man, who could be rehabilitated and could get back to work and so contribute to society [29]. Recommendations by Dr. Gottschalk's committee and public attention brought about by stories such as the "God Committee" raised public awareness, and the moral cost of withholding a life-saving treatment because of the financial cost was put into question. The 1972 amendment to Medicare entitlement extended support to the "disabled." A last-minute amendment to the bill included the provision that persons with CKD who required dialysis or kidney transplant "shall be deemed to be disabled" for the purposes of Medicare Parts A and B [27, 29]. In 1973, the Medicare ESRD program was approved, opening the door for Medicare to pay for dialysis and transplantation for almost all patients with ESKD [27, 30, 31].

This was a day-and-night change for the dialysis industry, going from tight funding and having to ration all expenses to near-universal government coverage for dialysis. At the time that the Medicare ESRD program was approved, 40% of the 10,000 current dialysis patients were on HHD [20, 31]. After Medicare ESRD, for-profit outpatient dialysis units popped up everywhere. These units had the advantage of standardized and efficient workflows, thus minimizing the cost of dialysis, while reducing variability in required care. Dialysis became available for older patients and those with multiple comorbidities. Between 1977 and 1992, for example, the median age of a dialysis patient increased from 54 to 63 years and the percentage of patients with diabetes went from 7.7% to 35.7% [20]. In addition to the physical reasons, more patients became not suitable for home dialysis because of social reasons. Provision of home dialysis became less attractive because it required more care and it was not compensated adequately, at least in comparison with in-center HD. Moreover, patients were no longer obligated to do home dialysis. All these factors contributed to a drop in utilization of home dialysis [20, 30].

Several healthcare policies and pay reforms were imposed since. These include adjusting the Medicare cover start date to first day of the month in which a patient starts training for home dialysis, different pay structures for drugs and injectables, payment for medical directorship, different pay schedules for in-center HD and home dialysis, among others. These policies had unintended negative effects on home dialysis utilization, and some, despite aiming to adjust for these consequences, had modest if any improvement in home dialysis uptake [32–36].

Success of Peritoneal Dialysis

PD, the other home dialysis modality, saw significant improvement in the early 1970s, giving it an edge over HHD [20, 30]. Boen and Tenckhoff developed a closed PD fluid supply system, reducing the risk of infection [37, 38]. The development of an indwelling PD catheter by Tenckhoff made it possible to provide intermittent PD, allowing PD to become sustainable as a long-term therapy [20, 38, 39]. Reverse osmosis was used for online preparation of sterile dialysate [20, 40]. Eventually, in 1976, the work of Robert Popovich and Jack Moncrief in Texas resulted in the development of continuous ambulatory PD (CAPD) [20, 38]. Subsequently, continuous cycler-assisted PD (CCPD) was developed by Diaz-Buxo and Nakayama in 1981, becoming the predominant type of PD in the United States [20, 38, 41]. PD became the most widely used form of home dialysis in the United States, growing from 1.6% to 15.5% of all maintenance dialysis patients in the period between 1980 and 1992, whereas HHD declined from 4.6% to 1.3% during the same period [20].

Renewed Interest in HHD

Recognition of some of the advantages of long and frequent dialysis renewed interest in HHD [20, 30]. In 1994, Robert Uldall from Toronto Western Hospital, Canada, demonstrated the feasibility and benefits of slow (8 h, blood flow 300 ml/min, dialysate flow 100 ml/min, 90% urea saturation), frequent (6 times per week) nocturnal dialysis. Dialysis was monitored remotely using a modem device. Patients reported better sleep and more energy, enabling them to have more active time during the day for work and other activities. Their blood pressure improved, and they no longer needed medications to control their phosphate levels [42, 43]. Several other groups demonstrated similar benefits leading to a renewed interest in HHD [20, 30].

The first FDA-approved device for HHD was the Aksys Personal HD machine (PHD, Aksys, Lincolnshire, IL), in March 2002. The device then acquired European Community approval in October 2002. The Aksys machine had a graphical user interface that provided clear guidance for the patient and a system for fluid generation of up to 50 L of ultrapure dialysate before each treatment. The dialyzer and lines were reusable for up to 30 days, a factor that made it easy for patients to set up and take down. Unfortunately, dialysate leaks and other technical issues with the device were common. The company ceased operations in early 2007 [44].

At the same time, Fresenius Medical Care North America made modifications to their 2008 K in-center HD machine and pushed it to market in 2003 as the 2008 K@ Home machine, with no clinical trials. The modifications included a reduction in height and inclusion of a touch screen. However, the device required installation of a typical water treatment at the patient's home [44].

In 2005, a new company, NxStage, developed a device, the System One for HHD. The device was small and portable, weighing 65 lb., and used four 5-L dialysate bags for each treatment. The use of a drop-down line cassette simplified setup and takedown. This machine was designed to make the most efficient use of the dialysate, by running a dialysate flow rate of 25–40% of the blood flow rate, maximizing the dialysate saturation. Given the limited dialysate volume, treatment was required 5 or 6 times per week. Consequently, NxStage developed the PureFlow system, which generated a batch of 60 L of dialysate (Sak). This became the primary use of the machine, with bags being mainly used when traveling [30, 44]. The popularity of the NxStage system contributed to growth of HHD [45].

Reconciling the Reasons for Fading Utilization of HHD

As discussed, the passage of the amendment to the Medicare bill in 1972 (Public Law 192) led to a rapid increase in the number of patients on maintenance hemodialysis in the United States. Over the next few years, there was a major decrease in the proportion of patients treated with HHD. The reasons for this change have been much debated. The financing provided by this bill allowed a tremendous expansion in the number of hemodialysis facilities, the majority of which did not have the ability to train patients for HHD . Blagg (2000) [46] and Maxwell (1987) [47] summarize the way in which reimbursement set up under Public Law 192 inadvertently penalized home dialysis training centers, their patients, and their nephrologists regarding reimbursement. This problem was recognized, and changes were made to reimbursement in 1978 under Public Law 95-292 [46], but by this time, the percentage of patients on HHD had fallen from more than 40% in 1972 to less than 16% in 1978 [47].

A second reason was that patients who previously had been unable to obtain access to dialysis were now being treated, including patients with significant other medical problems including cardiac disease and advanced diabetes which precluded HHD. Another large group were underprivileged patients who previously had no access to maintenance dialysis, and many of these did not have a home which had the space and storage required for HHD. These groups led to a major increase in the number of patients treated by in-center HD while contributing many fewer patients to HHD.

The role of freestanding for-profit dialysis facilities, first established by National Medical Care in 1968, in the decline in the percentage of patients on HHD is controversial and difficult to dissect out. However, given the business model whereby such centers were established without the facilities or staff to train patients for HHD, it would seem inevitable that the percentage of patients receiving HHD would fall, given the rapid increase in the number of patients dialyzed in these facilities. As of 2021, only 29.8% of all US facilities were certified to perform HHD, and of those certified, 37% had no active patients (USRDS 2021) [48]. A recent survey of the availability of dialysis treatment worldwide defined HHD as being "generally available" in >50% of centers (Htay 2020); the United States certainly does not meet this criterion.

A further result of this proliferation of in-center HD-only facilities was that many budding nephrologists received no training in HHD, and of course, this had a cascading effect on future generations. Hence, it is not surprising that in a survey of fellows in nephrology training programs in the United States, it was found that 67% of respondents felt that they were not prepared or were minimally prepared to manage HHD [49].

There has recently been a minor increase in HHD in the United States, as documented in the latest 2021 USRDS report. Although individuals initiating HHD in 2019 represented <1% of the total ESRD incident count, the percentage initiating HHD nevertheless increased by more than one-third (34.5%) between 2018 and 2019 so that the prevalence rate of HHD was 1.5% [48].

Many facilities are certified to offer home dialysis, but there is no assurance that a certified facility has an active home therapy program. According to data in Dialysis Facility Compare and Dialysis Facility Reports, 45.1% of Medicare-certified dialysis facilities in 2019 were not certified to offer either home dialysis modality; 8.0% were certified to offer at least 1 home dialysis modality but had no active patients; and 46.8% were certified to offer at least 1 home dialysis modality and had active patients [48]. Among facilities certified to offer HHD, 37% had no active patients. In contrast, among facilities certified to offer PD, only 17% had no active patients.

Countries much trumpeted as leading in the utilization of HHD include New Zealand, Australia, and Canada, yet the percentage of dialysis patients on HHD in those countries are 14%, 8%, and 5%, respectively. Denmark has 7% of patients on HHD, but the other Scandinavian countries Norway and Sweden have only 2% and 3%, respectively. Furthermore, the HHD numbers for England, Wales, and Northern Ireland are 5%, but for Scotland are only 3% [48]. These differences are hard to explain. All these countries have universal health care of various structures, so these numbers do not support the widely held belief that it is commercial pressures which inhibit the use of HHD.

Again, Hong Kong, which has a strong PD-first policy, has 69% of patients on PD but only 3% on HHD, so the idea that HHD can be a backup therapy to keep patients who fail PD on home dialysis is not supported.

In 2019, President Donald J. Trump issued an executive order "Advancing American Kidney Health" in order to promote the use of home dialysis and kidney transplantation. This order set the extremely ambitious goal of 80% of incident ESRD patients receiving a preemptive kidney transplant or initiating dialysis with a home therapy by 2025 [50].

In England, justice is open to all—like the Ritz Hotel.
~ Sir James Mathew

References

1. Kolff WJ, Berk HTJ, Welle NM, van der Ley AJW, van Dijk EC, van Noordwijk J. The artificial kidney: a dialyser with a great area. Acta Med Scand. 1944;117(2):121–34.
2. Kolff WJ. First clinical experience with the artificial kidney. Ann Intern Med. 1965;62:608–19.
3. Bywaters EG, Joekes AM. The artificial kidney; its clinical application in the treatment of traumatic anuria. Proc R Soc Med. 1948;41(7):420–6.
4. Fishman AP, Kroop IG, et al. Experiences with the Kolff artificial kidney. Am J Med. 1949;7(1):15–34.
5. NKM DL, Blaustein A. Studies of blood passed through an artificial kidney. Blood. 1949;4(5):653–66.
6. Teschan PE, Baxter CR, O'Brien TF, Freyhof JN, Hall WH. Prophylactic hemodialysis in the treatment of acute renal failure. Ann Intern Med. 1960;53:992–1016.
7. Alwall N, Norvitt L, Steins AM. Clinical extracorporeal dialysis of blood with artificial kidney. Lancet. 1948;1(6489):60–2.
8. Murray G, Delorme E, Thomas N. Development of an artificial kidney: experimental and clinical experiences. Arch Surg. 1947;55(5):505–22.
9. Alwall N. Historical perspective on the development of the artificial kidney. Artif Organs. 1986;10(2):86–99.
10. Quinton W, Dillard D, Scribner BH. Cannulation of blood vessels for prolonged hemodialysis. Trans Am Soc Artif Intern Organs. 1960;6:104–13.
11. Scribner BH, Buri R, Caner JE, Hegstrom R, Burnell JM. The treatment of chronic uremia by means of intermittent hemodialysis: a preliminary report. Trans Am Soc Artif Intern Organs. 1960;6:114–22.
12. Scribner BH, Caner JEZ, Buri R, Quinton W. The technique of continuous hemodialysis. ASAIO J. 1960;6(1):88–103.

13. Grimsrud L, Cole JJ, Lehman GA, Babb AL, Scribner BH. A central system for the continuous preparation and distribution of hemodialysis fluid. Trans Am Soc Artif Intern Organs. 1964;10:107–9.
14. Kolff WJ, Watschinger B, Vertes V. Results in patients treated with the coil kidney (disposable dialyzing unit). JAMA J Am Med Assoc. 1956;161(15):1433–7.
15. Alexander S. They decide who lives, who dies: medical miracle puts moral burden on small committee. Life. 1962:102–25.
16. Blagg CR. The early history of dialysis for chronic renal failure in the United States: a view from Seattle. Am J Kidney Dis. 2007;49(3):482–96.
17. Blagg CR, Hickman RO, Eschbach JW, Scribner BH. Home hemodialysis: six years' experience. N Engl J Med. 1970;283(21):1126–31.
18. Shaldon S, Oakley JJ. Experience with regular haemodialysis in the home. Br J Urol. 1966;38(6):616–20.
19. Merrill JP, Schupak E, Cameron E, Hampers CL. Hemodialysis in the home. JAMA. 1964;190:468–70.
20. Blagg CR. A brief history of home hemodialysis. Adv Ren Replace Ther. 1996;3(2):99–105.
21. Shaldon S. Independence in maintenance haemodialysis. Lancet. 1968;1(7541):520.
22. Baillod R, Comty C, Ilahi L, FID K-A, Sevitt L, Shaldon S. Overnight haemodialysis in the home. Proc Eur Dial Transplant Assoc. 1965;2:99–103.
23. Baillod R, Comty C, Crockett R, Shaldon S. Experience with regular haemodialysis in the home. Proc Eur Dial Transplant Assoc. 1966;3:121–6.
24. Shaldon S. National Kidney Centre. Br Med J. 1967;3(5559):241.
25. Eschbach JW Jr, Wilson WE Jr, Peoples RW, Wakefield AW, Babb AL, Scribner BH. Unattended overnight home hemodialysis. Trans Am Soc Artif Intern Organs. 1966;12:346–56.
26. DePalma JR, Pecker EA, Gordon A, Maxwell MH. A new compact automatic home hemodialysis system. Trans Am Soc Artif Intern Organs. 1968;14:152–9.
27. Rettig RA. Special treatment—the story of Medicare's ESRD entitlement. N Engl J Med. 2011;364(7):596–8.
28. Peitzman SJ. Chronic dialysis and dialysis doctors in the United States: a nephrologist-historian's perspective. Semin Dial. 2001;14(3):200–8.
29. Hanna KE, editor. Biomedical politics. Division of Health Sciences Policy, Committee to Study Biomedical Decision Making, Institute of Medicine. Washington, DC: National Academy Press; 1991.
30. Trinh E, Chan CT. The rise, fall, and resurgence of home hemodialysis. Semin Dial. 2017;30(2):174–80.
31. Moran J. The resurgence of home dialysis therapies. Adv Chronic Kidney Dis. 2007;14(3):284–9.
32. Miller BW. Reconciling the current status of home hemodialysis with the 2019 executive order-realistic or obtainable? Adv Chronic Kidney Dis. 2021;28(2):124–8.
33. Anumudu SJ, Eknoyan G. A historical perspective of how public policy shaped dialysis care delivery in the United States. Semin Dial. 2020;33(1):5–9.
34. Schreiber MJ, Chatoth DK, Salenger P. Challenges and opportunities in expanding home hemodialysis for 2025. Adv Chronic Kidney Dis. 2021;28(2):129–35.
35. Weinhandl ED. Economic impact of home hemodialysis. Adv Chronic Kidney Dis. 2021;28(2):136–42.
36. Erickson KF, Winkelmayer WC, Chertow GM, Bhattacharya J. Effects of physician payment reform on provision of home dialysis. Am J Manag Care. 2016;22(6):e215–23.
37. Tenckhoff H, Schechter H. A bacteriologically safe peritoneal access device. Trans Am Soc Artif Intern Organs. 1968;14:181–7.
38. Nobakht E, Mkrttchyan A, Nobakht N. History of peritoneal dialysis. In: Rastogi A, Lerma EV, Bargman JM, eds. Applied Peritoneal Dialysis: Improving Patient Outcomes. Springer. 2021:1–15. https://doi.org/10.1007/978-3-030-70897-9.
39. Tenckhoff H, Blagg CR, Curtis KF, Hickman RO. Chronic peritoneal dialysis. Proc Eur Dial Transplant Assoc. 1973;10(0):363–71.

40. Tenckhoff H, Meston B, Shilipetar G. A simplified automatic peritoneal dialysis system. Trans Am Soc Artif Intern Organs. 1972;18(0):436–40.
41. Diaz-Buxo JA, Farmer CD, Walker PJ, Chandler JT, Holt KL. Continuous cyclic peritoneal dialysis: a preliminary report. Artif Organs. 1981;5(2):157–61.
42. Pierratos A, Ouwendyk M, Francoeur R, et al. Nocturnal hemodialysis: three-year experience. J Am Soc Nephrol. 1998;9(5):859–68.
43. Uldall R, Ouwendyk M, Francoeur R, et al. Slow nocturnal home hemodialysis at the Wellesley Hospital. Adv Ren Replace Ther. 1996;3(2):133–6.
44. Moran J. Technical advances in home dialysis. Adv Chronic Kidney Dis. 2009;16(3):215–20.
45. Agar JWM, Barraclough KA, Piccoli GB. Home haemodialysis: how it began, where it went wrong, and what it may yet be. J Nephrol. 2019;32(3):331–3.
46. Blagg C. What went wrong with home hemodialysis in the United States and what can be done now? Hemodial Int. 2000;4(1):55–8.
47. Maxwell JH, Sapolsky HM. The first DRG: lessons from the end stage renal disease program for the prospective payment system. Inquiry. 1987;24(1):57–67.
48. 2021 USRDS annual data report: epidemiology of kidney disease in the United States. Bethesda: National Institutes of Health, National Institute of Diabetes and Digestive and Kidney Diseases; 2021.
49. Gupta N, Taber-Hight EB, Miller BW. Perceptions of home dialysis training and experience among US nephrology fellows. Am J Kidney Dis. 2021;77(5):713–718.e711.
50. Executive Order on Advancing American Kidney Health. The White House. https://www.whitehouse.gov/presidential-actions/executive-order-advancing-american-kidney-health/. Published 2019. Accessed 31 Dec 2020.

Dialysis Adequacy

3

Brent Miller

Initial Hemodialysis Prescriptions

Rarely do patients die of uremia in developed countries today. This is a remarkable achievement: hemodialysis has prevented hyperkalemia, refractory pulmonary edema, encephalopathy, neuropathy, bleeding, and pericarditis. In the initial development of chronic outpatient dialysis, equipment was rudimentary and scarce, few staff existed, and the finances of providing dialysis were tenuous, so home hemodialysis thrived in that environment. Further, the ability to provide peritoneal dialysis in the home had not yet arrived.

As resources improved, both the availability of outpatient center-based dialysis and an increase in the number of treatments were available for patients. With the increase in the number of dialysis days, improvements in uremic symptoms were noted [1]. When chronic outpatient hemodialysis was added as a Medicare Benefit in 1973, the standard practice of the innovators at the time was to perform dialysis three times a week in the outpatient center [2]. Thus, the practice at the time of thrice-weekly hemodialysis treatment was proposed by the United States Congress and signed into law by the Nixon administration. This guidance stands today. As is typical when a financing mechanism is available to a market, the market increases and innovation ensues. But as dialysis became widely available outside of academic centers doing research and moved away from the home setting to rigid schedules in a corporate environment, the question of how a dialysis treatment should be scientifically defined remained.

B. Miller (✉)
Division of Nephrology, Indiana University School of Medicine, Indianapolis, IN, USA
e-mail: bwm1@iu.edu

A. Shah et al. (eds.), *Applied Home Hemodialysis*,
https://doi.org/10.1007/978-3-031-77244-3_3

Urea Becomes "the" Uremic Solute

Urea is a 60 Dalton, water-soluble molecule that is produced by the urea cycle and is freely filtered at the glomerulus as a means of disposing of nitrogen derived from amino acids. The steady-state level increases with renal dysfunction and thus is a gross marker of renal function although its tubular absorption complicates this role. Further, protein restriction in advanced chronic kidney disease (CKD) lowered to 20–40 g daily lowered blood urea nitrogen levels and often improved uremic symptoms, suggesting that urea may be a major uremic toxin. Prior to readily available dialysis, advanced CKD patients were often given protein-restricted diets including "butterballs" (unsalted butter, powdered sugar, vanilla, and peppermint creamed, rolled into balls and frozen until eaten) to meet nutritional needs and to alleviate the symptoms of uremia [3]. Thus, removal of urea seemed a good standardized, easily measured target for measuring the success of dialysis therapy as large-scale dialysis emerged in the 1970s.

However, treatment for blood urea nitrogen levels (BUN) did not seem to correlate well with dialysis outcomes once hemodialysis treatments achieved the avoidance of major uremic consequences. In retrospect, the role of nutrition and urea generation in achieving the peak BUN concentration is obvious and must be considered along with the blood urea nitrogen levels surrounding a dialysis treatment. Thus, the concept of the amount of urea *removed* during a dialysis treatment crystallizes. The absolute reduction of blood urea nitrogen levels during a dialysis treatment was shown to be associated with improved clinical outcomes such as the need for less transfusions [4].

Development of a Hemodialysis "Dose" Using Urea Removal

Three subsequent landmark trials in the United States loom large over the development of the measurement of urea removal in dialysis and shaping clinical practice: National Cooperative Dialysis Study (NCDS) [5], Hemodialysis Study Group (HEMO) [6], and Frequent Hemodialysis Network (FHN) [7].

NCDS

Planning for a large trial on dialysis "adequacy" arose from a 1975 National Institutes of Health Conference (NIH) held just 2 years after Medicare began coverage of chronic outpatient hemodialysis. 151 patients were randomized into 4 treatment groups based upon dialysis time and a time-averaged BUN measurement—essentially a time of 4.5 or 3.25 h and a BUN concentration of 90 and 50 mg/dl—and then followed for treatment withdrawal or death. The common conclusion of this study—expressed in its 1981 abstract and carried forward for the subsequent 40 years and driving US policymakers toward a "urea-centric" view of dialysis quality—is that BUN concentration plays a much greater role than hemodialysis treatment time. However, several important points should be made when considering this conclusion particularly when the hard constraints of time and schedule are removed from home hemodialysis prescribed.

First, as Gotch and Sargent later demonstrated, the design of the study inextricably linked urea removal and nutrition [8]. Second, the NCDS patients are not representative of today's dialysis population—diabetic patients were excluded among other characteristics. Third, within each group, there was a trend toward better outcome as measured with first hospitalization with increasing dialysis time. Fourth, the dialysis prescription parameters utilized in the study are no longer commonly practiced. Fifth, this study is still done under the thrice-weekly, 2-day skip schedule. Lastly, to achieve the BUN targets, the investigators manipulated characteristics of the treatment such as dialysis membrane surface area, blood flow rate, dialysate flow rate, and the direction of flow to lower small molecule clearance, as measured by urea, in patients with longer dialysis times that are not done in common practice. Urea is a small, water-soluble, uncharged molecule. If the dialysis prescription is manipulated to decrease clearance of this molecule, then nearly every other uremic solute will be decreased no matter what the prescribed time. So the only real conclusion to be drawn from the NCDS is that nutrition and removal of urea matter to hemodialysis patient outcomes.

The Development of a Dialysis Dose: Kt/V and Urea Kinetics

The demonstration of the importance of urea removal and the subsequent discussion of the NCDS results led to the development of removal of urea as a quantum event in the dialysis prescription and the concepts of dialysis urea kinetics and dialysis adequacy as defined by removal urea ensued.

The estimate of removal of urea can be made by the clearance of urea by the dialysis membrane under treatment conditions (K) in ml/min multiplied by the dialysis treatment time (t) in minutes. This value is then divided by the patient's volume of distribution of urea (*Vurea*) to arrive at a unitless number representing the removal of urea during the dialysis treatment (Figs. 3.1 and 3.2). The various methods both to measure Kt/V in a dialysis treatment and to calculate V are beyond the discussion of this chapter. But by the mid-1980s, a measure for an isolated "dose" of dialysis is available and a reanalysis of the NCDS trial suggests that achieving a Kt/V_{urea} of 1–1.4 has dramatically better outcomes than lower Kt/V values.

HEMO Trial

The demonstration of the importance of urea removal to outcomes and the development of a mathematical method for quantitating urea removal set the stage for a trial to measure whether higher "doses" of dialysis improve mortality of hemodialysis patients. The belief in urea removal was so strong during this period that *hemodialysis time was not a variable in the study*; however, there was increasing interest in

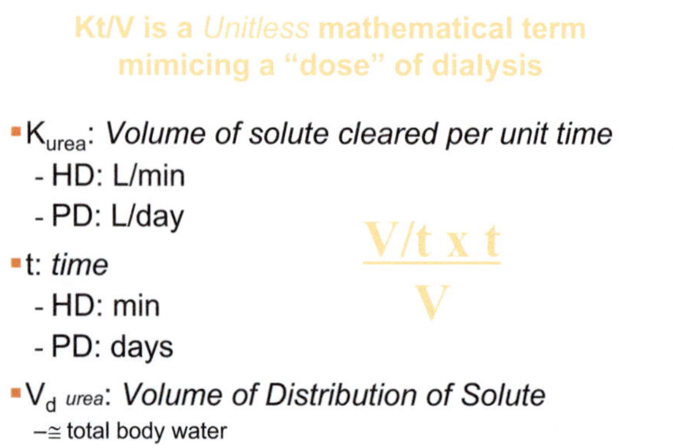

Fig. 3.1 Concept of urea removal during dialysis expressed as an amount of solute removed normalized to body mass

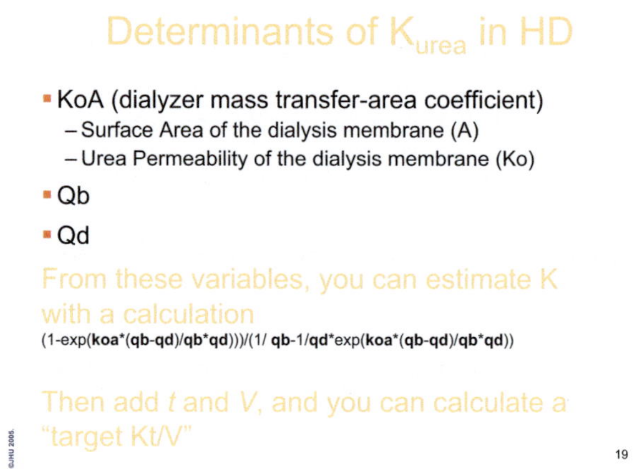

Fig. 3.2 Determinants of estimated urea clearance during hemodialysis. This value can be utilized to estimate a value of a prescribed treatment

removal of larger solutes, so-called "middle molecules." The development of "high-flux" membranes allowed this to be examined, so the participants were divided into low versus high Kt/V_{urea} (spKt/V 1.32 versus 1.71) and low versus high-flux dialysis membrane treatment groups.

That the HEMO study continues to generate academic work and discussion 2 decades after its conclusion speaks to the strength of its design and data collection. Unfortunately, its expense, complexity, and length have discouraged further such investments. 1846 patients were followed for 5 years, and no mortality difference was noted between the groups. Importantly, the time difference between the two groups was a mean of 29 min (190 versus 219 min). The surprise at this conclusion among nephrologists who had spent 30 years discussing urea as the uremic toxin and the connection between urea removal and dialysis outcomes was palpable. However, the question now arose among nephrologists interested in novel approaches to home hemodialysis about what defines an optimal treatment. If reasonable removal of urea is achieved, is dialysis frequency and/or time the next potential target for improving hemodialysis outcomes, and, how is this done in a clinical setting that has been carefully designed for efficiency of space, labor, and supplies?

Concomitantly with the publication of the HEMO study, a large, randomized trial in peritoneal dialysis (the ADEMEX trial) was completed and also showed no difference in mortality with higher urea removal in peritoneal dialysis [9]. Thus, urea as a stand-alone marker for optimal dialysis fails.

FHN

Another NIH-sponsored conference on novel approaches to hemodialysis was held in 2001 which led to the FHN trials. Two arms of the trial were held: one for daily, center-based hemodialysis versus standard of care and a second for nocturnal home hemodialysis versus standard of care. The funding for the studies did not allow for a hard outcome like the HEMO study; thus, a surrogate outcome of left ventricular hypertrophy was chosen. Further, the nocturnal hemodialysis arm fell markedly short of recruitment targets and is uninterpretable. However, the financially truncated, short daily arm randomized 247 patients for 1 year to 6-times-weekly dialysis versus thrice-weekly dialysis showed a significant improvement in patient outcomes with a treatment regimen under 3 hours for an average of 5.2 treatments weekly.

The advancement in understanding urea removal in dialysis leads to several different mathematical calculations and measurements. An *equilibrated* urea *Kt*/*V* value is introduced to differentiate from the older value which is considered a *single-pool* urea *Kt*/*V* (Fig. 3.3) [10]. To account for variable dialysis schedules, a *standardized* (generally to a week) urea *Kt*/*V* is also developed (Fig. 3.4) [11, 12]. Since the studies above have shown a clear negative impact on low urea removal in hemodialysis, when patients are placed on a home hemodialysis regimen, it is recommended to ensure the same weekly removal of urea is obtained on any home dialysis regimen that is prescribed.

TIME Trial

Given that the FHN trial showed a benefit if hemodialysis frequency, time, and urea removal are all increased, the next question would be if increasing dialysis time

$$spKt/V = -\mathrm{Ln}\left(\frac{BUN_{post}}{BUN_{pre}} - 0.008 \times t\right) + \left(4 - 3.5 \times \frac{BUN_{post}}{BUN_{pre}}\right) \times UF/W$$

Fig. 3.3 Single-pool *Kt*/*V* urea calculation that can be utilized during a hemodialysis session in the standard clinical setting. *BUN* blood urea nitrogen, *t* time in minutes, *UF* ultrafiltration during the treatment, *W* patient body weight in kg. (Adapted from Ref. [10])

Standardized Urea Kinetic Measurement

$$\mathrm{stdKt/V} = \frac{\dfrac{10080\,(1-e^{-eKt/V})}{t}}{\dfrac{(1-e^{-eKt/V})}{spKt/V} + \dfrac{10080}{N \times t} - 1}$$

Fig. 3.4 Standardized Kt/V urea calculation. This allows calculation for urea removal to be standardized over a period of time and account for different frequencies of hemodialysis. *N* number of treatments per week, *t* treatment time in minutes, *V* volume of distribution. (Adapted from Refs. [11, 12])

alone would lead to improved outcomes. To address the cost and complexity issues, a "pragmatic" clinical trial of 7035 patients in 266 dialysis centers was done in incident hemodialysis patients. This trial was an abject failure and was stopped at 1.1 years because a difference of only 9 min was achieved between the two groups [13]. The question of the optimal dialysis time remains unanswered.

Establishment of Urea Removal with Hemodialysis as a Regulatory Standard in the United States

Prior to the reporting of the HEMO trial in 2002, nephrology professionals in association with the National Kidney Foundation began a series of meetings to produce clinical practice guidelines, ultimately named KDOQI [14]. Although these were never intended to be used as a regulatory measure, KDOQI have been incorporated into various hemodialysis quality measures by governmental authorities and can even impact the facility payment for dialysis (Quality Incentive Program, QIP) to dialysis providers [15].

Residual Renal Function and Hemodialysis

In multiple hemodialysis and peritoneal dialysis studies, residual renal function has been noted to have more impact on mortality outcome than the dialysis treatment. Residual renal function is included in the measurement of dialysis adequacy in peritoneal dialysis; curiously, it has not been included in the measurement of dialysis adequacy in hemodialysis. No scientific explanation justifies this exclusion—the logistical complexity of collecting the specimens, the complexity of combining a continuous (urine) with a discontinuous (hemodialysis) variable, and the typical rapid loss of residual renal function in hemodialysis have been proposed for the omission. But mathematical models for combining the two components are widely available [16]. For patients with significant residual renal function making the effort and time to do their own hemodialysis treatments at home, adding extra time or treatments to meet an unproven metric cannot be justified. Recognizing this conundrum, CMS currently excludes patients doing more than three treatments a week from the QIP score for dialysis adequacy.

The Impact of Hemodialysis on Other Solutes

As the era of judging hemodialysis solely by small molecule removal with urea as the surrogate reaches its peak, significant attention is being devoted to other uremic solutes including those that are larger, charged, and significantly protein-bound. As this topic evolves, it is critical for the clinician to understand the impact of the hemodialysis prescription on other molecules. Nearly every aspect of the hemodialysis procedure impacts this topic, but two are particularly important to the nephrologist: dialysis time and dialysate volume. Although these are inseparable in the clinical setting (you often have to use more dialysate volume if you prescribe more time and vice versa), manipulation of these will affect clearance of various solutes.

For example, urea removal reaches maximum efficiency with a dialysate flow of approximately 1.5 times the blood flow and its clearance will increase proportionally up to this value. Conversely, increasing dialysis time but keeping the total dialysate volume constant (i.e., reducing dialysate flow) does *not* increase urea removal significantly. However, for other molecules such as phosphorus and beta-2 microglobulin, the opposite is true. Increasing dialysis time has a large impact on removal but increasing dialysate volume (i.e., increasing dialysate flow in a fixed time has a minimal impact) [17, 18].

As the era of metabolomics and transcriptomics begins, perhaps we will understand which biochemical pathways are responsible for an individual's clinical symptoms of uremia. For the clinical nephrologist prescribing home hemodialysis, understanding how the home hemodialysis prescription can be altered to respond to this data will be increasingly important.

Clinical Markers of Hemodialysis Efficacy

Solid clinical observations since the 1981 NCDS which implicated the link between nutrition and dialysis therapy have suggested that clinical markers could be better incorporated for adjusting the dialysis prescription (Table 3.1). There is some suggestion that this is being recognized by regulatory authorities (Table 3.2). Released from the confines of a rigid, center-based hemodialysis schedule, the nephrologist should be able to prescribe a home hemodialysis treatment regimen that addresses these clinical markers regardless of the biochemical measurement of urea removal.

Table 3.1 Potential clinical markers for adequate dialysis in addition to urea removal and nutritional status

Ultrafiltration rate < 10–13 ml/kg/h
Control of blood pressure with minimal antihypertensives
Control of phosphorus with minimal binders
Physical activity
Appetite
Neuromuscular irritability or restless legs
Pruritus
Sleep apnea

Table 3.2 Calendar year 2023 CMS quality incentive program metrics

Metric
Standardized hospitalization ratio
Standardized hospitalization readmission ratio
Long-term hemodialysis catheter rate
Consumer assessment of hemodialysis service
Kidney transplant waitlist
Urea Kt/V dialysis adequacy
Standardized fistula rate

https://www.cms.gov/newsroom/fact-sheets/calendar-year-2023-end-stage-renal-disease-esrd-prospective-payment-system-pps-final-rule-cms-1768-f

Summary

Both the optimal hemodialysis prescription and the optimal methodology for measuring the efficacy of hemodialysis remain elusive. Particularly in the United States, the development of treatment guidelines over the last 2 decades and the adoption of measurements of urea removal for quality metrics tied to financial reimbursement have placed the mathematical modeling of urea removal at the forefront of hemodialysis care. However, incorporation of other clinical data and understanding how to manipulate the home hemodialysis prescription to attain clinical results are the key to practical success of the home hemodialysis treatment.

Case Study #1

A 62-year-old man who weighs 270 pounds and is 71 inches tall with diabetic nephropathy starts home hemodialysis with a low dialysate volume prescription 5 days per week. His prescription is 25 L of dialysate over 2.5 h with a blood flow of 400 ml/min with a forearm arteriovenous fistula. His average ultrafiltration is 500 ml. His pre-dialysis BUN is 71 mg/dl and post-dialysis BUN is 50 mg/dl. His single-pool *Kt*/*V* is 0.41, and his weekly standardized *Kt*/*V* is 1.47. His phosphorus is 5.5 mg/dl; potassium, 4.0 mg/dl; and hemoglobin, 11.3 g/dl on a low-dose weekly erythropoietin-stimulating agent. His blood pressure is 128/82 on a low-dose angiotensin-converting enzyme inhibitor. He feels well and reports making significant urine that has not been quantitated. What is the next step?

Answer

This specific issue has not been addressed in a definitive study. Two unresolved issues are the solute removal targets for hemodialysis performed more than thrice weekly and the role of residual renal function in chronic outpatient hemodialysis.

In this patient, a subsequent 24-h urine collection demonstrated a creatinine clearance of 4.8 ml/min/1.73 m^2 and a urea clearance of 2.8 ml/min/1.73 m^2. When combined with his dialytic clearance, this yields a weekly standardized Kt/V_{urea} of 2.47, which is consistent with current recommendations of hemodialysis practice. Although one could adjust his prescription for other reasons, from both a clinical and a biochemical adequacy perspective, he is fine.

Case Study #2

A 58-year-old woman who weighs 82 kg with autosomal dominant polycystic disease has been on home hemodialysis for 2 years. She is anuric. With the loss of her residual renal function over the last 6 months, she has had some mild uremic symptoms, most notably pruritus and mild anorexia along with a decline in her weekly std. Kt/V_{urea} to 1.87 and an increase in her phosphorus to 6.5 mg/dl despite dietary restriction and phosphorous binder use. In addition to ensuring her vascular access is working well, dietary adherence, and binder adherence, what changes in the hemodialysis prescription would likely improve the following from most to least:

1. For her phosphorous level
2. For her symptoms of pruritus and anorexia
3. For her Kt/V_{urea}

Current Dialysis Prescription

- 4 days per week

25 L each Treatment
Qb 450 ml/min
Time 2.75 h

Proposed Changes in Dialysis Prescription

A. Increase the dialysate volume to 30 L; maintain time and dialysis frequency the same
B. Keep dialysate volume at 25 L; increase dialysis time to 3 h and frequency the same
C. Increase dialysate volume to 30 L; increase dialysis time to 3 h
D. Decrease dialysate volume to 20 L; keep dialysis time at 2.75 h; increase days to 5 days

Answer

1. D-C-B-A
2. D-C-B-A
3. D-C-A-B

References

1. Eschbach JW Jr, Wilson WE Jr, Peoples RW, Wakefield AW, Babb AL, Scribner BH. Unattended overnight home hemodialysis. Trans Am Soc Artif Intern Organs. 1966;12:346–56. PMID: 5960725
2. Eggers PW. Medicare's end stage renal disease program. Health Care Financ Rev. 2000;22(1):55–60. PMID: 25372768; PMCID: PMC4194691.
3. Borst JG. Protein katabolism in uraemia; effects of protein-free diet, infections, and blood-transfusions. Lancet. 1948;1(6509):824–9. PMID: 18860691.
4. Koch KM, Patyna WD, Shaldon S, Werner E. Anemia of the regular hemodialysis patient and its treatment. Nephron 1974; 12:405–19.
5. Lowrie EG, Laird NM, Parker TF, Sargent JA. Effect of the hemodialysis prescription of patient morbidity: report from the National Cooperative Dialysis Study. N Engl J Med. 1981;305(20):1176–81. https://doi.org/10.1056/NEJM198111123052003. PMID: 7027040.
6. Eknoyan G, Beck GJ, Cheung AK, Daugirdas JT, Greene T, Kusek JW, Allon M, Bailey J, Delmez JA, Depner TA, Dwyer JT, Levey AS, Levin NW, Milford E, Ornt DB, Rocco MV, Schulman G, Schwab SJ, Teehan BP, Toto R, Hemodialysis (HEMO) Study Group. Effect of dialysis dose and membrane flux in maintenance hemodialysis. N Engl J Med. 2002;347(25):2010–9. https://doi.org/10.1056/NEJMoa021583. PMID: 12490682.
7. FHN Trial Group, Chertow GM, Levin NW, Beck GJ, Depner TA, Eggers PW, Gassman JJ, Gorodetskaya I, Greene T, James S, Larive B, Lindsay RM, Mehta RL, Miller B, Ornt DB, Rajagopalan S, Rastogi A, Rocco MV, Schiller B, Sergeyeva O, Schulman G, Ting GO, Unruh ML, Star RA, Kliger AS. In-center hemodialysis six times per week versus three times per week. N Engl J Med. 2010;363(24):2287–300. https://doi.org/10.1056/NEJMoa1001593. Epub 2010 Nov 20. Erratum in: N Engl J Med. 2011 ;364(1):93. PMID: 21091062; PMCID: PMC3042140.
8. Gotch FA, Sargent JA. A mechanistic analysis of the National Cooperative Dialysis Study (NCDS). Kidney Int. 1985;28(3):526–34. https://doi.org/10.1038/ki.1985.160. PMID: 3934452
9. Paniagua R, Amato D, Vonesh E, Correa-Rotter R, Ramos A, Moran J, Mujais S. Effects of increased peritoneal clearances on mortality rates in peritoneal dialysis: ADEMEX, a prospective, randomized, controlled trial. J Am Soc Nephrol. 2002;13(5):1307–20. https://doi.org/10.1681/ASN.V1351307. PMID: 11961019.
10. Daugirdas JT. Second generation logarithmic estimates of single-pool variable volume Kt/V: an analysis of error. J Am Soc Nephrol. 1993;4(5):1205–13. https://doi.org/10.1681/ASN.V451205. PMID: 8305648.
11. Leypoldt JK. Urea standard Kt/V(urea) for assessing dialysis treatment adequacy. Hemodial Int. 2004;8(2):193–7. https://doi.org/10.1111/j.1492-7535.2004.01095.x. PMID: 19379417.
12. Gotch FA. The current place of urea kinetic modelling with respect to different dialysis modalities. Nephrol Dial Transplant. 1998;13(Suppl 6):10–4. https://doi.org/10.1093/ndt/13.suppl_6.10. PMID: 9719197.
13. Dember LM, Lacson E Jr, Brunelli SM, Hsu JY, Cheung AK, Daugirdas JT, Greene T, Kovesdy CP, Miskulin DC, Thadhani RI, Winkelmayer WC, Ellenberg SS, Cifelli D, Madigan R, Young A, Angeletti M, Wingard RL, Kahn C, Nissenson AR, Maddux FW, Abbott KC, Landis JR. The TiME trial: a fully embedded, cluster-randomized, pragmatic trial of hemodialysis session

duration. J Am Soc Nephrol. 2019;30(5):890–903. https://doi.org/10.1681/ASN.2018090945. Epub 2019 . PMID: 31000566; PMCID: PMC6493975.
14. National Kidney Foundation. KDOQI clinical practice guideline for hemodialysis adequacy: 2015 update. Am J Kidney Dis. 2015;66(5):884–930. https://doi.org/10.1053/j.ajkd.2015.07.015. Erratum in: Am J Kidney Dis 2016;67(3):534. PMID: 26498416.
15. Weiner D, Watnick S. The ESRD quality incentive program-can we bridge the chasm? J Am Soc Nephrol. 2017;28(6):1697–706. https://doi.org/10.1681/ASN.2016101079. Epub 2017 Mar 15. PMID: 28298324; PMCID: PMC5461804.
16. Daugirdas JT, Depner TA, Greene T, Silisteanu P. Solute-solver: a web-based tool for modeling urea kinetics for a broad range of hemodialysis schedules in multiple patients. Am J Kidney Dis. 2009;54(5):798–809. https://doi.org/10.1053/j.ajkd.2009.06.033. PMID: 19853198.
17. Eloot S, Van Biesen W, Dhondt A, Van de Wynkele H, Glorieux G, Verdonck P, Vanholder R. Impact of hemodialysis duration on the removal of uremic retention solutes. Kidney Int. 2008;73(6):765–70. https://doi.org/10.1038/sj.ki.5002750. Epub 2007 Dec 26. PMID: 18160958.
18. Bhimani JP, Ouseph R, Ward RA. Effect of increasing dialysate flow rate on diffusive mass transfer of urea, phosphate and beta2-microglobulin during clinical haemodialysis. Nephrol Dial Transplant. 2010;25(12):3990–5. https://doi.org/10.1093/ndt/gfq326. Epub 2010 Jun 13. PMID: 20543211; PMCID: PMC2989792.

Survival at Home

4

Matthew R. Lynch

Case
A 56-year-old woman with a past medical history of chronic kidney disease stage G5A3 from microvascular damage secondary to uncontrolled diabetes and hypertension presents to the hospital for evaluation of progressive shortness of breath and worsening lower extremity swelling. She was found to have an oliguric acute kidney injury, failing to respond to a diuretic challenge. She required initiation of kidney replacement therapy (KRT) during the hospital admission. Prior to discharge, she was given a brief introduction of various modes of KRT including peritoneal dialysis, in-center hemodialysis, home hemodialysis, and kidney transplantation. Understanding that she cannot immediately receive a kidney transplant, the patient asks which KRT modality may provide her the best chance for long-term survival.

Introduction

In general, data have demonstrated that for patients with end-stage kidney disease (ESKD), home hemodialysis (HHD) is associated with superior survival compared to other dialysis modalities. While this survival advantage of HHD is becoming accepted in nephrology circles, a more thorough examination of the data is necessary, particularly around the impact of bias, prescribed dialysis dose, and control for non-dialytic factors affecting mortality, in order to fully appreciate the potential and likely survival benefits of HHD.

The selection bias regarding who may be "eligible" for HHD versus PD versus in-center conventional hemodialysis (ICHD) makes examining differences in

M. R. Lynch (✉)
Department of Medicine, Warren Alpert Medical School of Brown University, Providence, RI, USA

Division of Nephrology, Brown Medicine, Providence, RI, USA
e-mail: mlynch7@lifespan.org

A. Shah et al. (eds.), *Applied Home Hemodialysis*,
https://doi.org/10.1007/978-3-031-77244-3_4

survival somewhat difficult. While this bias can be reduced by matching characteristics such as age and comorbidities, as many studies discussed in this chapter employ in their analyses, it is an imperfect solution. Furthermore, these retrospective analyses fail to consider the importance of non-dialytic factors that can contribute to mortality statistics, such as social determinants of health [1].

Another major limitation in interpreting these studies, as mentioned by Miller et al., is that the exact mechanism for the superior survival associated with HHD compared to other dialysis modalities is unknown [2]. While it is known that volume control strongly correlates with survival on dialysis, and more frequent dialysis with HHD allows better volume control, peritoneal dialysis (PD) also offers the opportunity for daily dialysis and enhanced volume control (with slower loss of residual renal function). Thus, differences between HHD and PD are unlikely to be explained by volume control alone.

Furthermore, HHD can be prescribed in various frequencies and treatment lengths. To examine whether HHD prescription is associated with mortality, a Canadian study compared survival between conventional HHD (3–6 h, 2–4 times per week), nocturnal HHD (6–8 h, 5–7 times per week), and short daily HHD (2–3 h, 5–7 times per week). It found no difference in overall mortality between the groups. Notably, however, those on nocturnal HHD had a statistically higher risk of treatment failure [3]. Additionally, a trial comparing survival in short daily HHD patients found that total weekly dialysis time was positively associated with better survival, but, somewhat surprisingly, *Kt/V* was not associated with survival [4].

HHD vs. ICHD

Comparison between mortality in patients on HHD or its research surrogate, intensive hemodialysis, and conventional thrice-weekly in-center dialysis has generally shown favorable results for HHD in retrospective studies using data from large databases. However, the results of randomized controlled trials (RCTs), albeit with small sample sizes, did not completely agree with this finding. Thus, the true mortality benefit of HHD may not yet be fully appreciated.

The major trials of the Frequent Hemodialysis Network (FHN)—the Daily Trial and Nocturnal Trial—are among the most influential in how we think about the benefits of HHD, as they represent rare, prospective, randomized clinical trials in this area [5, 6]. In the Daily Trial, 245 patients were randomized to either six-times-weekly in-center hemodialysis ($n = 125$) or conventional thrice-weekly in-center dialysis ($n = 120$). The Daily Trial found that more frequent dialysis had a superior composite outcome of death and change in left ventricular mass. Importantly, survival was not examined independently due to underpowering. Additionally, the more intensive regimen is extrapolated to equivalency for increased intensity of HHD.

In the Nocturnal Trial, 87 patients were randomized to either six-times-weekly nocturnal HD ($n = 45$) or thrice-weekly conventional HD. While there was improved hypertension control with nocturnal HD, the trend toward a superior composite outcome of death and change in left ventricular mass was not statistically significant, as the study underenrolled [6]. A consequence of this underenrollment was significant variability in the intervention and control group characteristics. A 1-year follow-up of participants after the study concluded suggested higher mortality in the nocturnal HD group. However, the authors caution that the mortality rate in the conventional dialysis arm was particularly low at 0.03 deaths per patient-year and there was significant crossover between arms, potentially skewing results [7].

While RCTs have somewhat conflicting outcomes for HHD mortality benefit, retrospective trials do not—all have demonstrated an HHD mortality benefit or benefit for its surrogate, intensive HD. Three representative examples of these trials are described below. One early study compared patients on home or in-center short daily hemodialysis in the United States, France, the UK, and Italy to conventional thrice-weekly hemodialysis controls from the USRDS database. Both short daily dialysis cohorts had superior 5-year survival compared to matched conventional dialysis patients. Additionally, those on short daily HHD had better survival than short daily in-center dialysis [8]. In a second study, Weinhandl et al. matched 1873 HHD and 9365 conventional HD patients for demographics (except insurance) and comorbidities in a 1:5 intention-to-treat analysis. They concluded those on HHD had 13% lower all-cause mortality than in-center counterparts [9]. A third study matched 338 patients from the International Quotidian Dialysis Registry of patients on intensive (home and in-center) dialysis with 1388 patients on the Dialysis Outcomes and Practice Patterns Study on conventional, in-center HD. After matching for age, country of origin, ESKD vintage, and comorbid conditions, those on intensive dialysis were shown to associate with decreased mortality rates. Interestingly, subgroup analysis of those older than the median age of the cohort (52 years) revealed a tendency toward improved mortality with intensive dialysis, but this trend did not reach statistical significance [10].

HHD vs. PD

Mortality comparisons between HHD and PD are intriguing, as they compare the two home modalities directly, providing salient data for those considering home dialysis but undecided between modalities. As described below, studies comparing HHD and PD have shown either a slight mortality advantage for HHD or no difference in mortality outcomes between the modalities.

In a large retrospective study of incident home dialysis patients in Australia and New Zealand, Nadeau-Fredette et al. compared overall and on-treatment survival of over 10,000 PD patients with that of 706 HHD patients. Using a multivariable Cox proportional hazard analysis, HHD patients had superior overall and on-treatment survival. However, the PD population was significantly older, and had more cardiovascular comorbidities, higher diabetes rates, and different ESKD etiology [11].

Similarly, a retrospective USRDS study from 2004 to 2011 found, after matching for age, race, comorbidities, and dialysis initiation year, lower mortality for HHD versus PD. This HHD benefit was seen in nearly all subgroups (age, weight, heart failure presence). However, no difference was seen in patients with diabetes, although a trend toward lower HHD mortality existed [12].

A Canadian study of incident dialysis patients choosing HHD or PD between 2000 and 2013 found that patients on HHD had lower mortality than those in the PD cohort. Intriguingly, in the most modern of the cohorts—those initiating dialysis between 2011 and 2013—there was no difference in morality, when adjusted for age, comorbid conditions, and dialysis unit size, perhaps due to either change in patient selection or shorter follow-up [13].

Echoing the theme of a likely but non-definitive HHD mortality benefit versus PD, Weinhandl et al. matched over 4000 HHD and PD patients by dialysis vintage, ESKD etiology, comorbidities, and insurance. In an intention-to-treat analysis, 3-year HHD mortality was lower than PD. However, in patients starting HHD or PD as the primary modality (excluding modality switches), the trend toward improved HHD survival was not statistically significant [14].

To provide a counterbalance, a matched cohort study of 1915 incident HHD and 1915 incident PD patients in the United States followed patients from dialysis day 90 through modality change, transplant, or death. The cohorts were matched for comorbidities, race, insurance, ESKD etiology, BMI, serum creatinine, and albumin. Although there was a trend toward better HHD survival, at the 3-year analysis end point, there was no difference in all-cause mortality between groups [15].

HHD vs. Transplant

Kidney transplant is the superior KRT when available, as dialysis cannot fully replicate kidney clearance or metabolic functions. Thus, transplant recipients unsurprisingly have lower mortality than HHD patients. However, as detailed below, certain HHD prescriptions and populations may find HHD may bridge this gap for those who are not candidates for kidney transplant.

Ethier and colleagues conducted a study comparing the survival rates of patients undergoing HHD and those receiving their first kidney transplant, beyond the initial 90 days post-procedure. They analyzed 20 years of data from Australia and New Zealand, involving 1411 HHD patients and 13,406 transplant recipients. Unsurprisingly, they found that kidney transplant recipients generally had better survival rates. However, a notable observation emerged when considering the type of transplant received: living donor, standard criteria donor, or expanded criteria donor. The mortality rates of patients receiving kidneys from expanded criteria donors were found to be comparable to those of HHD patients. This might be attributed to the recipients of expanded criteria donor kidneys often being older and having a higher prevalence of cardiovascular comorbidities, compared to recipients of kidneys from other types of donors [16].

A study conducted at a single center in the United States analyzed the survival rates of 116 patients on intensive HHD and 3073 kidney transplant recipients. The intensive HHD group underwent an average of 40 h of dialysis per week, with a mean weekly *Kt*/*V* of 5.25. Similar to previous findings, recipients of living donor transplants exhibited the highest survival rates. However, when adjustments were made for age and comorbidities, the survival rates of the intensive HHD cohort and those who received a deceased donor transplant were found to be statistically similar [17]. In contrast, a retrospective matched cohort study, involving nearly 500 elderly patients (aged 65 or older), compared the survival rates of HHD patients and kidney transplant recipients. The transplant recipients displayed superior survival rates. It is important to note that the *Kt/V* values for the HHD group in this latter study were not reported [18].

HHD in Multiple Comparison with Other KRT Modalities

Studies that comprehensively compare all KRT modalities within a population have been conducted by a few investigators. In these studies, HHD has consistently been associated with improved survival outcomes.

A substantial cohort of over 40,000 patients with incident ESKD from Australia and New Zealand was analyzed over a nearly 16-year period to compare the mortality rates associated with various kidney replacement therapies. Hemodialysis, including both home and in-center, was categorized into three groups: conventional (three or fewer weekly sessions lasting less than 6 h each), quasi-intensive (four sessions weekly or three or fewer sessions lasting more than 6 h each), and intensive (five or more sessions weekly). PD and kidney transplantation were also evaluated. The study found that quasi-intensive HHD was associated with better survival rates compared to conventional, in-center hemodialysis. Intensive HHD, while not conclusively superior, showed a trend toward improved survival. The study also revealed that PD had the highest mortality rate among the KRT modalities, while kidney transplantation exhibited the lowest mortality rate [19].

A retrospective study using data from Sweden compared survival between 152 HHD, 456 PD, and 608 conventional HD patients. The cohorts were matched for gender, comorbidities, age, and date of dialysis initiation; furthermore, the analysis was adjusted for rate of transplant, as patients were followed after transplant to death. Using an intention-to-treat analysis, those on HHD had superior survival (18.5 years from the start of dialysis) compared to those on PD (15 years) and conventional HD (11.9 years) [20].

Conclusion

Numerous retrospective studies have investigated the relationship between dialysis modality and mortality, with the majority suggesting that HHD is associated with similar or superior survival outcomes. However, it's crucial to note that RCTs conducted on this topic have not reached the same conclusion, indicating a need for further research in this area. For instance, emerging research underscores the significance of social determinants of health in individuals with chronic kidney disease (CKD), but these crucial factors are not captured in the extensive databases used for retrospective analyses of dialysis populations. Consequently, these influential variables remain absent from current analyses exploring the associations between dialysis modality and mortality. Moreover, while theories suggest that improved hypertension and volume management, reduced progression of left ventricular hypertrophy, and enhanced weekly *Kt/V* could explain the potentially superior survival rates associated with HHD, existing research has yet to clarify the mechanisms responsible for these observed benefits.

Back to the Case

The patient was particularly struck by the mortality data surrounding intensive HHD when compared to transplant, and she chose to initiate this as a bridge to eventual kidney transplant.

References

1. Norton JM, Moxey-Mims MM, Eggers PW, et al. Social determinants of racial disparities in CKD. J Am Soc Nephrol. 2016;27(9):2576–95. https://doi.org/10.1681/ASN.2016010027.
2. Miller AJ, Perl J, Tennankore KK. Survival comparisons of intensive vs. conventional hemodialysis: pitfalls and lessons. Hemodial Int. 2018;22(1):9–22. https://doi.org/10.1111/hdi.12559.
3. Tennankore KK, Na Y, Wald R, Chan CT, Perl J. Short daily-, nocturnal- and conventional-home hemodialysis have similar patient and treatment survival. Kidney Int. 2018;93(1):188–94. https://doi.org/10.1016/j.kint.2017.06.014.
4. Kjellstrand C, Buoncristiani U, Ting G, et al. Survival with short-daily hemodialysis: association of time, site, and dose of dialysis. Hemodial Int. 2010;14(4):464–70. https://doi.org/10.1111/j.1542-4758.2010.00475.x.
5. Group FHNT, Chertow GM, Levin NW, et al. In-center hemodialysis six times per week versus three times per week. N Engl J Med. 2010;363(24):2287–300. https://doi.org/10.1056/NEJMoa1001593.
6. Rocco MV, Lockridge RS Jr, Beck GJ, et al. The effects of frequent nocturnal home hemodialysis: the Frequent Hemodialysis Network Nocturnal Trial. Kidney Int. 2011;80(10):1080–91. https://doi.org/10.1038/ki.2011.213.
7. Rocco MV, Daugirdas JT, Greene T, et al. Long-term effects of frequent nocturnal hemodialysis on mortality: the Frequent Hemodialysis Network (FHN) Nocturnal Trial. Am J Kidney Dis. 2015;66(3):459–68. https://doi.org/10.1053/j.ajkd.2015.02.331.
8. Kjellstrand CM, Buoncristiani U, Ting G, et al. Short daily haemodialysis: survival in 415 patients treated for 1006 patient-years. Nephrol Dial Transplant. 2008;23(10):3283–9. https://doi.org/10.1093/ndt/gfn210.
9. Weinhandl ED, Liu J, Gilbertson DT, Arneson TJ, Collins AJ. Survival in daily home hemodialysis and matched thrice-weekly in-center hemodialysis patients. J Am Soc Nephrol. 2012;23(5):895–904. https://doi.org/10.1681/ASN.2011080761.
10. Nesrallah GE, Lindsay RM, Cuerden MS, et al. Intensive hemodialysis associates with improved survival compared with conventional hemodialysis. J Am Soc Nephrol. 2012;23(4):696–705. https://doi.org/10.1681/ASN.2011070676.
11. Nadeau-Fredette AC, Hawley CM, Pascoe EM, et al. An incident cohort study comparing survival on home hemodialysis and peritoneal dialysis (Australia and New Zealand Dialysis and Transplantation Registry). Clin J Am Soc Nephrol. 2015;10(8):1397–407. https://doi.org/10.2215/CJN.00840115.
12. Nesrallah GE, Li L, Suri RS. Comparative effectiveness of home dialysis therapies: a matched cohort study. Can J Kidney Health Dis. 2016;3:19. https://doi.org/10.1186/s40697-016-0105-x.

13. Nadeau-Fredette AC, Tennankore KK, Perl J, Bargman JM, Johnson DW, Chan CT. Home hemodialysis and peritoneal dialysis patient and technique survival in Canada. Kidney Int Rep. 2020;5(11):1965–73. https://doi.org/10.1016/j.ekir.2020.08.020.
14. Weinhandl ED, Gilbertson DT, Collins AJ. Mortality, hospitalization, and technique failure in daily home hemodialysis and matched peritoneal dialysis patients: a matched cohort study. Am J Kidney Dis. 2016;67(1):98–110. https://doi.org/10.1053/j.ajkd.2015.07.014.
15. Choi SJ, Obi Y, Ko GJ, et al. Comparing patient survival of home hemodialysis and peritoneal dialysis patients. Am J Nephrol. 2020;51(3):192–200. https://doi.org/10.1159/000504691.
16. Ethier I, Cho Y, Hawley C, et al. Multicenter registry analysis comparing survival on home hemodialysis and kidney transplant recipients in Australia and New Zealand. Nephrol Dial Transplant. 2021;36(10):1937–46. https://doi.org/10.1093/ndt/gfaa159.
17. Nishio-Lucar AG, Bose S, Lyons G, Awuah KT, Ma JZ, Lockridge RS Jr. Intensive home hemodialysis survival comparable to deceased donor kidney transplantation. Kidney Int Rep. 2020;5(3):296–306. https://doi.org/10.1016/j.ekir.2019.12.019.
18. Molnar MZ, Ravel V, Streja E, et al. Survival of elderly adults undergoing incident home hemodialysis and kidney transplantation. J Am Geriatr Soc. 2016;64(10):2003–10. https://doi.org/10.1111/jgs.14321.
19. Marshall MR, Polkinghorne KR, Kerr PG, Hawley CM, Agar JW, McDonald SP. Intensive hemodialysis and mortality risk in Australian and New Zealand populations. Am J Kidney Dis. 2016;67(4):617–28. https://doi.org/10.1053/j.ajkd.2015.09.025.
20. Rydell H, Ivarsson K, Almquist M, Segelmark M, Clyne N. Improved long-term survival with home hemodialysis compared with institutional hemodialysis and peritoneal dialysis: a matched cohort study. BMC Nephrol. 2019;20(1):52. https://doi.org/10.1186/s12882-019-1245-x.

Cardiovascular Outcomes Associated with Frequent Hemodialysis

5

Justin Cheng and Christopher T. Chan

Introduction

Case Presentation: Sam is a 49-year-old man with ESKD from diabetic nephropathy. He has recently transitioned to in-center hemodialysis, after peritoneal membrane failure. He has a history of well-controlled hypertension and type 1 diabetes. He has a family history of premature coronary artery disease (CAD). He was working as an accountant, but took time off after peritoneal dialysis (PD) failure. What can you tell Sam regarding cardiovascular (CV) benefits of home hemodialysis to justify transitioning from in-center hemodialysis.

Hemodialysis (HD) is the most common treatment modality worldwide for patients with ESKD. A recent review showed that 89% of all dialysis patients receive HD [2]. Chronic maintenance HD is offered mainly in high-income countries due to its high cost to the healthcare system, especially when considering that a relatively small fraction of the population requires this treatment [3]. Nevertheless, HD remains an important life-sustaining modality [4].

In addition to a lower quality of life, HD patients also have an inappropriately high mortality rate despite decades of research and process improvement [5]. According to USRDS 2018 (Fig. 5.1), the majority of mortality is associated with CV diseases [1]. There are many interlinked factors between renal and cardiac disease, as shown in Fig. 5.2. First, kidney disease and ischemic heart disease share similar risk factors for disease progression, such as hypertension and diabetes. Among numerous pathways, both hypertension and diabetes are pro-inflammatory, which augments a positive feedback loop of both renal and cardiac disease progression [6, 7]. Chronic kidney disease can precipitate volume overload and resistant hypertension in later stages, both detrimental to optimal cardiac function.

J. Cheng · C. T. Chan (✉)
Division of Nephrology, University Health Network, Toronto and the University of Toronto, Toronto, ON, Canada
e-mail: Christopher.chan@uhn.ca

A. Shah et al. (eds.), *Applied Home Hemodialysis*,
https://doi.org/10.1007/978-3-031-77244-3_5

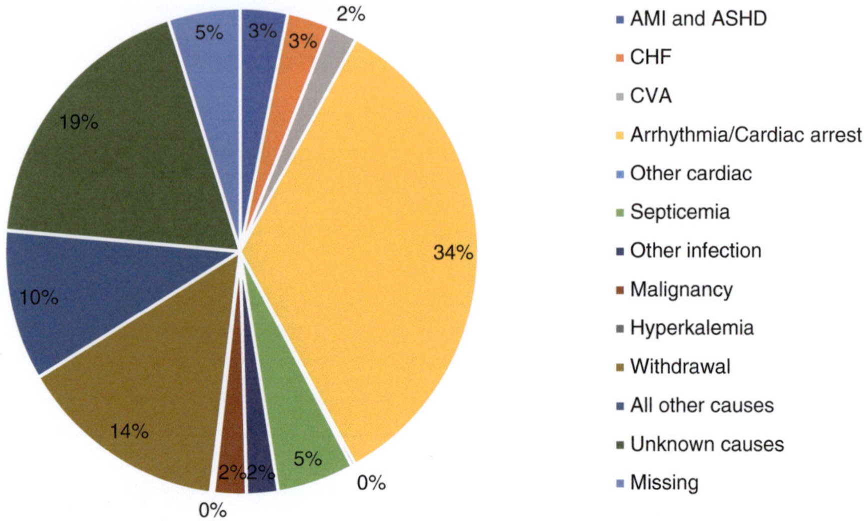

Fig. 5.1 USRDS data demonstrating distribution of known causes of mortality in hemodialysis population in 2018

Due to the aforementioned positive feedback loop, patients often develop ESKD and cardiomyopathy. Even worse, advanced kidney disease often prohibits pharmaceutical agents that effectively treat hypertension, diabetes, proteinuric kidney disease, and congestive heart failure. With advanced cardiac and renal disease, patients may require aggressive ultrafiltration (UF) in order to control symptoms from congestive heart failure. However, myocardial stunning associated with UF further causes cardiac injury. Eventually, cardiac and renal disease may lead to death as a result of pump failure and sudden cardiac death due to ischemic events or arrhythmias.

There is of great interest as to whether frequent hemodialysis (FHD) and increased clearance will decrease CV-related mortality in the HD population. The National Cooperative Dialysis Study (NCDS) was the first randomized controlled trial (RCT) that demonstrated a relationship between time spent on HD and patient outcomes [8]. Targeting a lower time-averaged concentration of urea led to fewer incidence of withdrawal from the trial due to death or medical reasons ($P < 0.0001$). However, only a signal was found to favor longer duration of dialysis at 4.5 h, compared to 3 h with $P = 0.06$. This statistically nonsignificant result was likely a consequence of limited recruitment, with 155 participants split into four groups with 2 × 2 design. Subsequently, in a follow-up analysis in 1985, the authors demonstrated that Kt/V_{Urea} had a significant association with patient outcomes, to a certain ceiling effect [9]. Another major landmark trial guiding current HD practices is the HEMO study, published in 2002 [10]. In this study, high or low Kt/V_{Urea} targets did not demonstrate any significant difference in all-cause mortality, hospitalization for cardiac causes, or CV mortality. Despite limitations such as newer evidence to suggest CV itself independently predicting mortality as a surrogate for body mass and nutritional status, conventional hemodialysis (CHD) consisting of three sessions each week, 4 h each time, is widely practiced [11].

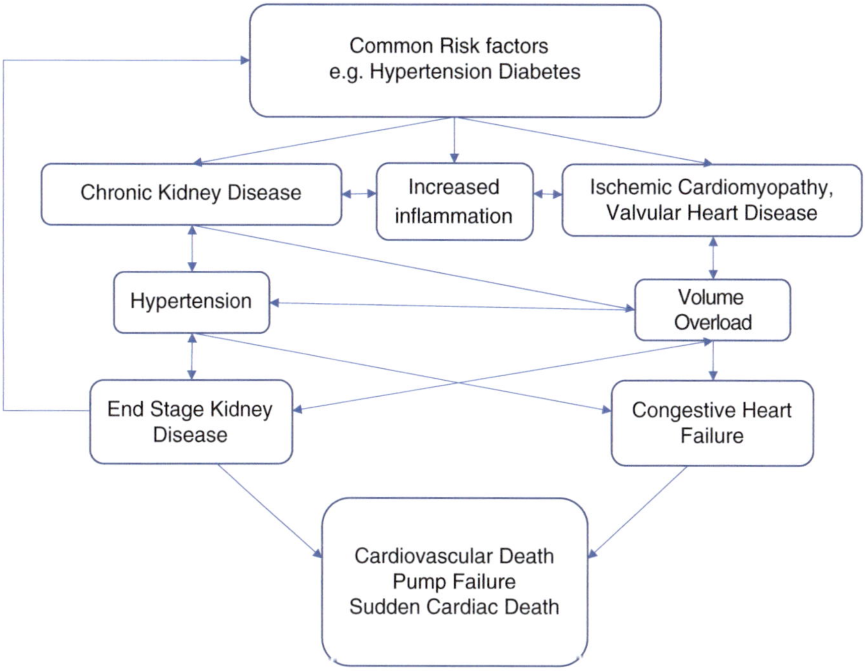

Fig. 5.2 Interplay between cardiac and renal disease

However, CHD mimics native kidney function poorly, and the nature of in-center CHD often demands a fixed and rigid schedule from patients. An alternative to HD is FHD, which consists of many variants as patients are able to choose their own treatment schedule. One of these is termed short daily hemodialysis (SDHD). Often, patients perform HD approximately six times a week, 2 h each time, or with other combinations that result in total treatment time similar to CHD. Another option is nocturnal hemodialysis (NHD), where dialysis is performed over extended hours at night, at variable frequency throughout the week.

This chapter will serve as a review of existing evidence regarding more FHD and CV outcomes. In this chapter, FHD and evidence supporting its use is discussed as an entire entity, rather than specific SDHD or NHD regimens, as we believe FHD regimens should be dictated by patient preference with clinician guidance. Achieving a good understanding of this chapter will be paramount in patient advocacy and counseling.

Ultrafiltration and Myocardial Stunning

Extracellular fluid (ECF) volume homeostasis is maintained by the sum of residual urine output and UF on HD. However, some patients may have normal residual urine output at the time of dialysis initiation, and this value often decays with time, especially with CHD [12]. As residual urine output diminishes with repeated prerenal insults on HD, UF becomes the outlet for ECF homeostasis. Studies have demonstrated that UF rates greater than 10 ml/h/kg are associated with higher CV mortality [13]. For Sam, a 70-kg anuric patient receiving 12 h of dialysis weekly with CHD, this translates to a maximum fluid gain of 1.19 L per day. Unsurprisingly, approximately 37% of patients on CHD exceed this rather restrictive target from a recent retrospective study, and they were found to have worse CV outcomes irrespective of heart failure or diabetes status [14].

One explanation may be related to the magnitude of interdialytic weight gain (IDWG), as UF only occurs three times a week. This then leads to sustained refractory hypertension, left ventricular (LV) remodeling, and greater risk of arrhythmias [15]. During dialysis for these patients, a higher rate of fluid results in a rapid drop in coronary perfusion pressure, and leads to myocardial stunning [16]. As a form of ischemic cardiac injury, myocardial stunning has been visualized as regional or global wall motion abnormalities on echocardiography or magnetic resonance imaging (MRI) [17]. Myocardial injury is proportional to UF rate and intradialytic hypotension. While marked wall motion abnormalities are temporary during HD as blood pressure recovers post-dialysis, myocardial stunning results in long-term loss of systolic function and higher cardiac mortality [18].

The benefit of improved ECF control and UF in FHD is twofold. First, IDWG is attenuated with an increase in HD frequency. This results in a lesser degree of ECF overload and improved blood pressure control, two major risk factors for LV dysfunction. Most importantly, the UF rate is often lower in FHD, especially in the form of NHD with extended hours of HD. This allows for a balance between plasma refill and UF, even in patients with autonomic dysfunction. To illustrate the importance of continued plasma refill in UF, we will use Sam as an example. He weighs 70 kg and is 170 cm tall. With a pre-dialysis hematocrit of 35%, Sam has a total blood volume of 4.7 L and a plasma volume of 3029 ml according to the Nadler formula [19]. Even a modest UF goal of 2.38 L in CHD is 79% of his total plasma volume. However, if Sam performs FHD six times a week, then the UF goal is only 39% of his total plasma volume. In addition, time between FHD sessions allows further equilibrium of total body water to all compartments. Taken together, FHD reduces the harmful cycle of ECF volume overload coupled with rapid fluid removal leading to myocardial stunning and adverse cardiac outcomes.

Blood Pressure Control and Heart Rate Variability

Refractory hypertension affects 80% of patients with ESKD [20]. Treatment of hypertension with pharmacological agents may perpetuate the vicious cycle of intradialytic hypotension, inability to reach target weight followed by ECF overload, and interdialytic hypertension despite a higher pill burden.

Hypertension in ESKD is a resultant of ECF overload and increased peripheral resistance [21]. As discussed above, ECF overload can be better controlled with FHD due to increased total treatment time. The Frequent Hemodialysis Network (FHN) trial has demonstrated that FHD is associated with a significant reduction in pre-dialysis systolic and diastolic blood pressure, as well as the number of antihypertensives [22]. This trial enrolled 245 patients randomized to CHD or six-times-weekly HD in FHD. At the end of the 12-month-long trial, patients received on average 2.88 and 5.17 treatments per week, respectively. Patients with FHD achieved a 10-mmHg reduction in pre-dialysis systolic blood pressure compared to the CHD group. The CHD group required 2.8 antihypertensives on average in the beginning of the study and 2.58 at the end of the trial; on the other hand, the FHD group required 2.69 and 1.87 antihypertensives, respectively.

In an observational crossover study, NHD was associated with better blood pressure control compared to CHD despite no change in patients' target weight or stroke volume, suggesting that the hypotensive effect of longer HD is mediated through a reduction in total peripheral resistance [23]. In addition, the authors demonstrated the feasibility of restoring endothelial-independent vasodilation. The above observations have led to the hypothesis that vasoconstrictive uremic toxins are removed preferentially during NHD due to enhanced clearance of small and middle molecules.

A closely related concept is heart rate variability (HRV). As an emerging concept, it is a noninvasive assessment of autonomic modulation typically achieved via 24-h Holter monitors. Rapid adaptation of the heart rate by the sympathetic and parasympathetic systems is a normal physiologic response to stress. Analysis of HRV allows a noninvasive and continuous monitoring of sympathetic versus parasympathetic balance [24]. A lower HRV, from reduced parasympathetic activation or sympathetic system overactivation, is associated with increased CV events, including hospitalization and sudden cardiac death [25]. Observations from the FHN trial demonstrated that patients with FHD had higher HRV compared to patients on CHD [26].

Left Ventricular Hypertrophy and Cardiac Function

Left ventricular hypertrophy (LVH) affects 70–90% of patients established on HD [27, 28], and may lead to congestive heart failure among HD patients. Left ventricular mass (LVM) can be expressed as left ventricular mass index (LVMi), when it is standardized to the total body surface area of the patient. ECF overload and hypertension are both identified as major culprits for causing maladaptive changes in the myocardium. In patients with declining renal function, these risk factors are more challenging to manage due to limited pharmacological options and result in worsening LVH [29]. In a prospective cohort of CHD patients followed for 18 months, an increase in LVMi appears to correlate with progression of time on CHD; an elevated LVMi is observed to be an independent risk factor for CV events in the HD population [30].

Reversal of these drivers for myocardium maladaptation has been shown to halt the progression of LVH and achieve regression in certain cases [31]. To this end, high-quality evidence in the form of independent RCTs conducted in NHD vs CHD showed a mean reduction in LVM of approximately 14 g at 1 year [32, 33]. This is surprisingly close to the 13.8 g reported in the FHN trial [34]. These results are compiled in Table 5.1. An observational study showed that a 10% reduction in LVM

Table 5.1 LV mass change with intensive HD

	n	HD intervention	Duration of follow-up	LVM change (g)	*p*
Culleton et. al	52	NHD, 6 times per week	6 months	15.3	0.04
Wald et. al	67	NHD, 3 times per week	12 months	14.2	0.03
FHN trial group	125	FHD, 6 times per week	12 months	13.8	<0.001

was associated with a 22% reduction in all-cause mortality and 28% in CV-related mortality after adjustment among HD patients [35].

Ongoing research suggests that hormonal and toxic factors may also contribute to LVH. One such factor is the homeostasis of calcium and phosphate through parathyroid hormone and FGF-23, among others. Studies have shown that an elevated level of FGF-23 among HD patients is an independent risk factor for increased LVMi and CV mortality [36]. The serum FGF-23 level has a direct relationship to its co-receptor in the proximal tubule, klotho. Low serum klotho levels have been observed with increased mortality related to CV events, after adjusting for other risk factors [37]. As a result, it is hypothesized that improved homeostasis of the bone mineral metabolism axis leads to a reduction in LVM and CV mortality via intermediary hormonal effects [38].

FHD has been shown to be beneficial in addressing hormonal contributors to LVH. First, improved pre-dialysis phosphate levels are reported in patients on FHD [39]. Increased time on dialysis leads to increased removal, as with other dialyzable toxins [40]. Furthermore, increased frequency allows greater equilibrium between the accessible intravascular compartment and the intracellular compartment. Post hoc analysis of the FHN trial also demonstrated increased levels of klotho which had led to LVH regression, suggesting a role from intermediary hormones [41–45].

Coronary Calcification and FHD

While CAD and acute myocardial infarction (AMI) only account for 3% of total deaths among HD patients, a past history of both CAD and AMI is risk factors for heart failure, arrhythmias, and sudden cardiac death. The high prevalence of CAD in the HD population may be partially explained by the shared risk factors between atherosclerosis and ESKD [46]. In addition, increased oxidative stress and inflammation associated with uremic toxins and abnormal bone mineral metabolism also contribute to accelerated CAD [47]. Computed tomography (CT) is used as a non-invasive alternative to assess for coronary artery calcification (CAC), and has been shown previously to correlate with the extent and severity of lesions identified in invasive angiography [48]. A cohort study among patients enrolled in FHD noted that patients with established CAC seen on CT had a 9% increase in the CAC score at 12 months [49]. In comparison, another cohort study following patients on CHD had demonstrated a doubling of CAC score at a mean follow-up time of 20 months [50]. However, the two cohorts differ significantly with respect to age, a major risk factor for CAD. A direct comparison between similar or randomized cohorts is needed in the future.

Arrhythmias and Sudden Cardiac Death

Among HD patients, arrhythmias and sudden cardiac death make up 38% among all mortality from USRDS data in 2018. While many disease entities result in life-threatening arrhythmias, HD patients are especially at risk due to rapid shifts of fluid and electrolytes with intermittent HD. In a novel study, implantable loop recorders were provided to patients who underwent CHD [51]. In a follow-up period of 6 months, 20% of patients experienced bradycardia, and 9% of patients had asystole episodes. The highest event rate of non-atrial fibrillation, clinically significant arrhythmias, was during the dialysis session 72 h after the last treatment. In other words, CHD patients are at the highest risk for significant arrhythmias during a Monday or Tuesday dialysis session, where rapid changes in electrolytes including potassium and total body water distribution are expected. The second most significant time interval was 12 h prior to the aforementioned HD treatment. Interestingly, analysis of pre-HD electrolyte levels did not find any significant associations with event rates. As such, the absolute level of serum electrolytes pre-HD is not as important as the rate and magnitude of change after a long period without HD treatment. This is supported by data from the DOPPS with 37,765 patients, where it was found that dialysate potassium lower than 3 mEq/L was associated with a 17–39% higher likelihood of sudden death [52]. FHD is associated with a lower potassium gradient between the serum and dialysate and may lead to lower rates of clinically significant arrhythmias [53].

Limitations and Future Directions

In this chapter, we presented several observational and cohort studies in FHD patients and compared them to results from similar studies in CHD patients. We acknowledge that there are likely to be significant fundamental differences with respect to both patient populations. Generally, FHD patients are younger than CHD cohorts. One would postulate that FHD cohorts are less frail and comorbid than CHD cohorts, given the inherent need to undergo training for FHD at home or more frequent travel for in-center FHD. Fortunately, we do have evidence from several RCTs that demonstrate benefits of FHD in randomized cohorts. To optimize this therapy further, large RCTs need to be carried out over longer observational periods. However, it is acknowledged that FHD as a modality is as much a medical decision as well as a lifestyle decision. Significant challenges are anticipated with respect to recruitment and randomization for such studies.

Table 5.2 FHD results

Beneficial outcome in FHD	References
Blood pressure control	[22, 23]
Heart rate variability (HRV)	[26]
Left ventricular (LV) mass reduction	[32–34]
Phosphate control	[39]
Klotho level	[41]
Coronary artery calcification (CAC) assessment with computed tomography	[49]
Potassium gradient	[53]

Conclusion

HD patients suffer significant morbidity and mortality from CV-related causes. The etiology of CV disease among the HD population includes hypertension, volume overload, myocardial stunning, and rapid electrolyte and fluid shifts during CHD. Other dialysis-related CV risk factors include accumulation of uremic toxins, dysregulation of the sympathetic and parasympathetic system, and deranged calcium, phosphate, and bone metabolism. FHD results in smaller deviations from homeostasis and increased uremic toxin clearance compared to CHD. These results are summarized in Table 5.2.

Despite the above, there has not been a definitive RCT that demonstrates improved CV or all-cause mortality among HD patients with FHD. Nephrologists should have regular discussions with patients regarding their values and goals of dialysis, in the context of potential CV benefits while recognizing the higher treatment burden with home dialysis.

References

1. United States Renal Data System. 2020 USRDS Annual Data Report: epidemiology of kidney disease in the United States. Bethesda: National Institutes of Health, National Institute of Diabetes and Digestive and Kidney Diseases; 2020.
2. Himmelfarb J, Vanholder R, Mehrotra R, Tonelli M. The current and future landscape of dialysis. Nat Rev Nephrol. 2020;16:573–85.
3. Vanholder R, Davenport A, Hannedouche T, Kooman J, Kribben A, Lameire N, Lonnemann G, Magner P, Mendelssohn D, Saggi S, Shaffer R, Moe S, Biesen M, van der Sande F, Mehrotra R. Reimbursement of dialysis: a comparison of seven countries. J Am Soc Nephrol. 2012;23:1291–8.
4. Brown E, Zhao J, McCullough K, Fuller D, Figueiredo A, Bieber B, Finkelstein F, Shen J, Kanjanabuch T, Kawanishi H, Pisoni R, Perl J. Burden of kidney disease, health-related quality of life, and employment among patients receiving peritoneal dialysis and in-center hemodialysis: findings from the DOPPS Program. Am J Kidney Dis. 2021;78(4):489–501.
5. Pozzoni P, Del Vecchio L, Pontoriero G, Di Filippo S, Locatelli F. Long-term outcome in hemodialysis: morbidity and mortality. J Nephrol. 2004;17(Suppl 8):S87–95.
6. Petrie JR, Guzik TJ, Touyz RM. Diabetes, hypertension, and cardiovascular disease: clinical insights and vascular mechanisms. Can J Cardiol. 2018;34:575–84.
7. Amdur RL, Feldman HI, Gupta J, Yang W, Kanetsky P, Shlipak M, Rahman M, Lash JP, Townsend RR, Ojo A, Roy-Chaudhury A, Go AS, Joffe M, He J, Balakrishnan VS, Kimmel PL, Kusek JW, Raj DS. Inflammation and progression of CKD: the CRIC Study. Clin J Am Soc Nephrol. 2016;11:1546–56.

8. Lowrie E, Laird N, Parker T, Sargent J. Effect of the hemodialysis prescription on patient morbidity. N Engl J Med. 1981;305(20):1176–81.
9. Gotch F, Sargent J. A mechanistic analysis of the National Cooperative Dialysis Study (NCDS). Kidney Int. 1985;28(3):526–34.
10. Eknoyan G, Beck G, Cheung A, Daugirdas J, Greene T, Kusek J, Allon M, Bailey J, Delmez J, Depner T, Dwyer J, Levey A, Levin N, Milford E, Ornt D, Rocco M, Schulman G, Schwab S, Teehan B, Toto R. Effect of dialysis dose and membrane flux in maintenance hemodialysis. N Engl J Med. 2002;347(25):2010–9.
11. Himmelfarb J. Success and challenge in dialysis therapy. N Engl J Med. 2002;347:2068–70.
12. Jansen M, Hart A, Korevaar J, Dekker F, Boeschoten E, Krediet RT. Predictors of the rate of decline of residual renal function in incident dialysis patients. Kidney Int. 2002;62(3):1046–53.
13. Assimon M, Wenger J, Wang L, Flythe J. Ultrafiltration rate and mortality in maintenance hemodialysis patients. Am J Kidney Dis. 2016;68(6):911–22.
14. Cabrera C, Brunelli S, Rosenbaum D, Anum E, Ramakrishnan K, Jensen D, Stålhammar N, Stefánsson B. A retrospective, longitudinal study estimating the association between interdialytic weight gain and cardiovascular events and death in hemodialysis patients. BMC Nephrol. 2015;16(113):1–9.
15. Inrig J, Patel U, Gillespie B, Himmelfarb J, Hasselblad V, Reddan D, Lindsay R, Winchester J, Stivelman J, Toto R, Szczech L. Relationship between interdialytic weight gain and blood pressure among prevalent hemodialysis patients. Am J Kidney Dis. 2007;50(1):108–18.
16. Chou J, Kalantar-Zadeh K, Mathew A. A brief review of intradialytic hypotension with a focus on survival. Semin Dial. 2017;30(6):473–80.
17. Buchanan C, Mohammed A, Cox E, Köhler K, Canaud B, Taal M, Selby N, Francis S, McIntyre C. Intradialytic cardiac magnetic resonance imaging to assess cardiovascular responses in a short-term trial of hemodiafiltration and hemodialysis. J Am Soc Nephrol. 2017;28(4):1269–77.
18. Jefferies H, Virk B, Schiller B, Moran J, McIntyre C. Frequent hemodialysis schedules are associated with reduced levels of dialysis-induced cardiac injury (myocardial stunning). Clin J Am Soc Nephrol. 2011;6(6):1326–32.
19. Nadler S, Hidalgo JH, Bloch T. Prediction of blood volume in normal human adults. Surgery. 1962;51(2):224–32.
20. Chan C, Floras J, Miller J, Richardson R, Pierratos A. Regression of left ventricular hypertrophy after conversion to nocturnal hemodialysis. Kidney Int. 2002;61:2235–9.
21. Kundhal K, Pierratos A, Chan C. Newer paradigms in renal replacement therapy: will they alter cardiovascular outcomes? Cardiol Clin. 2005;23(3):385–91.
22. Kotanko P, Garg A, Depner T, Pierratos A, Chan C, Levin N, Greene T, Larive B, Beck G, Gassman J, Kliger A, Stokes J. Effects of frequent hemodialysis on blood pressure: results from the randomized frequent hemodialysis network trials. Hemodial Int. 2015;19:386–401.
23. Chan C, Harvey P, Picton P, Pierratos A, Miller J, Floras J. Short-term blood pressure, noradrenergic, and vascular effects of nocturnal home hemodialysis. Hypertension. 2003;42(5):925–31.
24. Shaffer F, Ginsberg JP. An overview of heart rate variability metrics and norms. Front Public Health. 2017;5(258):1–17.
25. Drawz P, Babineau D, Brecklin C, He J, Kallem R, Soliman E, Xie D, Appleby D, Anderson A, Rahman M, Investigators CS. Heart rate variability is a predictor of mortality in chronic kidney disease: a report from the CRIC Study. Am J Nephrol. 2013;38(6):517–28.
26. Chan C, Chertow G, Daugirdas J, Greene T, Kotanko P, Larive B, Larive B, Pierratos A, Stokes J. Effects of daily hemodialysis on heart rate variability: results from the Frequent Hemodialysis Network (FHN) Daily Trial. Nephrol Dial Transplant. 2014;29(1):168–78.
27. Lopez-Gomez J, Verde E, Perez-Garcia R. Blood pressure, left ventricular hypertrophy and long-term prognosis in hemodialysis patients. Kidney Int. 1998;54:S92–8.
28. Levin A, Singer J, Thompson C, Ross H, Lewis M. Prevalent left ventricular hypertrophy in the predialysis population: Identifying opportunities for intervention. Am J Kidney Dis. 1996;27(3):347–54.
29. House A, Wanner C, Sarnak MJ, Piña IL, McIntyre CW, Komenda P, Kasiske BL, Deswal A, deFilippi CR, Cleland JGF, Anker SD, Herzog CA, Cheung M. Heart failure in chronic

kidney disease: conclusions from a Kidney Disease: Improving Global Outcomes (KDIGO) Controversies Conference. Kidney Int. 2019;95:1304–17.
30. Zoccali C, Benedetto F, Mallamaci F, Tripepi G, Giacone G, Stancanelli B, Cataliotti A, Malatino L. Left ventricular mass monitoring in the follow-up of dialysis patients: prognostic value of left ventricular hypertrophy progression. Kidney Int. 2004;65(4):1292–498.
31. Shenasa M, Shenasa H. Hypertension, left ventricular hypertrophy, and sudden cardiac death. Int J Cardiol. 2017;237:60–3.
32. Wald R, Goldstein M, Perl J, Kiaii M, Yuen D, Wald R, Harel Z, Weinstein J, Jakubovic B, Leong-Poi H, Kirpalani A, Leipsic J, Dacouris N, Wolf M, Yan A. The association between conversion to in-centre nocturnal hemodialysis and left ventricular mass regression in patients with end-stage renal disease. Can J Cardiol. 2016;32(3):369–77.
33. Culleton B, Walsh M, Klarenbach S, Mortis G, Scott-Douglas N, Quinn R, Tonelli M, Donnelly S, Friedrich M, Kumar A, Mahallati H, Hemmelgarn BR, Manns BJ. Effect of frequent nocturnal hemodialysis vs conventional hemodialysis on left ventricular mass and quality of life a randomized controlled trial. JAMA. 2007;298(11):1291–9.
34. The FHN Trial Group. In-center hemodialysis six times per week. N Engl J Med. 2010;363(24):2287–300.
35. London G, Pannier B, Guerin A, Blacher J, Marchais S, Darne B, Metivier F, Adda HSM. Alterations of left ventricular hypertrophy in and survival of patients receiving hemodialysis: follow-up of an interventional study. J Am Soc Nephrol. 2001;12(12):2759–67.
36. Unver S, Kavlak E, Gumusel H, Celikbilek F, Esertas K, Muftuoglu T, Kirilmaz A. Correlation between hypervolemia, left ventricular hypertrophy and Correlation between hypervolemia, left ventricular hypertrophy and. Ren Fail. 2015;37(6):951–6.
37. Memmos E, Sarafidis P, Pateinakis P, Tsiantoulas A, Faitatzidou D, Giamalis P, Vasilikos V, Papagianni A. Soluble Klotho is associated with mortality and cardiovascular events in hemodialysis. BMC Nephrol. 2019;20(217):1–10.
38. Erben R. Physiological actions of fibroblast growth factor-23. Front Endocrinol. 2018;9(267):1–7.
39. Copland M, Komenda P, Weinhandl E, McCullough P, Morfin J. Intensive hemodialysis, mineral and bone disorder, and phosphate binder use. Am J Kidney Dis. 2016;68(5):S24–32.
40. Twardowski Z. Treatment time and ultrafiltration rate are more important in dialysis prescription than small molecule clearance. Blood Purif. 2007;25:90–8.
41. Chan C, Kaysen G, Beck G, Li M, Lo J, Rocco M, Kliger A, Trials F. Changes in biomarker profile and left ventricular hypertrophy regression: results from the Frequent Hemodialysis Network Trials. Am J Nephrol. 2018;47(3):208–17.
42. Gutierrez O, Mannstadt M, Isakova T, Rauh-Hain J, Tamez H, Shah A, Smith K, Lee H, Thadhani R, Jüppner H, Wolf M. Fibroblast growth factor 23 and mortality among patients undergoing hemodialysis. N Engl J Med. 2008;359(6):584–92.
43. Hu M, Kuro-o M, Moe O. Klotho and chronic kidney disease. Contrib Nephrol. 2013;180:47–63.
44. Smith K, deFilippi C, Isakova T, Gutiérrez O, Laliberte K, Seliger S, Kelley W, Duh S, Hise M, Christenson R, Wolf M, Januzzi M. Fibroblast growth factor 23, high-sensitivity cardiac troponin. Am J Kidney Dis. 2013;61(1):67–73.
45. Yang K, Wang C, Nie L, Zhao X, Gu J, Guan X, Wang S, Xiao T, Xu X, He T, Xia X, Wang J, Zhao J. Klotho protects against indoxyl sulphate-induced myocardial hypertrophy. J Am Soc Nephol. 2015;26:2434–46.
46. Burlacu A, Genovesi S, Basile C, Ortiz A, Mitra S, Kirmizis D, Kanbay M, Davenport A, van der Sande F, Covic A. Coronary artery disease in dialysis patients: evidence synthesis, controversies and proposed management strategies. J Nephrol. 2021;34:39–51.
47. Sarnak M, Amann K, Bangalore S, Cavalcante J, Charytan D, Craig J, Gill J, Hlatky M, Jardine A, Landmesser U, Newby L, Herzog C, Cheung M, Wheeler DC, Winkelmayer WC, Marwick T. Chronic kidney disease and coronary artery disease. J Am Coll Cardiol. 2019;74(14):1823–38.

48. Mautner S, Mautner G, Froehlich J, Feuerstein IM, Proschan MA, Roberts WC, Doppman JL. Coronary artery disease: prediction with in vitro electron beam CT. Radiology. 1994;192:625–30.
49. Yuen D, Pierratos A, Richardson R, Chan C. The natural history of coronary calcification progression in a cohort of nocturnal haemodialysis patients. Nephrol Dial Transplant. 2006;21(5):1407–12.
50. Goodman W, Goldin J, Kuizon B, Yoon C, Gales B, Sider D, Wang Y, Chung J, Emerick A, Greaser L, Elashoff R, Salusky I. Coronary-artery calcification in young adults with end-stage renal disease who are undergoing dialysis. N Engl J Med. 2000;342(20):1478–83.
51. Roy-Chaudhury P, Tumlin J, Koplan B, Costea A. Primary outcomes of the Monitoring in Dialysis Study indicate that clinically significant arrhythmias are common in hemodialysis patients and related to dialytic cycle. Kidney Int. 2018;93:941–51.
52. Jadoul M, Thumma J, Fuller D, Tentori F, Li Y, Morgenstern H, Mendelssohn D, Tomo T, Ethier J, Port F, Robinson B. Modifiable practices associated with sudden death among hemodialysis patients in the dialysis outcomes and practice patterns study. CJASN. 2012;7:765–4.
53. Brunelli S, Spiegel D, Du Mond C, Oestrreicher N, Winkelmayer W, Kovesdy C. Serum-to-dialysate potassium gradient and its association with short-term outcomes in hemodialysis patients. Nephrol Dial Transplant. 2018;33:1207–14.

Complications of Home Hemodialysis

6

Heedeok Han and Sean Kalloo

These complications can be categorized into five main categories: procedure-related, vascular-access-related, medical, nutritional, and psychosocial. The major procedure-related complications include hemorrhage, air embolism, and water-system-related problems. Patients and their caregivers should be trained properly with clear instructions on securing the needles and being knowledgeable and attentive to alarms. Machines should be tested before use to ensure that the monitor and alarm system is working properly. When performing dialysis, dialysis access and tubing, screens, alarms, and monitoring devices should be visible throughout the duration of the treatment. The water system should be monitored on a regular basis for adequacy. Due to the increased frequency of cannulation compared to conventional hemodialysis, patients and care partners should also be aware that there is a higher risk of developing vascular-access-related complications.

Lastly, although home hemodialysis can empower patients to perform dialysis treatment independently at home, it can place an additional burden on patients and care partners alike. Psychosocial stressors are overlooked and can lead to burnout, poor compliance, and discontinuation of therapy.

Patient Case

The patient is a 66-year-old male with a history of end-stage renal diseases on home hemodialysis 5 days a week who presented with a fever of 103.7 at home and lethargy. The patient did not endorse erythema or purulence of the arteriovenous (AV)

H. Han
Division of Nephrology, Columbia University Medical Center, New York, NY, USA
e-mail: hh2868@cumc.columbia.edu

S. Kalloo (✉)
Division of Nephrology, Department of Medicine, Columbia University Medical Center, New York, NY, USA
e-mail: sk3382@cumc.columbia.edu

A. Shah et al. (eds.), *Applied Home Hemodialysis*,
https://doi.org/10.1007/978-3-031-77244-3_6

fistula. The patient's vital signs on arrival to the emergency room were notable for temperature of 37.3, heart rate of 93, blood pressure of 95/69, respiration rate of 16, and oxygen saturation of 96% on room air. Physical examination was notable for normal heart sounds without murmurs, AV fistula was without erythema or drainage, and the absence of splinter hemorrhage, Osler's nodes, or Janeway's lesion was noted. Laboratories were notable for white blood cell counts of 8300 per microliter elevated CRP of 189 mg/L, ESR of 60 mm/h, and peripheral blood cultures that grew methicillin-resistant *Staphylococcus aureus* in 2 out of 2 bottles. The patient was initiated on IV vancomycin. Subsequent workup was notable for MRI brain without contrast demonstrating subacute infarctions spanning multiple vascular territories, compatible with central embolic etiology. The transesophageal echocardiogram obtained showed 1.6 × 2.1 cm highly mobile vegetation from the mitral valve with mild mitral regurgitation. The ultrasound of the AV fistula did not show any evidence of fluid collection; however, no other sources were identified during the hospitalization. The cardiothoracic surgery team was consulted for surgical intervention, but the patient declined intervention. The patient was discharged with 6 weeks of IV vancomycin.

- *Introduction*
- There are many potential benefits of home hemodialysis compared to conventional in-center hemodialysis [1–7]. However, there are unique complications that patients and the healthcare team need to be aware of due to the absence of direct supervision from medical professionals. These complications can be categorized into five main categories: procedure-related, vascular-access-related, medical, nutritional, and psychosocial. Managing these complications can be challenging for patients, caregivers, and healthcare providers.
- Providers who lack the experience working with home hemodialysis have expressed safety concerns about home hemodialysis [8]. Despite these concerns, serious adverse events in home hemodialysis are infrequent [9, 10]. A single-center report from a program in Canada that included 202 patients with a total follow-up of 757 patients-years reported that the rate of serious adverse events was 0.009 per patient-year and 0.038 per 1000 dialysis treatments [11]. Similarly, reports from 2 adult home hemodialysis programs that included 190 patients and approximately 500 patient-years of treatment noted 1 death and 6 potentially fatal adverse events, yielding a crude rate of 0.060 events per 1000 dialysis treatments [12].
- In terms of mortality, 9 cases of death related to adverse events have been reported in the literature. The most common adverse event was blood loss (7 out of 9 cases), followed by one episode of air embolism and one episode of hypercalcemia. Although rare, these adverse events can be fatal, and it is critical to review the most common complications and adverse events in home hemodialysis (Table 6.1).
- *Procedure-Related Complications*
- The most common procedure-related complications of home hemodialysis include major bleeding, air embolism, and water-system-related complications.
  - *Major Bleeding*

Table 6.1 Complications of Home Hemodialysis

Procedure-related complications	
Major bleeding	Bleeding can occur from needle dislodgement, disconnection from the catheter, bleeding from the dialysis circuit, and bleeding into the dialysis circuit
Air embolism	Common air entry points are between the patient and the blood pump due to high negative pressure and leaks in the circuit, air in the dialysate fluid, and during connection and disconnection to the dialysis circuit
Water-related events	Chemical contaminations, presence of bacteria and endotoxins, and varying water pressure and temperature are common water-related complications
Vascular access	More frequent access procedures, access failure, and access-related infections have been noted in more frequent hemodialysis
Medical complication	
Cardiovascular	Intradialytic hypotension (IDH) can occur due to machine dysfunction or when the patient does not follow ultrafiltration recommended by supervising staff. IDH can also occur if antihypertensive medications are not appropriately down-titrated
Loss of residual renal function	Lower urine volume, kidney urea, and creatinine clearance at 4 and 12 months have been reported in the FHN nocturnal trial
Mineral bone diseases	Hypophosphatemia has been associated with more frequent hemodialysis
Nutrition and psychosocial complications	
Nutrition complications	Lower thiamine, pyridoxine, and vitamin C have been reported in home hemodialysis patients, as well as lower levels of L-carnitine and acetylcarnitine
Psychosocial complications	Anxiety due to self-delivering medical therapy, illness intrusiveness, increased financial burden, and care partner burnout have been noted

- Major bleeding due to unobserved blood loss can be life-threatening. Blood loss can occur during hemodialysis mainly through the following mechanisms: needle dislodgement, disconnection from the catheter, bleeding from the dialysis circuit, and bleeding into the dialysis circuit. In a single-center study that reported 22 first events and 7 recurrent events, 18 out of 29 (62%) events were related to AV fistula or graft needle dislodgements. Four of these events led to blood loss, three of which led to blood loss requiring transfusion [11]. In another study that included two home hemodialysis programs, 6 out of the 7 events reported during the studies were related to blood loss [12]. In both of these studies, the majority of the events were attributed to patient error, such as incorrect taping or cannulation technique, improper threading, misuse of machine alarms, and misalignment of an arterial clamp.
- *Air Embolism*
- Air embolism is rare due to recent advancements in technology and equipment that have built-in sensors to detect and terminate treatment in the presence of air in the dialysis circuit. In the previously mentioned single-center Canadian study, air embolism accounted for 6 out of 29 reported adverse events. However, it was still less than one occurrence per 30,000 dialysis treatments [11]. Another study only reported one episode of air embolism in approximately 500 patient-years of treatment and less than one episode per 100,000 dialysis treatments [12]. In the Frequent Hemodialysis Network

(FHN) Nocturnal Trial, one patient died from the frequent nocturnal arm. In all cases, air embolism was attributed to patient error [13].

- Air entry can occur in three susceptible areas: (1) between the patient and the blood pump due to high negative pressure and leaks in the circuit, (2) air in the dialysate fluid, and (3) during connection and disconnection to the dialysis circuit [12]. Air embolism can also occur during insertion or removal of a central venous catheter. Venous air embolism occurs when air is introduced into the systemic venous circulation. The air in the venous circulation can travel to the pulmonary circulation via right side of the heart and cause acute respiratory failure, circulatory collapse from obstructive shock, and cardiac arrest. Arterial air embolism occurs less frequently but can have serious consequences such as end-organ ischemia. It can occur via direct introduction of air into the systemic arterial circulation, incomplete filtration of venous air emboli at the pulmonary capillaries, and paradoxical embolization through septal defect, patent foramen ovale, or pulmonary AV malformation.
- The patient should immediately clamp and disconnect to prevent further air entry into the circuit. Patients with venous air embolism should be placed in the left lateral decubitus position, Trendelenburg position, or left lateral decubitus head-down position. Patients with arterial embolism should be placed in the supine position [14]. Emergency medical services should be contacted by the patient's caregiver.
- *Prevention*
- There are several methods that can be utilized to prevent or reduce the incidence of procedure-related adverse events. First and foremost, the patients and their caregivers should be trained properly with clear instructions on securing the needles and being knowledgeable and attentive to alarms. Machines should be tested before use to ensure that the monitor and alarm system is working properly. When performing dialysis, dialysis access and tubing, screens, alarms, and monitoring devices should be visible throughout the duration of the treatment. When adverse events do occur, retraining the patients has shown some promise as recurrent adverse events only occurred in 32% of the patients. Remote monitoring, supplementary visits using telehealth, and using catheters or cannulation needles with integrated warning devices can also be utilized to mitigate the risk of unobserved adverse events [15]. Lastly, all patients and caregivers need clear instructions on when and how to contact emergency medical services.
- *Water-Related Events*
- A typical dialysis patient is exposed to 300 to 600 L of water per week. Due to more prolonged and frequent dialysis, home hemodialysis patients will often be exposed to more water when compared to that of in-center hemodialysis. Therefore, maintaining water quality that meets the best standard practice is quintessential to home hemodialysis. Guidelines that are adapted by many agencies around the world on water quality and treatment can be located in the International Standards Organization (ISO) catalog.

- Problems that arise due to contaminants in water used for home hemodialysis are similar to those of in-center hemodialysis. Table 6.2, adapted from a paper published in 2013 by Layman et al., shows signs and symptoms related to its respective water contaminants [16]. Most of these chemicals are removed via the reverse osmosis (RO) machine, but chlorine and chloramine that are added to the water as a disinfectant are not well removed by the RO and can damage the RO membrane. Therefore, activated carbon beds or filters are used to remove chlorine from the water. It is crucial to ensure removal of chlorine and chloramine as excess in these contaminants can cause hemolysis, hemolytic anemia, and methemoglobinemia [17–19]. It has also been associated with erythropoietin resistance [20].
- In addition to the chemical contaminants that were previously mentioned, bacteria and endotoxin can also be present in the water. RO membranes, ultrafilter, and ultraviolet light can be utilized to remove these particles from the water system. If bacteria and endotoxin enter the bloodstream from the blood compartment, it can cause bacteremia and pyrogenic reactions.
- As municipal water supply can vary day to day, monitoring for quality is important. Before treatment or every batch, a simple test strip can be used to detect the presence of excess chlorine or chloramines in the water. The presence of bacteria and other chemicals can be detected by sending a sample of treatment water to the laboratory for safety evaluation.
- A technical problem with the water supply that can become an issue in home hemodialysis is low water pressure. If the pressures from main water supply are low, it can cause an issue with the reverse osmosis machines, as it requires a certain level of pressure to function. Low pressure could be inherently low from water mains, but other factors such as HD site being geographically located above ground level (i.e., high-rise building) can cause the water pressure to be lower than the required level. The use of a booster pump at the feed waterline, installation of a header tank, or use of a "flow-fed" RO unit instead of a "pressure-fed" RO unit can be used to overcome low water pressures.

Table 6.2 Signs and symptoms associated with exposure to water contaminants

Symptoms	Possible water contaminants
Anemia	Aluminum, chloramine, copper, zinc
Bone disease	Aluminum, fluoride
Hemolysis	Copper, nitrates, chloramine
Hypertension	Calcium, sodium
Hypotension	Bacteria, endotoxin, nitrates
Metabolic acidosis	Low pH, sulfates
Neurological deterioration	Aluminum
Nausea and vomiting	Bacteria, calcium, copper, endotoxin, low pH, magnesium, nitrates, sulfates, zinc, microcystins
Death	Aluminum, fluoride, endotoxin, bacteria, chloramine, microcystins
Visual disturbances	Microcystins
Liver failure	Microcystins

- Water temperature can vary depending on location—and extremes of temperature can make RO units inefficient or inoperative. A thermostatic mixing valve can be used to mix hot and cold water when the feed water is too cold. When the feed water is too hot, the heat exchanger can be used to cool the water. A higher water pH will reduce the efficiency of carbon filters and RO membrane. Machine malfunctions resulting in machine shutdown are power failure and compromise in water supply. The dialysis session should be terminated in this instance, and the dialysis center should be contacted for service [21].
- Lastly, there was a case report of life-threatening hypercalcemia due to a technical error due to the drain port of the reverse osmosis machine being connected to the dialysis machine.

- *Vascular-Access-Related Complications*
- AV fistulas remain the optimal dialysis access for more frequent hemodialysis [22, 23]. However, due to the increased frequency of cannulation compared to conventional hemodialysis, it is at a higher risk of developing complications.
- In the two randomized controlled trials from the FHN, there was evidence of more access-related events in the frequent hemodialysis group [13]. In the FHN Daily Trial, 47% of the patients undergoing short daily hemodialysis (SDHD) required at least one procedure related to vascular access, compared to only 29% in the conventional hemodialysis group. The frequent hemodialysis group also had a higher hazard ratio (HR) in the analysis of time to first intervention (HR 1.71; 95% CI, 1.08–2.73) and had trend toward requiring multiple interventions (HR 1.35; 95% CI, 0.84–2.18). Daily hemodialysis patients also had significantly more total AV access repairs than the conventional hemodialysis patients ($P = 0.011$) [24]. Hospitalization between the groups did not differ. Likewise, in the FHN Nocturnal Trial, there was a trend toward the frequent nocturnal group having more access-related complications. In the frequent nocturnal group, there were a total of 34 vascular access events (17 failure and 17 access procedures) compared to 21 events (13 failures and 8 access procedures) in the conventional group ($P = 0.10$). 51% of patients in the nocturnal group compared to 36% of the patients in the conventional hemodialysis group suffered vascular access failure or underwent at least one vascular access procedure.
- In a large case series from Australia that included 286 patients undergoing extended-hours dialysis, Kaplan-Meier curves showed the group that received more frequent dialysis (>3.5 sessions/week) had an increased incidence of access-related events than the lesser dialysis frequency group (≤3.5 sessions/week; log-rank $P < 0.001$). An increase in dialysis frequency remained a significant predictor of access-related events on multivariate analysis [25].
- As with mechanical complications, access-related infections are also common in home hemodialysis due to frequent cannulation. In a large observational cohort study using US Renal Data System data that matched 3480 home hemodialysis patients to 17,400 conventional dialysis patients, home dialysis cohort had a higher rate of hospitalization due to vascular access infection than the conventional hemodialysis cohort with a HR of 1.39 (1.28–1.5) [26]. In the previously

mentioned Australian case series that reported outcomes from extended-hours dialysis patients, the most frequent access-related adverse event in the study group was infection (59.5%) [25].

- The use of a central venous catheter for dialysis access has been associated with an increased risk of infection, hospitalization, and death [27, 28]. The buttonhole cannulation technique also seems to be associated with an increased risk of infection compared to rope-ladder cannulation [29–31].
- *Medical Complications*
  - *Cardiovascular*
  - Intradialytic hypotension (IDH) is a common and significant complication of in-center hemodialysis. It is worse with worse cardiac function and mortality [32]. Although cardiovascular stability has consistently been reported to be better with longer and more frequent dialysis, IDH can occur if there is machine dysfunction and the patient does not follow ultrafiltration recommended by supervising staff. IDH can also occur if antihypertensive medications are not appropriately down-titrated. Patients frequently require less antihypertensive therapy with more frequent/longer dialysis sessions.
  - *Loss of residual renal function*
  - With a lower rate of ultrafiltration and lower frequency of IDH, one would expect that residual renal function (RRF) would be more preserved in patients that choose home dialysis as their dialysis modality. However, in the FHN Nocturnal Trial, patients in the nocturnal group who received dialysis 6 times per week had lower urine volume, kidney urea, and creatinine clearance at 4 and 12 months [13]. It is possible that overall lower blood pressure in patients with home dialysis may decrease renal perfusion, leading to an increased rate of decline of RRF.
  - *Mineral Bone Disease*
  - Longer and more frequent dialysis sessions have shown to significantly reduce phosphorous levels leading to the discontinuation of phosphate binders [13]. However, it can also lead to clinically significant electrolyte abnormalities. Longer dialysis can lead to an increased risk of post-dialysis hypophosphatemia, and the addition of phosphate to the dialysate should be considered. Calcium in dialysate should be adjusted according to the therapy prescription as inappropriate dialysate calcium can cause detrimental effects on bone mineral disease [33]. An observational study that was published in 2003 noted that there was a negative calcium balance in nocturnal dialysis patients who dialyzed against 1.25 mmol/L calcium for 8 h when compared to calcium balances of conventional hemodialysis and SDHD. The nocturnal group also had significantly elevated bone alkaline phosphatase levels and intact parathyroid hormone levels [34]. Markers of bone turnover were normalized by 21 months when 1.75 mmol/L calcium bath was used in this group.
- *Nutrition and Psychosocial Complications*
  - *Nutrition*
  - There have been few observational studies and reports that have described loss of nutrients with longer dialysis. In a study that compared water-soluble

vitamin levels in 26 extended dialysis (>15 h/week) to the conventional group, the extended dialysis group was noted to have significantly lower thiamine and vitamin C levels [35]. Lower levels of pyridoxine have also been reported in home hemodialysis patients [36]. A recent observational study from Canada also reported that L-carnitine and acetylcarnitine levels were also noted to be decreased in patients after conversion from conventional hemodialysis to nocturnal hemodialysis [37].

- *Psychosocial*
- Home hemodialysis can empower patients to perform dialysis treatments independently at home by providing increased autonomy and flexibility in daily schedule. However, doing dialysis at home can place a strain or be a source of an additional burden on patients and care partners alike. Psychosocial stressors are overlooked and can lead to burnout, poor compliance, and discontinuation of therapy.
- Although many home dialysis patients enjoy the flexibility offered by home hemodialysis, it can be a source of anxiety in patients and care partners due to the complexity of therapy, machine maintenance and complications, medical catastrophes, and self-cannulation [38]. Some patients also fear lack of close monitoring by medical staff and experience social isolation [12, 39]. In addition to these factors, patients who perform home hemodialysis at night may experience sleep disturbances due to machine alarms. Other psychosocial stressors that have been noted are illness intrusiveness due to ongoing daily therapy and the presence of dialysis machines and supplies at home and increased direct financial burden to the patients due to higher water and electricity cost and home renovation [38, 40].
- Care partners are instrumental members of the home treatment team, and increased support has been associated with improved adherence, quality of life, and survival in dialysis patients [41, 42]. However, care partners can be affected by increased responsibilities in home hemodialysis. Analysis of effects of frequent hemodialysis on perceived caregiver burdens in the FHN Daily and FHN Nocturnal Trials showed that 70% and 92% of the caregivers, respectively, were unpaid at baseline or during follow-up. In this analysis, it was noted that there was no difference between in-center conventional dialysis and in-center daily dialysis. However, there was a significant increase in the caregiver burden score by the Cousineau scale with home nocturnal dialysis +9.4 (95% ZCI, 0.55–18.3; $P = 0.04$) when relative to home conventional dialysis after multiple imputations for missing data in the nocturnal study. In the Nocturnal Trial, there was an inverse correlation between change in perceived caregiver burden and adherence to prescribed dialysis treatments [43].
- It is paramount that the patients and their care partners undergo adequate training prior to starting or transitioning to home hemodialysis. Training must be done as early as possible and should be individualized as patients have different levels of functioning, social support, financial stability, and employment. Patients and care partners should be informed about not only the benefits of home hemodialysis but also its complications. Any concerns raised

during the training period should be addressed not only prior to initiation of dialysis but on a regular basis afterward [44].

- Group meeting with other home hemodialysis patients, providing extra training even after initiation of home hemodialysis, and offering remote monitoring, can also alleviate the concerns associated with home hemodialysis. Lastly, using other helpers and short-term respite care can assist in easing the burden on the care partners [45, 46].

References

1. Culleton BF, Walsh M, Klarenbach SW, Mortis G, Scott-Douglas N, Quinn RR, et al. Effect of frequent nocturnal hemodialysis vs conventional hemodialysis on left ventricular mass and quality of life: a randomized controlled trial. JAMA. 2007;298(11):1291–9.
2. Group FHNT, Chertow GM, Levin NW, Beck GJ, Depner TA, Eggers PW, et al. In-center hemodialysis six times per week versus three times per week. N Engl J Med. 2010;363(24):2287–300.
3. Hall YN, Larive B, Painter P, Kaysen GA, Lindsay RM, Nissenson AR, et al. Effects of six versus three times per week hemodialysis on physical performance, health, and functioning: Frequent Hemodialysis Network (FHN) randomized trials. Clin J Am Soc Nephrol. 2012;7(5):782–94.
4. Hladunewich MA, Hou S, Odutayo A, Cornelis T, Pierratos A, Goldstein M, et al. Intensive hemodialysis associated with improved pregnancy outcomes: a Canadian and United States cohort comparison. J Am Soc Nephrol. 2014;25(5):1103–9.
5. Lockridge RS, Kjellstrand CM. Nightly home hemodialysis: outcome and factors associated with survival. Hemodial Int. 2011;15(2):211–8.
6. McFarlane PA, Bayoumi AM, Pierratos A, Redelmeier DA. The quality of life and cost utility of home nocturnal and conventional in-center hemodialysis. Kidney Int. 2003;64(3):1004–11.
7. Weinhandl ED, Liu J, Gilbertson DT, Arneson TJ, Collins AJ. Survival in daily home hemodialysis and matched thrice-weekly in-center hemodialysis patients. J Am Soc Nephrol. 2012;23(5):895–904.
8. Tong A, Palmer S, Manns B, Craig JC, Ruospo M, Gargano L, et al. Clinician beliefs and attitudes about home haemodialysis: a multinational interview study. BMJ Open. 2012;2(6):e002146.
9. Kraus M, Burkart J, Hegeman R, Solomon R, Coplon N, Moran J. A comparison of center-based vs. home-based daily hemodialysis for patients with end-stage renal disease. Hemodial Int. 2007;11(4):468–77.
10. Sands JJ, Lacson E Jr, Ofsthun NJ, Kay JC, Diaz-Buxo JA. Home hemodialysis: a comparison of in-center and home hemodialysis therapy in a cohort of successful home hemodialysis patients. ASAIO J. 2009;55(4):361–8.
11. Tennankore KK, d'Gama C, Faratro R, Fung S, Wong E, Chan CT. Adverse technical events in home hemodialysis. Am J Kidney Dis. 2015;65(1):116–21.
12. Wong B, Zimmerman D, Reintjes F, Courtney M, Klarenbach S, Dowling G, et al. Procedure-related serious adverse events among home hemodialysis patients: a quality assurance perspective. Am J Kidney Dis. 2014;63(2):251–8.
13. Rocco MV, Lockridge RS Jr, Beck GJ, Eggers PW, Gassman JJ, Greene T, et al. The effects of frequent nocturnal home hemodialysis: the Frequent Hemodialysis Network Nocturnal Trial. Kidney Int. 2011;80(10):1080–91.
14. Jorens PG, Van Marck E, Snoeckx A, Parizel PM. Nonthrombotic pulmonary embolism. Eur Respir J. 2009;34(2):452–74.

15. Abra G, Schiller B. Public policy and programs—missing links in growing home dialysis in the United States. Semin Dial. 2020;33(1):75–82.
16. Layman-Amato R, Curtis J, Payne GM. Water treatment for hemodialysis: an update. Nephrol Nurs J. 2013;40(5):383–404. 65 quiz 5
17. Tipple MA, Shusterman N, Bland LA, McCarthy MA, Favero MS, Arduino MJ, et al. Illness in hemodialysis patients after exposure to chloramine contaminated dialysate. ASAIO Trans. 1991;37(4):588–91.
18. Junglee NA, Rahman SU, Wild M, Wilms A, Hirst S, Jibani M, et al. When pure is not so pure: chloramine-related hemolytic anemia in home hemodialysis patients. Hemodial Int. 2010;14(3):327–32.
19. de Torres JP, Strom JA, Jaber BL, Hendra KP. Hemodialysis-associated methemoglobinemia in acute renal failure. Am J Kidney Dis. 2002;39(6):1307–9.
20. Fluck S, McKane W, Cairns T, Fairchild V, Lawrence A, Lee J, et al. Chloramine-induced haemolysis presenting as erythropoietin resistance. Nephrol Dial Transplant. 1999;14(7):1687–91.
21. Agar JW, Perkins A, Heaf JG. Home hemodialysis: infrastructure, water, and machines in the home. Hemodial Int. 2015;19(Suppl 1):S93–S111.
22. Suri RS, Nesrallah GE, Mainra R, Garg AX, Lindsay RM, Greene T, et al. Daily hemodialysis: a systematic review. Clin J Am Soc Nephrol. 2006;1(1):33–42.
23. Shurraw S, Zimmerman D. Vascular access complications in daily dialysis: a systematic review of the literature. Minerva Urol Nefrol. 2005;57(3):151–63.
24. Suri RS, Larive B, Sherer S, Eggers P, Gassman J, James SH, et al. Risk of vascular access complications with frequent hemodialysis. J Am Soc Nephrol. 2013;24(3):498–505.
25. Jun M, Jardine MJ, Gray N, Masterson R, Kerr PG, Agar JW, et al. Outcomes of extended-hours hemodialysis performed predominantly at home. Am J Kidney Dis. 2013;61(2):247–53.
26. Weinhandl ED, Nieman KM, Gilbertson DT, Collins AJ. Hospitalization in daily home hemodialysis and matched thrice-weekly in-center hemodialysis patients. Am J Kidney Dis. 2015;65(1):98–108.
27. Rivara MB, Soohoo M, Streja E, Molnar MZ, Rhee CM, Cheung AK, et al. Association of vascular access type with mortality, hospitalization, and transfer to in-center hemodialysis in patients undergoing home hemodialysis. Clin J Am Soc Nephrol. 2016;11(2):298–307.
28. Mustafa RA, Zimmerman D, Rioux JP, Suri RS, Gangji A, Steele A, et al. Vascular access for intensive maintenance hemodialysis: a systematic review for a Canadian Society of Nephrology clinical practice guideline. Am J Kidney Dis. 2013;62(1):112–31.
29. Van Eps CL, Jones M, Ng T, Johnson DW, Campbell SB, Isbel NM, et al. The impact of extended-hours home hemodialysis and buttonhole cannulation technique on hospitalization rates for septic events related to dialysis access. Hemodial Int. 2010;14(4):451–63.
30. Muir CA, Kotwal SS, Hawley CM, Polkinghorne K, Gallagher MP, Snelling P, et al. Buttonhole cannulation and clinical outcomes in a home hemodialysis cohort and systematic review. Clin J Am Soc Nephrol. 2014;9(1):110–9.
31. Lok CE, Sontrop JM, Faratro R, Chan CT, Zimmerman DL. Frequent hemodialysis fistula infectious complications. Nephron Extra. 2014;4(3):159–67.
32. Burton JO, Jefferies HJ, Selby NM, McIntyre CW. Hemodialysis-induced cardiac injury: determinants and associated outcomes. Clin J Am Soc Nephrol. 2009;4(5):914–20.
33. Rickers H, Christensen M, Christiansen C, Rodbro P. Bone mineral loss during centre and home haemodialysis. Influence of vitamin D metabolites and serum parathyroid hormone. Proc Eur Dial Transplant Assoc Eur Ren Assoc. 1985;21:435–40.
34. Al-Hejaili F, Kortas C, Leitch R, Heidenheim AP, Clement L, Nesrallah G, et al. Nocturnal but not short hours quotidian hemodialysis requires an elevated dialysate calcium concentration. J Am Soc Nephrol. 2003;14(9):2322–8.
35. Coveney N, Polkinghorne KR, Linehan L, Corradini A, Kerr PG. Water-soluble vitamin levels in extended hours hemodialysis. Hemodial Int. 2011;15(1):30–8.
36. Hawley CM, Jeffries J, Nearhos J, Van Eps C. Complications of home hemodialysis. Hemodial Int. 2008;12(Suppl 1):S21–5.

37. Kalim S, Wald R, Yan AT, Goldstein MB, Kiaii M, Xu D, et al. Extended duration nocturnal hemodialysis and changes in plasma metabolite profiles. Clin J Am Soc Nephrol. 2018;13(3):436–44.
38. Pipkin M, Eggers PW, Larive B, Rocco MV, Stokes JB, Suri RS, et al. Recruitment and training for home hemodialysis: experience and lessons from the Nocturnal Dialysis Trial. Clin J Am Soc Nephrol. 2010;5(9):1614–20.
39. Walker RC, Hanson CS, Palmer SC, Howard K, Morton RL, Marshall MR, et al. Patient and caregiver perspectives on home hemodialysis: a systematic review. Am J Kidney Dis. 2015;65(3):451–63.
40. Fong E, Bargman JM, Chan CT. Cross-sectional comparison of quality of life and illness intrusiveness in patients who are treated with nocturnal home hemodialysis versus peritoneal dialysis. Clin J Am Soc Nephrol. 2007;2(6):1195–200.
41. Ibrahim N, Teo SS, Che Din N, Abdul Gafor AH, Ismail R. The role of personality and social support in health-related quality of life in chronic kidney disease patients. PLoS One. 2015;10(7):e0129015.
42. Ahrari S, Moshki M, Bahrami M. The relationship between social support and adherence of dietary and fluids restrictions among hemodialysis patients in Iran. J Caring Sci. 2014;3(1):11–9.
43. Suri RS, Larive B, Hall Y, Kimmel PL, Kliger AS, Levin N, et al. Effects of frequent hemodialysis on perceived caregiver burden in the Frequent Hemodialysis Network trials. Clin J Am Soc Nephrol. 2014;9(5):936–42.
44. Jacquet S, Trinh E. The potential burden of home dialysis on patients and caregivers: a narrative review. Can J Kidney Health Dis. 2019;6:2054358119893335.
45. Yu ZL, Seow YY, Seow PS, Tan BL. Effectiveness of a day care program in supporting patients on peritoneal dialysis and their caregivers. Int Urol Nephrol. 2016;48(5):799–805.
46. Karkar A, Hegbrant J, Strippoli GF. Benefits and implementation of home hemodialysis: a narrative review. Saudi J Kidney Dis Transpl. 2015;26(6):1095–107.

Vascular Access at Home

7

Sindhuri Prakash-Polet and Sean Kalloo

Case

A 73-year-old male with a history of ischemic cardiomyopathy, gout, recurrent nephrolithiasis, and chronic kidney disease due to multiple episodes of obstructive uropathy progressed to renal failure. He has been under excellent nephrology care and has been well counseled on his impending need for renal replacement therapy. He opted for a home modality as he had a great support system at home. He initiated peritoneal dialysis. However, the patient developed recurrent peritonitis within the first year of initiation, resulting in peritoneal dialysis failure. The decision to start hemodialysis was made. Given his excellent support system at home, and his desire to maintain his quality of life, the patient wants to continue a home modality. The option of home hemodialysis was considered. The patient and family want to know more about his vascular access options, cannulation techniques, and safety concerns to adequately perform home hemodialysis.

Introduction

Home hemodialysis as a modality has been steadily increasing since 2000s. According to the USRDS, about 9% of patients with end-stage kidney disease were on home modalities by the end of 2018 [1]. This statistic has been reinforced by the "Advancing American Kidney Health" executive order signed in 2019, evidenced

S. Prakash-Polet (✉)
Department of Medicine, Division of Nephrology, Columbia University Irving Medical Center, College of Physicians and Surgeons, New York, NY, USA
e-mail: sp2518@cumc.columbia.edu

S. Kalloo
Department of Radiology, Columbia University Irving Medical Center, College of Physicians and Surgeons, New York, NY, USA
e-mail: sk3382@cumc.columbia.edu

A. Shah et al. (eds.), *Applied Home Hemodialysis*,
https://doi.org/10.1007/978-3-031-77244-3_7

by an incident increase of home modality usage to 20% in 2021, with the majority of patients (about 80%) undergoing peritoneal dialysis [2]. Moreover, patients on home hemodialysis have higher rates of survival [3], decreased ventricular mass [4], improved blood pressure, improved nutritional status, and better overall quality of life when compared to patients undergoing in-center hemodialysis [5]. Despite this, factors that affect expansion of home hemodialysis are complex, involving clinical, operational patient and caregiver barriers. Apprehension surrounding the equipment, vascular access maintenance, and self-cannulation represent a few of the psychological barriers that affect the decision to pursue home hemodialysis. It is well known that early pre-dialysis care and optimal access placement with adequate training can promote home hemodialysis [6, 7]. In this book chapter, we address types of vascular access, cannulation techniques, and safety concerns of vascular access in home hemodialysis.

Types of Vascular Access

Home hemodialysis can be accomplished by all three types of vascular access including central venous catheters, arteriovenous fistulas, and arteriovenous grafts (Table 7.1). As with in-center hemodialysis, the preferred access for home

Table 7.1 Vascular access types—features of the different types of vascular access with advantages and disadvantages of each type

Vascular access types			
	Arteriovenous fistula (AVF)	*Arteriovenous grafts (AVG)*	*Central venous cuffed catheters (CVC)*
Features			
Longevity	5–10 years	2–3 years	Weeks–months
Mortality risk	Lowest mortality rate	Higher mortality rate than fistula, but lower than CVC	High mortality
Infection risk	Lowest infection rate	Higher infection rate than AVF	Highest infection rate
Time to use	6–12 months	2–3 weeks	Immediate
Ease of cannulation	More difficult to cannulate, requires extensive training	Easily identified by the patient for cannulation, requires extensive training	No cannulation required
Risk of pain on cannulation	Pain expected	Pain expected	No pain
Risk of bleeding	High risk of bleeding and bruising	High risk of bleeding & bruising	Lower risk of bleeding
Risk of failure	High primary failure rate	High secondary failure rate	NA
Rate of interventions	Might require interventions for primary patency	Requires more number of interventions for secondary patency	Requires high number of interventions and exchanges

Overall, arteriovenous fistula is the most superior type of vascular access when compared to the other types; however, the access type should be personalized for each patient depending on their ESKD life plan hemodialysis is arteriovenous fistula given the lower mortality risk, lower complication rates, decreased hospitalization, and need for intervention. These features render the fistulae as the most optimal access as patients have longer periods of successful maintenance dialysis making them the access type with the highest longevity [8]. Although they are the ideal type of vascular access and have prompted many initiatives to increase their creation and maintenance over the years, several barriers exist that prevent ubiquitous use. Fistulae can only be placed in patients with permissive vascular anatomy. In addition, they have high primary failure rates due to early thrombosis or inability to mature and are susceptible to increased pain and bruising early on. Fistulae are also susceptible to developing vascular steal syndrome. Arteriovenous grafts are less ideal than arteriovenous fistulae, due to increased rates of thrombosis and infection requiring frequent interventions for patency, altogether affecting secondary patency rates. Nevertheless, they are a good alternative when the fistula fails to mature or when the vascular anatomy precludes creation of arteriovenous fistula. Both fistulae and grafts have increased risk of aneurysms and bleeding, thus making it less ideal in elderly, sick patients [9]. Interestingly, patient survival is superior in patients with fistulae and grafts when treatment was performed at home when compared to in-center hemodialysis [10].

Central venous catheters are associated with higher rates of adverse outcomes in the home setting similar to the rates encountered at in-center hemodialysis. These include infection, hospitalization, need for intervention, arrhythmias, cardiac perforation, and even death [11, 12].

Theoretically, patients receiving home hemodialysis are less at risk for nosocomial infection, but central venous catheters are still foreign bodies that are prone to infection and inflammation that are associated with a higher risk of death and technique failure [13, 14]. Due to these reasons, the use of central venous catheters is considered suboptimal although technically easier to use for patients and caregivers and is reserved for a select group of patients for long-term use. These include situations when a central venous catheter is the only option after many attempts at arteriovenous fistula or graft creation have failed or are prohibitive, patients with a limited lifespan, or situations when the central venous catheter is preferred access and contributes to the patient's quality of life [15].

Although arteriovenous fistulas remain the most ideal vascular access for home hemodialysis, the decision on the type of vascular access should involve consideration of various factors. Planning should start as soon as the estimated glomerular filtration rate falls below the threshold of 15–20 ml/min/m^2, or when patients have rapidly declining renal function at a rate exceeding 10 ml/min/year as fistulas are usually ready to be used 6–12 months after creation and might require maturation procedures to facilitate the process [16]. In addition, advanced chronic kidney disease patients have higher rates of peripheral arterial disease and venous stenosis, which makes fistula creation challenging [17, 18]. Access must be placed in the nondominant arm to reduce the impact of their quality of life ideally. The anatomy of the vasculature needs to be evaluated as the blood vessels must be capable of delivering blood flow that can support dialysis without compromising perfusion to the hand. Physical examination characteristics that are ideal for fistula placement are adequate upper extremity arterial pressure, absence of collateral veins, and differential arm size that indicate good arterial and venous systems. In practice, the minimum arterial diameter is 2 cm, and the venous diameter at the planned venous anastomotic site is 2.5 cm for fistula creation with high maturation rate, and blood vessels that do not meet this minimum requirement should be evaluated for feasibility for arteriovenous fistula creation. Secondary patency rates are higher in patients who undergo duplex ultrasonography than with fistula creation after physical examination alone, but early fistula failure is not different among patients who routinely undergo vein mapping and patients who are preoperatively selected for imaging [19, 20]. Patients that need to be risk-stratified for individuals who need additional imaging studies or interventions are elderly age, existence of peripheral vascular disease, or ipsilateral vessel damage (e.g., individuals with prior peripherally inserted central catheters), or individuals who are suspected to have central venous stenosis may not have a favorable arteriovenous fistula outcome [15]. In patients where vascular anatomy is a precluding factor to arteriovenous fistula creation or if patients are considered to have a higher likelihood of failure of arteriovenous fistula, or low life expectancy, arteriovenous grafts can be created. While central venous catheters should ideally be only used in a transition period, in the acute phase before arteriovenous fistulas or grafts, there are some situations when they can be used especially when an arteriovenous fistula or graft is not feasible. These include patients who have low life expectancy, severe peripheral vascular disease, and low cardiac output that impacts fistula flow, patients who have had multiple vascular surgeries, or have a higher risk of thrombosis or bleeding, and obese patients [21]. Other factors include functional status of the individual patient, dexterity, caregiver support, and patient's overall preference [22]. Studies have shown that adequate educational programs that are initiated in the pre-dialysis phase have shown to promote patient choice in favor of home hemodialysis and arteriovenous access placement, evidenced by arteriovenous access use in about 60% of patients undergoing hemodialysis in the United States and Canada [14, 23, 24]. Thus, starting the conversation of an end-stage kidney disease life plan earlier can benefit the patient in having enough time to choose wisely with all factors considered.

Patient and Safety Concerns in Vascular Access

Concerns of procedural complications, pain, and lack of technical skills predominate the decisions against self-cannulation, which can be mitigated by good training and education [25, 26]. When informed about improved survival, increased flexibility, and improved quality of life, patients actually tended to choose home hemodialysis when given unlimited nursing support and extended training periods [27]. Patients should be allowed to self-cannulate in their training period which can ease fears surrounding self-cannulation, with a training pace individualized for the comfort level of each patient. The use of warm compress for vasodilation, topical analgesics, and psychological therapy (including talk therapy, hypnotherapy, and anti-anxiolytics) can be used to mitigate pain and fear experienced during access cannulation. This can be done not only with hands-on training, but also with the use of training videos, and support groups that can be helpful. Psychological mechanisms can be used to overcome the fears that arise in the self-cannulation process that incorporates reframing the self-cannulation process as a vital part of staying alive with acceptance and normalization of the process [28]. Patients also harbor fear of being able to perform dialysis adequately and fear of social isolation [29]. The traditional in-center hemodialysis center is not equipped for training of this magnitude as patients need individual training plan with one-on-one attention. Thus, transitional care units can serve to provide this service as patients learn to accept and thrive in their new lifestyle. Patients have more support from dedicated staff with family engagement, peer mentoring, familiarity with home dialysis machines in an environment akin to the home setting, and education on complications of vascular access at a pace that is comfortable for the patient with as much training as needed to become independent operators [30].

Home hemodialysis renders itself to more personalized care and can involve more frequent dialysis sessions ad libitum than in-center hemodialysis. Given that the goal of home hemodialysis is to ensure that patients become proficient enough to perform dialysis without supervision, patients and their caregivers should be briefed on the potential dialysis and access-related adverse events with a plan of action with frequent training refreshers. Although discussed in detail in the chapter dedicated to complications of hemodialysis, some of the major access-related adverse events are presented here. Increased frequency of hemodialysis is associated with access dysfunction that requires interventions due to frequent cannulation impacting overall vascular access survival. In addition, infection is the most common vascular access-related adverse event type even among patients with arteriovenous fistulae dialyzed at home [31, 32]. Although relatively rare, serious and potentially catastrophic events include needle dislodgement that can lead to fatal hemorrhage and air embolism that can result in cardiopulmonary arrest [33, 34]. In an analysis of serious adverse events during home hemodialysis, needle dislodgements that were most commonly due to patient error with incorrect taping technique or cannulation, however, also occurred due to equipment malfunction and defective needles. Similarly, air embolism not only occurred due to incorrect procedure during retransfusion and priming but also occurred due to lack of clamp on the dialysis catheter [33]. Air embolism has also occurred with the use of a central venous catheter without a closed connector device which has prompted the use of these devices in patients being dialyzed at home [35, 36].

The rate of these adverse events occurs 1 in 11,000–20,000 home hemodialysis sessions which is more frequent than conventional hemodialysis which is reportedly 1 in 60,000–70,000. Knowledge that a fatal hemorrhage from vascular access cannulation is a rare event can help assuage worries, and patients should be taught to have close monitoring of vascular access during dialysis to be able to respond to adverse events. Such measures include mandating the use of wetness detectors at the venous needle sites, proper procedure for needle stabilization after cannulation, and use of closed connector devices to reduce needle dislodgement and prevent air embolism [37]. In addition, patients who have more frequent dialysis sessions should be taught to observe signs of aneurysmal dilation and bacterial infection that weaken the vascular wall and make it prone to bleeding [38]. Patients should be educated on the elements of access dysfunction, and should be coupled with an access management team that involves an interventionalist to have routine examination and maintenance of their vascular access.

Cannulation Techniques

The two types of cannulation techniques recommended for arteriovenous fistulas are the rope ladder technique (using rotating sites throughout the entire length of the fistula or graft) or buttonhole technique (use of a constant site only in an arteriovenous fistula) (Table 7.2). There is no difference in primary patency after 1 year and no difference in quality of life between the two techniques [39]. The rope ladder technique requires a large fistula or graft which can be cannulated at various sites with a sharp needle. The buttonhole technique involves the development of a tract after cannulation with a sharp needle about 8–10 times, which can then be accessed by a blunt needle. The technique involves precision and requires that a single operator with the same angle with the same tourniquet pressure be used prior to tract formation. Scabs must be removed with a separate needle to reduce the risk of infection, and diligent hand washing is required [22]. Buttonholes are associated with an increased risk of infection and bacteremia [40, 41], but may reduce fistula infiltration, hematoma, and aneurysm formation [42, 43] without increasing the life of the fistula [44]. The use of the buttonhole technique can increase ease of cannulation, increase hemostasis time, improve pain, and comfort level of self-cannulation [45]. The use of topical mupirocin as prophylaxis has shown to reduce rates of staphylococcus bacteremia in patients using buttonhole cannulation and may mitigate the observed infection-related complications although studies with larger cohorts and longer observation periods are needed [46]. A third method called the area

Table 7.2 Cannulation techniques: advantages and disadvantages of the two types of cannulation techniques available for home dialysis

Cannulation techniques =		
	Rope Ladder	*Buttonhole*
Features		
Types of access	Arteriovenous fistulas and grafts	Arteriovenous fistula only
Pain on cannulation	Increased pain on cannulation	Decreased pain on cannulation
Infection rate	Lower rate of infection	Higher rate of infection
Access length	Requires long fistula length	No impact of length on ability to have a site of cannulation
Aneurysm formation	Decreased risk of aneurysm formation	
Patient + caregiver engagement	Requires constant decision on site of cannulation	Site of cannulation is constant and prepared for use

Buttonhole cannulation although easier for patients increases the risk of infection affecting morbidity

Fig. 7.1 Buttonhole cannulation—example of an arteriovenous fistula with buttonholes

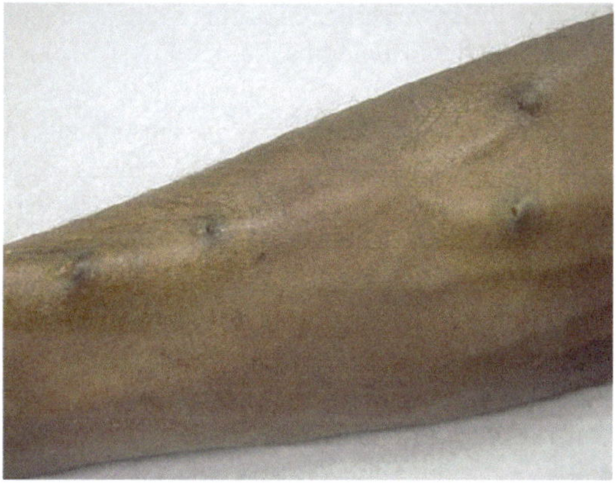

Buttonhole cannulation
Photo courtesy of Dr. Brent Miller

technique is not recommended for cannulation, as it frequently increases the risk of stenosis and aneurysmal formation due to damage to the fistula in a concentrated area thus reducing the life of the fistula (Fig. 7.1).

Patients should be trained in aseptic technique, with meticulous hand washing, followed by access cleansing with soap and water followed by cleansing with chlorhexidine or povidone-iodine solution. Needles should be inserted bevel up, and needles should be placed 3 inches apart if antegrade and 1 inch apart if placed in opposite directions, with a good distance (at least 1.5 cm away from the site of venous anastomosis). The typical angle used for arteriovenous fistulas is 25–30° and for the arteriovenous graft is about 15°. Needles should be securely tapped without tension on lines to avoid needle dislodgement. Central venous catheters must be locked with either heparin or sodium citrate after use to maintain patency, and the exit site should be covered with an antimicrobial ointment and dressed with gauze carefully. It is important to note that each patient has a self-appointed caregiver who also undergoes the same training as the patient to ensure that the protocol for cannulation is followed and can help with troubleshooting and any issues that arise.

Maintenance of Vascular Access in Home HD

Regular surveillance of vascular access either in-person or remotely should be conducted at regular intervals and at the time of any signs of vascular access dysfunction. Any overlying ulceration or discoloration over the skin of a fistula or a graft should be interrogated for possible infection. In patients with a central venous catheter, the exit site should be monitored for signs of infection. Signs of arteriovenous fistula or graft dysfunction that patients can report include prolonged bleeding of the fistula after decannulation (bleeding after 10 mins of hemostasis), swelling of the arm with the fistula, enlarging veins or aneurysms, difficulty with cannulation, and pain in the ipsilateral shoulder. Physical examination conducted by the nephrologist or interventionalist should involve inspection, palpation, and auscultation, and the presence of bruits, decrease in pulse augmentation, and failure to collapse with arm elevation indicate arterial and venous stenoses. Dialysis parameters such as changes in venous pressures, changes in blood flow, and decreased dialysis adequacy indicate problems with the access that warrant intervention [47].

Maintenance of stable hemodialysis at home involves the use of anticoagulation to prevent circuit clotting like in-center hemodialysis. Heparin is the mainstay of treatment in dialysis with fewer bleeding complications when compared to warfarin [48] and is currently dosed in a similar fashion as with in-center hemodialysis. Unfractionated heparin is administered as a bolus dose at the start of the treatment, and an additional bolus is given during the treatment as needed to prevent clotting in the dialysis circuit and excessive bleeding post-dialysis. The dose is modified in patients with an increased risk of bleeding and can be monitored at home using activated coagulation time. In situations with excessive bleeding from the use of anticoagulation with unfractionated heparin, protamine sulfate can be administered to control the bleed. Low molecular weight heparin has been used for anticoagulation; however, long half-life can lead to their accumulation and theoretically cause major bleeding during home dialysis [49]. Short-acting low molecular weight heparin such as dalteparin has been shown to have no major adverse effects in pediatric patients [50] undergoing home hemodialysis and in adult patients [51] although the sample size was small and it needs to be tested in larger cohorts of different age groups.

New Directions in Home HD

New needles and cannulation techniques are underway to improve home hemodialysis. Single-needle hemodialysis was previously deemed to provide inadequate hemodialysis [52]. With newer pump systems, both two-pump system and single-pump systems are shown to provide adequate dialysis and will reduce vascular access trauma during cannulation [53]. Patients who have difficulty with cannulation can be trained in using ultrasound guidance for finding an appropriate window for cannulation. In addition, newer tools called the venous window needle guide can be placed subcutaneously over the fistula that can allow the buttonhole cannulation technique for dialysis in fistulas that are deemed difficult to cannulate, extending the life of the arteriovenous access [54]. The use of patients that have exhausted vascular access options with SVC occlusion can be evaluated for hemodialysis reliable outflow (HeRO) catheters that can bypass venous outflow obstruction, giving direct access to central venous circulation. These catheters are placed as a last resort in patients that have catheter dependence, with a patency rate of 30% [55].

Home hemodialysis provides a patient freedom, better quality of life, and convenience, and allows personalized care with improved volume and electrolyte control. Decisions on access type and techniques of self-cannulation can be individualized, and frequent monitoring of access by a team can allow for the successful use of home hemodialysis.

References

1. System USRD. 2020 USRDS Annual Data Report: epidemiology of kidney disease in the United States. 2020. https://adr.usrds.org/2020.
2. Weinhandl ED, Gilbertson D.T., Wetmore, J.B., Johansen, K.L. Recent trends in utilization of home dialysis modalities, overall and by duration of ESKD. Kidney Week. 2021;Abstract PO0956.
3. Weinhandl ED, Liu J, Gilbertson DT, Arneson TJ, Collins AJ. Survival in daily home hemodialysis and matched thrice-weekly in-center hemodialysis patients. J Am Soc Nephrol. 2012;23(5):895–904. https://doi.org/10.1681/ASN.2011080761.
4. Trinh E, Chan CT. Intensive home hemodialysis results in regression of left ventricular hypertrophy and better clinical outcomes. Am J Nephrol. 2016;44(4):300–7. https://doi.org/10.1159/000449452.
5. Miller BW, Himmele R, Sawin DA, Kim J, Kossmann RJ. Choosing home hemodialysis: a critical review of patient outcomes. Blood Purif. 2018;45(1–3):224–9. https://doi.org/10.1159/000485159.
6. Chan CT, Wallace E, Golper TA, et al. Exploring barriers and potential solutions in home dialysis: an NKF-KDOQI conference outcomes report. Am J Kidney Dis. 2019;73(3):363–71. https://doi.org/10.1053/j.ajkd.2018.09.015.
7. Lockridge R, Weinhandl E, Kraus M, et al. A systematic approach to promoting home hemodialysis during end stage kidney disease. Kidney360. 2020;1:993.
8. Al Shakarchi J, Day C, Inston N. Vascular access for home haemodialysis. J Vasc Access. 2018;19(6):593–5. https://doi.org/10.1177/1129729818764135.
9. Blake PG, Quinn RR, Oliver MJ. The risks of vascular access. Kidney Int. 2012;82(6):623–5. https://doi.org/10.1038/ki.2012.181.
10. Kasza J, Wolfe R, McDonald SP, Marshall MR, Polkinghorne KR. Dialysis modality, vascular access and mortality in end-stage kidney disease: a bi-national registry-based cohort study. Nephrology. 2016;21(10):878–86. https://doi.org/10.1111/nep.12688.
11. Rivara MB, Soohoo M, Streja E, et al. Association of vascular access type with mortality, hospitalization, and transfer to in-center hemodialysis in patients undergoing home hemodialysis. Clin J Am Soc Nephrol: CJASN. 2016;11(2):298–307. https://doi.org/10.2215/CJN.06570615.
12. Hayes WN, Tennankore K, Battistella M, Chan CT. Vascular access-related infection in nocturnal home hemodialysis. Hemodial Int. 2014;18(2):481–7. https://doi.org/10.1111/hdi.12140.
13. Perl J, Wald R, McFarlane P, et al. Hemodialysis vascular access modifies the association between dialysis modality and survival. J Am Soc Nephrol. 2011;22(6):1113–21. https://doi.org/10.1681/ASN.2010111155.
14. Perl J, Nessim SJ, Moist LM, et al. Vascular access type and patient and technique survival in home hemodialysis patients: the Canadian Organ Replacement Register. Am J Kidney Dis. 2016;67(2):251–9. https://doi.org/10.1053/j.ajkd.2015.07.032.
15. Lok CE, Huber TS, Lee T, et al. KDOQI clinical practice guideline for vascular access: 2019 update. Am J Kidney Dis. 2020;75(4 Suppl 2):S1–S164. https://doi.org/10.1053/j.ajkd.2019.12.001.
16. Asif A, Cherla G, Merrill D, Cipleu CD, Briones P, Pennell P. Conversion of tunneled hemodialysis catheter-consigned patients to arteriovenous fistula. Kidney Int. 2005;67(6):2399–406. https://doi.org/10.1111/j.1523-1755.2005.00347.x.
17. Arinze NV, Gregory A, Francis JM, Farber A, Chitalia VC. Unique aspects of peripheral artery disease in patients with chronic kidney disease. Vasc Med. 2019;24(3):251–60. https://doi.org/10.1177/1358863X18824654.

18. Tedla FM, Clerger G, Distant D, Salifu M. Prevalence of Central Vein Stenosis in Patients Referred for Vein Mapping. Clin J Am Soc Nephrol: CJASN. 2018;13(7):1063–8. https://doi.org/10.2215/CJN.14001217.
19. Smith GE, Barnes R, Chetter IC. Randomized clinical trial of selective versus routine preoperative duplex ultrasound imaging before arteriovenous fistula surgery. Br J Surg. 2014;101(5):469–74. https://doi.org/10.1002/bjs.9435.
20. Ferring M, Claridge M, Smith SA, Wilmink T. Routine preoperative vascular ultrasound improves patency and use of arteriovenous fistulas for hemodialysis: a randomized trial. Clin J Am Soc Nephrol: CJASN. 2010;5(12):2236–44. https://doi.org/10.2215/CJN.02820310.
21. Drew DA, Lok CE. Strategies for planning the optimal dialysis access for an individual patient. Curr Opin Nephrol Hypertens. 2014;23(3):314–20. https://doi.org/10.1097/01.mnh.0000444815.49755.d9.
22. Agarwal AK, Boubes KY, Haddad NF. Essentials of vascular access for home hemodialysis. Adv Chronic Kidney Dis. 2021;28(2):164–9. https://doi.org/10.1053/j.ackd.2021.06.008.
23. Lacson E Jr, Wang W, DeVries C, et al. Effects of a nationwide predialysis educational program on modality choice, vascular access, and patient outcomes. Am J Kidney Dis. 2011;58(2):235–42. https://doi.org/10.1053/j.ajkd.2011.04.015.
24. Rocco MV, Larive B, Eggers PW, et al. Baseline characteristics of participants in the Frequent Hemodialysis Network (FHN) daily and nocturnal trials. Am J Kidney Dis. 2011;57(1):90–100. https://doi.org/10.1053/j.ajkd.2010.08.024.
25. Jayanti A, Foden P, Wearden A, et al. Self-cannulation for haemodialysis: patient attributes, clinical correlates and self-cannulation predilection models. PLoS One. 2015;10(5):e0125606. https://doi.org/10.1371/journal.pone.0125606.
26. Walker RC, Hanson CS, Palmer SC, et al. Patient and caregiver perspectives on home hemodialysis: a systematic review. Am J Kidney Dis. 2015;65(3):451–63. https://doi.org/10.1053/j.ajkd.2014.10.020.
27. Walker RC, Morton RL, Palmer SC, Marshall MR, Tong A, Howard K. A discrete choice study of patient preferences for dialysis modalities. Clin J Am Soc Nephrol: CJASN. 2018;13(1):100–8. https://doi.org/10.2215/CJN.06830617.
28. Moore C, Majeed-Ariss R, Jayanti A, Mitra S, Skevington S, Wearden A. How an ordeal becomes the norm: a qualitative exploration of experiences of self-cannulation in male home haemodialysis patients. Br J Health Psychol. 2018;23(3):544–60. https://doi.org/10.1111/bjhp.12303.
29. McLaughlin K, Manns B, Mortis G, Hons R, Taub K. Why patients with ESRD do not select self-care dialysis as a treatment option. Am J Kidney Dis. 2003;41(2):380–5. https://doi.org/10.1053/ajkd.2003.50047.
30. Hussein WF, Bennett PN, Schiller B. Innovations to increase home hemodialysis utilization: the transitional care unit. Adv Chronic Kidney Dis. 2021;28(2):178–83. https://doi.org/10.1053/j.ackd.2021.02.009.
31. Group FHNT, Chertow GM, Levin NW, et al. In-center hemodialysis six times per week versus three times per week. N Engl J Med. 2010;363(24):2287–300. https://doi.org/10.1056/NEJMoa1001593.
32. Jun M, Jardine MJ, Gray N, et al. Outcomes of extended-hours hemodialysis performed predominantly at home. Am J Kidney Dis. 2013;61(2):247–53. https://doi.org/10.1053/j.ajkd.2012.08.032.
33. Tennankore KK, d'Gama C, Faratro R, Fung S, Wong E, Chan CT. Adverse technical events in home hemodialysis. Am J Kidney Dis. 2015;65(1):116–21. https://doi.org/10.1053/j.ajkd.2014.08.013.
34. Ouwendyk M, Pierratos A, Francoeur R, Wallace L, Sit W, Vas S. Slow nocturnal home hemodialysis (SNHHD)—one year later. J CANNT. 1996;6(2):26–8.
35. Rocco MV, Lockridge RS Jr, Beck GJ, et al. The effects of frequent nocturnal home hemodialysis: the Frequent Hemodialysis Network Nocturnal Trial. Kidney Int. 2011;80(10):1080–91. https://doi.org/10.1038/ki.2011.213.

36. Suri RS, Larive B, Sherer S, et al. Risk of vascular access complications with frequent hemodialysis. J Am Soc Nephrol. 2013;24(3):498–505. https://doi.org/10.1681/ASN.2012060595.
37. Nesrallah GE, Mustafa RA, MacRae J, et al. Canadian Society of Nephrology guidelines for the management of patients with ESRD treated with intensive hemodialysis. Am J Kidney Dis. 2013;62(1):187–98. https://doi.org/10.1053/j.ajkd.2013.02.351.
38. Jose MD, Marshall MR, Read G, et al. Fatal dialysis vascular access hemorrhage. Am J Kidney Dis. 2017;70(4):570–5. https://doi.org/10.1053/j.ajkd.2017.05.014.
39. Chan MR, Shobande O, Vats H, et al. The effect of buttonhole cannulation vs. rope-ladder technique on hemodialysis access patency. Semin Dial. 2014;27(2):210–6. https://doi.org/10.1111/sdi.12143.
40. Allon M. Is it time to abandon buttonhole cannulation of arteriovenous fistulas? Kidney Med. 2019;1(5):235–7. https://doi.org/10.1016/j.xkme.2019.07.009.
41. O'Brien FJ, Kok HK, O'Kane C, et al. Arterio-venous fistula buttonhole cannulation technique: a retrospective analysis of infectious complications. Clin Kidney J. 2012;5(6):526–9. https://doi.org/10.1093/ckj/sfs135.
42. Vaux E, King J, Lloyd S, et al. Effect of buttonhole cannulation with a polycarbonate PEG on in-center hemodialysis fistula outcomes: a randomized controlled trial. Am J Kidney Dis. 2013;62(1):81–8. https://doi.org/10.1053/j.ajkd.2013.01.011.
43. van Loon MM, Goovaerts T, Kessels AG, van der Sande FM, Tordoir JH. Buttonhole needling of haemodialysis arteriovenous fistulae results in less complications and interventions compared to the rope-ladder technique. Nephrol Dial Transplant. 2010;25(1):225–30. https://doi.org/10.1093/ndt/gfp420.
44. Macrae JM, Ahmed SB, Hemmelgarn BR, Alberta Kidney Disease Network. Arteriovenous fistula survival and needling technique: long-term results from a randomized buttonhole trial. Am J Kidney Dis. 2014;63(4):636–42. https://doi.org/10.1053/j.ajkd.2013.09.015.
45. Kim MK, Kim HS. Clinical effects of buttonhole cannulation method on hemodialysis patients. Hemodial Int. 2013;17(2):294–9. https://doi.org/10.1111/j.1542-4758.2012.00753.x.
46. Nesrallah GE, Cuerden M, Wong JH, Pierratos A. Staphylococcus aureus bacteremia and buttonhole cannulation: long-term safety and efficacy of mupirocin prophylaxis. Clin J Am Soc Nephrol. 2010;5(6):1047–53.
47. Salman L, Beathard G. Interventional nephrology: physical examination as a tool for surveillance for the hemodialysis arteriovenous access. Clin J Am Soc Nephrol: CJASN. 2013;8(7):1220–7. https://doi.org/10.2215/CJN.00740113.
48. Biggers JA, Remmers AR Jr, Glassford DM, Sarles HE, Lindley JD, Fish JC. The risk of anticoagulation in hemodialysis patients. Nephron. 1977;18(2):109–13.
49. Davenport A. What are the anticoagulation options for intermittent hemodialysis? Nat Rev Nephrol. 2011;7(9):499–508. https://doi.org/10.1038/nrneph.2011.88.
50. Lutkin M, Stronach L, Yadav P, Hothi DK. Dalteparin anticoagulation in paediatric home haemodialysis. Pediatr Nephrol. 2018;33(12):2337–41. https://doi.org/10.1007/s00467-018-4032-1.
51. Beijering RJR, ten Cate H, Stevens P, et al. Randomised long-term comparison of tinzaparin and dalteparin in haemodialysis. Clin Drug Investig. 2003;23(2):85–97. https://doi.org/10.2165/00044011-200323020-00002.
52. Huang SH, Shah S, Thomson BK, Laporte S, Filler G, Lindsay RM. What is single needle cannulation hemodialysis: is it adequate? Blood Purif. 2014;38(1):13–7. https://doi.org/10.1159/000363049.
53. Bieser W, Welsch M, Jakob M, et al. Effectiveness of a new single-needle single-pump dialysis system with simultaneous monitoring of dialysis dose. Artif Organs. 2018;42(8):814–23. https://doi.org/10.1111/aor.13149.
54. Jennings WC, Galt SW, Shenoy S, et al. The Venous Window Needle Guide, a hemodialysis cannulation device for salvage of uncannulatable arteriovenous fistulas. J Vasc Surg. 2014;60(4):1024–32. https://doi.org/10.1016/j.jvs.2014.04.016.
55. Davis KL, Gurley JC, Davenport DL, Xenos ES. The use of HeRo catheter in catheter-dependent dialysis patients with superior vena cava occlusion. J Vasc Access. 2016;17(2):138–42. https://doi.org/10.5301/jva.5000493.

Patient Training and Preparation of the Home for Dialysis

8

Brent Miller

The Structure of Nephrology Practice and HHD in the United States

Many of the difficulties this chapter will address are the result of home hemodialysis (HHD) being a single-digit prevalent therapy in an already small disease state residing within a health system that manages neither chronic illness nor transitions of care well (Fig. 8.1) [1, 2]. Hopefully, this will change as the system moves toward "value-based care." In the early days of outpatient hemodialysis (HD) therapy in the United States and prior to the development of outpatient peritoneal dialysis (PD) in the 1970s, HHD accounted for approximately 40% of the overall dialysis treatments [3]. That story is worth studying and is discussed in an earlier chapter in this book.

In most nephrology practices, most patients with chronic kidney disease (CKD) in the United States start dialysis without adequate preparation or planning and a shocking number of prevalent center-based HD patients report not being aware of home dialysis as an option [4]. Many even start via an emergency admission process to a hospital with a quick placement of an HD catheter followed by a first dialysis experience in a hospital acute dialysis setting or even an intensive care unit and a prompt discharge to an outpatient facility. Addressing this systematic problem is the first step to improving HHD training.

The staffing of HHD centers also impacts performance. Many of the skills of a proficient outpatient center-based HD nurse or technician are not the same as an HHD nurse or technician. Patient education and the ability to triage problems are critical to the HHD nurse. The majority of HHD centers are small with limited staff (Fig. 8.2); thus, there is often not the ability to "specialize" such as having specific HHD trainers nor the ability to offload many of the other non-nursing tasks that may interfere with patient training.

B. Miller (✉)
Division of Nephrology, Indiana University School of Medicine, Indianapolis, IN, USA
e-mail: Bwm1@iu.edu

A. Shah et al. (eds.), *Applied Home Hemodialysis*,
https://doi.org/10.1007/978-3-031-77244-3_8

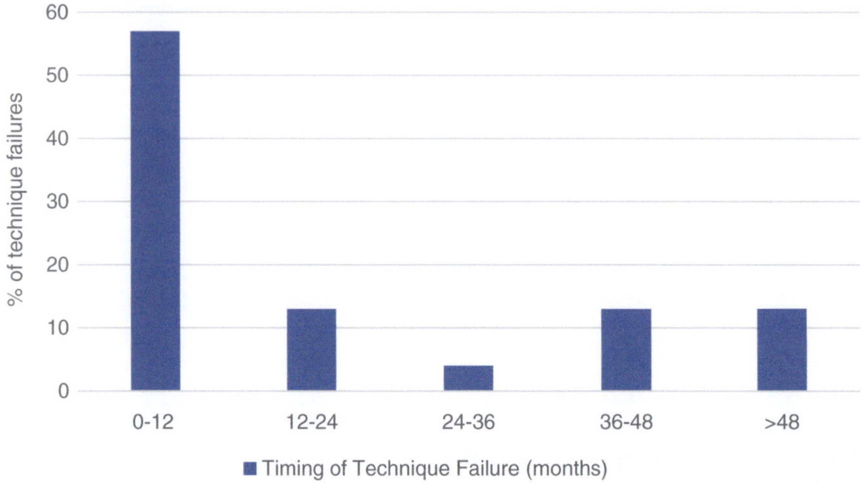

Fig. 8.1 Timing of technique failure for home hemodialysis patients. Most of the technique failure occurs in the first year and is largely for nonmedical reasons. This is the opposite of the results of the other home dialysis modality, peritoneal dialysis. (Chart adapted from data in reference [1])

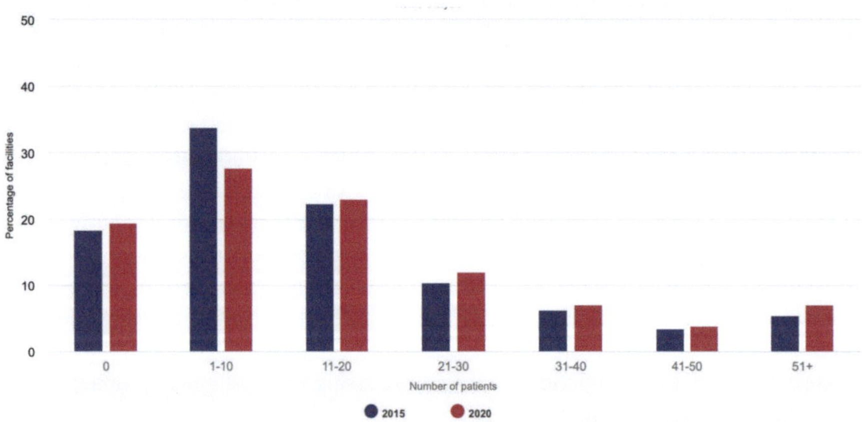

Fig. 8.2 Size of certified home dialysis programs in the United States from the USRDS database, reference [5, Fig. 2.5]. Most dialysis providers utilized a nurse:patient ratio of approximately 1:15–20; thus, most home dialysis programs have a single dialysis nurse

Lastly, home dialysis represents less than 20% of dialysis therapy in the United States, and HHD, just a few percent [5]. In contrast, over 7000 center-based dialysis facilities take care of the overwhelming number of patients in the United States. Each center has a fixed capital cost and ongoing investment and expenses, similar to an airline business model. So, both the inertia of nephrology practice and efficient allocation of capital may unintendedly impair optimal HHD training. HHD also has a large upfront cost in training, largely due to the time allocated to nursing effort

Fig. 8.3 Rough estimate of per treatment cost in US dollars of dialysis therapies in the United States based on author's experience in multiple home hemodialysis programs over 2 decades. Note relative fixed costs of in-center HD which would increase per treatment cost of census decreases

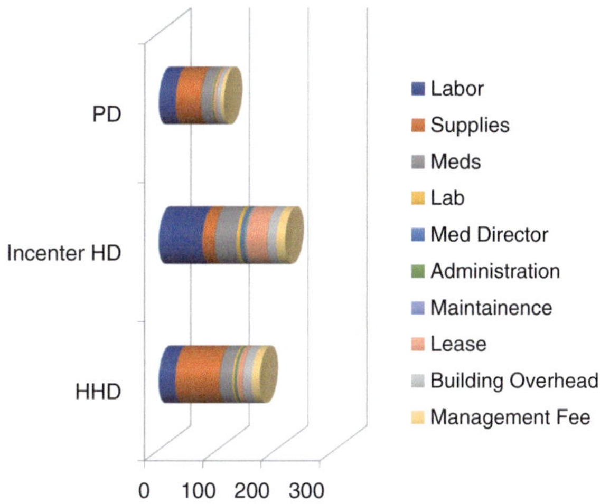

over multiple weeks. From a business standpoint for the dialysis provider, the "break-even" period is several months after HHD training. If the HHD practice has a high technique failure rate, the business of HHD becomes unprofitable and unsustainable for the entity. Most studies have shown a transplant and death-censored technique failure rate of HHD of slightly more or less than 20% at 1 year [6], but training is a critical concern if the practitioner wants to keep a vibrant HHD program (Fig. 8.3).

Patient Journey to Home Hemodialysis

Another difference between HHD and PD is that most PD patients are incident, but the majority of HHD patients are prevalent, including some who transfer from PD to HHD. This dichotomy may make practical and scientific sense. PD is the simplest form of dialysis therapy; thus, it represents a reasonable starting point for most patients. Similarly, PD works best with residual renal function, which most incident patients possess and is also preserved longer on PD than any form of HD.

HHD represents the most complex form of dialysis, and it offers the potential for the most intensive dialysis therapy. So, it may be viewed as a destination for many dialysis patients rather than a starting point. HD patients lose residual renal function sooner than PD patients, and there is some concern that intensive HD regimens cause even faster loss of residual renal function [7].

For the patient interested in HHD, there are many online resources and support groups. Additionally, identifying another patient who has gone through the journey of HHD can provide a perspective for the potential HHD patient.

Preparation for Home Hemodialysis Training

Time Commitment

A frank discussion with the patient to prepare them for beginning home dialysis training should occur before training (Table 8.1) [8]. Typically, the HHD training time is 4 weeks with 4–5 sessions per week. So, the patient will need to plan for time away from work or family accordingly. Since the HD treatment is provided during training, a typical training day will last 5–6 h. Generally, the training occurs in the dialysis center so additional travel time for the patient may be required. Many programs have instituted some in-home training, particularly near the end of training.

To account for this intensive commitment by the dialysis provider, the Centers for Medicare and Medicaid Services (CMS) reimburses the dialysis provider for up to 25 training sessions (082X). Additionally, similar to PD, CMS also reimburses the nephrologist for supervision of home dialysis training (Current Procedural Terminology Code® (CPT) 90989). Furthermore, the US Congress has intentionally encouraged financial incentives to promote home dialysis for over 40 years, including Medicare coverage beginning on day 1 of dialysis for the home dialysis patient.

Home Suitability and Support

Since the dialysis treatment will be performed in the patient's home, a careful review of the home environment should be completed prior to training. The specific requirements will depend upon the HHD machine and water source utilized, but standardized checklists are available. Currently, most HHD patients have a person who assists with the treatment, often called a "caregiver" or "care partner." The relative amount of involvement of the care partner and patient varies, but it should be understood prior to training.

Table 8.1 Tips for patients beginning home hemodialysis

1.	Plan ahead for the approximately month-long training with things such as grocery shopping and meal planning
2.	Preview the training materials
3.	Stay rested
4.	Take notes
5.	Ask questions
6.	Find a good hand lotion for hand washing
7.	Overcome the anxiety of cannulation
8.	Express a small amount of grief and anger
9.	Have a plan for the trash such as using supply boxes

Adapted from Ref. [7]

Vascular Access and Cannulation

Special attention is required on the topic of vascular access training. Trepidation and anxiety of the cannulation procedure are repeatedly mentioned as a concern by patients considering or starting HHD. Additionally, several serious complications including excess bleeding, damage to the access, and infection can occur with poor management of the vascular access in the home. To this end, several practices specific to vascular access should be considered. First, since the overwhelming majority of HHD patients start with center-based HD, beginning the journey to self-cannulation prior to training is helpful. Second, considering topical anesthesia such as lidocaine/prilocaine 45 min before self-cannulation removes one barrier. If severe anxiety presents, bypassing technical cannulation training the first week may be necessary and instead concentrate on the intellectual component of the vascular access. Lastly, embracing the use of low-cost, hand-held ultrasound devices can assist in successful training.

Best Training Practices

Much HHD training literature and complete programs are available [9–11]. Regardless of the methodology selected, a consistent approach with the nephrology staff and nursing staff in the home dialysis center is critical. This does not mean that each patient and caregiver should be taught in the same way. To the contrary, HHD training staff must understand principles of adult learning and adjust training techniques to incorporate the best methods for each patient.

Lastly, the examples set by the training nurse will mirror what the patient performs[12]. So, it is critical that the training be precise.

Key Points

- Home hemodialysis has a high technique failure in the first year that can be ameliorated by a careful approach to patient training.
- Vascular access training is the most time-consuming and complex part of home hemodialysis training.
- Home hemodialysis training should include specific preparations for the patient's home environment.

References

1. Jayanti A, Nikam M, Ebah L, Dutton G, Morris J, Mitra S. Technique survival in home haemodialysis: a composite success rate and its risk predictors in a prospective longitudinal cohort from a tertiary renal network programme. Nephrol Dial Transplant. 2013;28(10):2612–20. https://doi.org/10.1093/ndt/gft294. PMID: 24078644.

2. Trinh E, Hanley JA, Nadeau-Fredette AC, Perl J, Chan CT. A comparison of technique survival in Canadian peritoneal dialysis and home hemodialysis patients. Nephrol Dial Transplant. 2019;34(11):1941–9. https://doi.org/10.1093/ndt/gfz075. PMID: 31329952.
3. Blagg CR. A brief history of home hemodialysis. Adv Ren Replace Ther. 1996;3(2):99–105. https://doi.org/10.1016/s1073-4449(96)80048-3. PMID: 8814931.
4. Golper TA, Saxena AB, Piraino B, Teitelbaum I, Burkart J, Finkelstein FO, Abu-Alfa A. Systematic barriers to the effective delivery of home dialysis in the United States: a report from the Public Policy/Advocacy Committee of the North American Chapter of the International Society for Peritoneal Dialysis. Am J Kidney Dis. 2011;58(6):879–85. https://doi.org/10.1053/j.ajkd.2011.06.028. Epub 2011 Sep 8. PMID: 21903316.
5. United States Renal Data System. 2022 USRDS Annual Data Report: epidemiology of kidney disease in the United States. Bethesda: National Institutes of Health, National Institute of Diabetes and Digestive and Kidney Diseases; 2022.
6. Weinhandl ED, Gilbertson DT, Collins AJ. Mortality, hospitalization, and technique failure in daily home hemodialysis and matched peritoneal dialysis patients: a matched cohort study. Am J Kidney Dis. 2016;67(1):98–110. https://doi.org/10.1053/j.ajkd.2015.07.014. Epub 2015 Aug 28. PMID: 26319755.
7. Daugirdas JT, Greene T, Rocco MV, Kaysen GA, Depner TA, Levin NW, Chertow GM, Ornt DB, Raimann JG, Larive B, Kliger AS, FHN Trial Group. Effect of frequent hemodialysis on residual kidney function. Kidney Int. 2013;83(5):949–58. https://doi.org/10.1038/ki.2012.457. Epub 2013 Jan 23. PMID: 23344474; PMCID: PMC3855839.
8. https://homedialysis.org/life-at-home/care-partners/ten-tried-true-tips-for-home-dialysis-training. Accessed 27 Feb 2022.
9. https://nxsteps2.fmcna.com/nxlevel/portal/#/. Accessed 3 Feb 2023.
10. Rioux JP, Marshall MR, Faratro R, Hakim R, Simmonds R, Chan CT. Patient selection and training for home hemodialysis. Hemodial Int. 2015;19(Suppl 1):S71–9. https://doi.org/10.1111/hdi.12254. PMID: 25925826.
11. Mitra S, Cress C, Goovaerts T. Workforce development and models of care in home hemodialysis. Hemodial Int. 2015;19(Suppl 1):S43–51. https://doi.org/10.1111/hdi.12291. PMID: 25925823.

Technique Survival, Psychosocial Aspects, Respite Care, and Discontinuation in Home Hemodialysis

9

Nupur Gupta

Introduction

Recent policy changes have renewed the nephrology community's interest in home hemodialysis (HHD). Most of these policies focus on increasing the uptake of HHD [1]. More granular data is needed on best practices to achieve clinical and quality outcomes within the United States. There is an increased emphasis on patient modality education, technological advances, and physician training to escalate the incidence of HHD. Various aspects of technique survival need exploration as they contribute to morbidity and mortality [2]. The USRDS reports are increasing both the incidence and prevalence of HHD [3]. The rates of technique survival vary among home dialysis centers and countries [3, 4]. The experience of a large dialysis organization in the United States demonstrated the average census across 323 clinics offering HHD was four patients per clinic, and the 1-year technique failure rate was 24.9% [5]. There is evidence of higher 90-day mortality among patients who experience technique failure than those who stay on therapy [5]. The journey of HHD patients begins with modality education, training, adjusting to therapy, and working toward transplant, although some may not be eligible. The patient referral and training increase for HHD is crucial to understanding factors and strategies to improve outcomes and make the journey less burdensome.

N. Gupta (✉)
Division of Nephrology, Indiana University School of Medicine, Indianapolis, IN, USA
e-mail: nugupta@iu.edu

A. Shah et al. (eds.), *Applied Home Hemodialysis*,
https://doi.org/10.1007/978-3-031-77244-3_9

Patient Education and Training

A significant proportion of patients crash start in dialysis from the hospital or coping with the news of starting dialysis in the kidney clinic. They are experiencing fear, denial, and anxiety while making these life-changing decisions [6]. Common themes described by patients and their care partners include fear of needle cannulation, machine complications, handling alarms, and disconnection [7]. These can be further complicated by frequent physician appointments, travel to the home dialysis unit, or hospitalization. In addition, patients may be concerned about how home dialysis fits into their daily schedule, which may require adjustments to their daily activities such as employment, scholarly activities, social engagements, or hobbies. The alleviation of concerns and setting of expectations begins with pre-dialysis modality education.

The multidisciplinary team does the modality education in the pre-dialysis stage or transitional care units. Although the team educates the patient on the benefits of home dialysis, it is imperative to discuss the risk and set expectations for training. The complexity of training and emotions increases their risk of discontinuation. The patients are advised to get a care partner to attend the education sessions to understand their dynamics, alleviate their fears, and share an HHD training sample. In training, the trainer should assess patients' progress individually and tailor the training accordingly. Allowing the patients flexibility of days and treatment timing helps decrease the burden both on patients and on care partners. Shafi and Jaar suggested starting patients with incremental HHD to help with the patient or caregiver burnout, frequently linked to treatment frequency or length [8]. To complete training, the patient and care partner should independently perform treatments, including collecting supplies and disposing of biohazardous waste, and mirror the treatments at home. This allows the trainer to intervene on any issues of concern. After thorough review and education, if patients are not convinced that home dialysis is the best option, home dialysis should not be pushed further. There may be risks of significant psychosocial stress and burden.

Machine-Related Issues

The fear of potential adverse events and inadequately performing the treatment persists among patients even after training [9]. These apprehensions are reduced as the time on HHD increases, although the constant responsibility and time required to prepare and finish the treatment is an essential contributor to the burden. The patients and care partners both fear adverse events despite the low incidence. They fear misjudgment of machine alarms, infection-related complications with arteriovenous (AV) access, needle dislodgement, disconnection, air embolism, and machine and water source maintenance. In a retrospective quality improvement study of two adult HHD programs in Canada, one death and six potentially fatal adverse events occurred: crude rate of 0.060 events/1000 dialysis treatments. Six out of seven events were related to significant blood loss (one including exsanguination) [10]. While adverse event rates are low, outcomes can be lethal and scare the patient and care partner.

During the training, quizzes or demonstrations should assess the understanding of machine setup and emergency procedures. If deficiencies are identified, the patients/care partner should be retrained. Many patients develop time-saving habits or "shortcuts" over time without realizing the implications of such practices. Some practices include lack of wetness sensor devices, dialyzing solo without appropriate training, and not recording vitals during the treatments. The clinic should re-emphasize emergency procedures during visits, utilize a machine setup checklist, and review remote patient data, which may be valuable strategies to decrease adverse outcomes.

Access-Related Complications

The AV access complications in HHD include fear of needle cannulation, dislodgement, infection, bleeding, infiltrations, and stenosis. There is a higher incidence of infectious and mechanical complications in HHD than in-center as they dialyze more frequently. Data from the Frequent Hemodialysis Network (FHN) trial has also shown a higher incidence of interventions on AV access with a higher frequency of use as occurs with HHD. An alternative to cannulation of AV access is using tunneled central venous catheters (CVCs) as long-term vascular access for patients treated with HHD [11]. In an extensive study of patients on incident HHD, CVC was associated with a higher risk for death and hospitalization but not transfer to in-center HD than treatment with AV access [12]. Contrastingly, in patients undergoing in-center HD, the use of CVCs is associated with a greater risk of adverse clinical outcomes, including higher mortality and hospitalization rates, at least partly because of the greater incidence of infection-related complications. The incidence of dislodgement and air embolism has been reduced by using a wetness alarm and a closed connector [12]. It is crucial to educate patients on the importance of these practices during monthly clinics as the adverse events could be lethal.

Buttonhole cannulation for arteriovenous fistula (AVF) is popular in HHD patients due to ease of needling and reduced pain. The drawback is increased infections as compared to rope ladder cannulation. In an observational study comparing the incidence of bacteremia and local infection, buttonhole-related bacteremia in HHD was 0.196/1000 fistula days, while five related hospitalizations and three metastatic infections [13]. A study that retrospectively analyzed AVF infection data and compared results with existing literature showed an increased risk of infection with buttonholes along with significantly greater demands on staff time [14]. Therefore, the buttonhole should be avoided as much as possible. However if using buttonholes, strict aseptic precautions should be undertaken to create and maintain them including mupirocin cream and using blunts only for cannulation [15].

Psychosocial Aspects of HHD

Home hemodialysis (HHD) provides flexibility and autonomy to patients in directing their treatment. The ability to perform treatment at home while continuing with daily activities and managing the supplies can be stressful for both patient and care partner. The burden of therapy, fear of isolation, and not being monitored can cause distress. They also may be financially burdened with increased electricity and water bills, home renovation, and loss of employment. While the patient and care partner undergo training, they also struggle to adapt to HHD in their social life and hobbies. All the factors described above could cause psychosocial distress. In a study cohort, the inability to cope with the burden of therapy and inappropriate home conditions were cited as the most common reasons for discontinuation of the HHD [16].

Supporting the Patient

The multidisciplinary team, including the nephrologist, nurses, and social workers, should ensure that patient and care partner are adequately supported. Peer-to-peer, professional, respite, financial, and travel assistance is needed from the team. The feeling of isolation can set in as the patient performs treatments at home. Support groups locally, web-based, or even peer matching "buddy system" can reduce the feeling of isolation for both patient and care partner. Local support groups provide a platform for patients and care partners to discuss concerns with people facing similar challenges. Health professionals could lead these meetings to facilitate discussion and interactions. The buddy system includes matching patients with whom they can share concerns and discuss the journey of training and day-to-day troubleshooting. The buddy should be cautious in answering questions and direct all the medical questions to the clinic staff. The buddy system could be patients at the local dialysis unit level, national level like NKF PEERS, and social media groups [17, 18].

Many times, psychosocial illnesses are also unrecognized, impacting their ability to train and perform the treatment. In the FREEDOM study, participants had a significant decrease in their depressive symptoms [19]. However, the patients enrolled in the FHN trial receiving short daily in-center did not experience improvement in depression [20]. In a cross-sectional survey of patients enrolled in the FHN trial, more than half of 236 patients on HHD with caregivers worried that their caregivers were overextended and felt guilty about the demands their illness had on their caregivers. It was also noticed that the highest perception of burden was in patients with unpaid caregivers, and this increased with deterioration in the functional ability of patients. This overall perceived burden by patients on their caregivers was associated with worse depression and quality of life [21].

Each team member should assess the patient for depression and anxiety during training and clinic visits. In the United States, KDQOL-36 is assessed annually for each patient undergoing dialysis [22]. A self-reported distress thermometer is also being utilized for screening for depression and anxiety [23]. Overall, the health-related quality is improved in HHD, but the team should refer the patient for appropriate diagnosis and treatment to healthcare professionals if signs and symptoms are recognized. It may be even prudent to proactively involve the counselor or psychologist with certain high-risk patients to avoid discontinuation. Other strategies, like identifying high-risk patients and monitoring them closely to intervene early, may be of value.

Care Partner Burden

A patient can dialyze solo or with a care partner aiding, who can be family or friend. The involvement of the care partner can be from ultimately assisting the patient to minimal assistance. The partner's support could vary from time to time depending on the patient's confidence or clinical condition. The clinical team, especially the training staff, should encourage self-care to minimize partner burnout. The cannulation could be the most challenging part; patient learning to self-cannulate helps alleviate the stress. The training staff encourages self-care for the patient, and providing feedback for each step aids both partner and patient to succeed. There should be open communication between patient, care partner, and clinical staff in setting expectations and strategies to succeed. "Burnout" and resources like respite, shifting responsibility to patient, should be extensively discussed in training. As the patient continues to be treated at home, proactively monitoring the patient and care partner stressors avoids fatigue and offering respite reduces withdrawal from therapy.

In another analysis of 87 patients in the FHN trial, 92% reported having an unpaid caregiver at baseline or follow-up. Relative to conventional home dialysis, the 12-month change in the mean perceived caregiver burden score (by the Cousineau scale) with nocturnal home dialysis was +6.1 (95% CI, −0.8 to +13.1; $p = 0.08$). Changes in the Cousineau questionnaire scores from baseline to 12 months were inversely correlated with overall adherence to the prescribed HD treatment ($p = 0.02$) [24]. These results were in sharp contrast to the FHN Daily Trial, where in-center daily dialysis did not result in higher perceptions of caregiver burden. The in-center daily dialysis provided socialization and support from the nursing staff, which likely reduces the caregiver burden. As socialization is needed for the patient, the care partner also may benefit from a buddy system. The buddy system could be in the form of support groups or individuals. These support groups could be local or national, or even on social media. The clinic staff needs to develop open communication with care partners to discuss their concerns and ask for help comfortably.

Respite Care

Respite care, also called back-up care for patients and care partners, enables technique survival by decreasing burnout. The respite care allows freedom for care partner to travel and care for their needs. It could be provided by trained health professionals or paid respite care partners in place of the care partner. Respite could also be for patients dialyzing solo, and they come to the center to dialyze. The best model would be continuing treatments at home, but in some cases, the patient may have to go to the center for treatments depending on the availability of resources. The timing and frequency of respite are other attributes. This could be on-demand by the patient or care partner or planned yearly. On-demand care is requested either by patient or care partner when they are unable to perform treatments. The inability could be deteriorations in health or travel or burnout. The planned respite is when a patient uses respite to just provide break to the care partner or self. However, there is not much data on which model works better.

Remote Patient Monitoring

Telehealth involves all health-related services like education, remote monitoring, patient care, and provider-to-provider communication. Telehealth can be done via telephone, real-time audio-visual communication, and asynchronous and remote patient monitoring (RPM). Telemedicine is defined as "the exchange of medical information from one site to another via electronic communication to improve patients health status" [25]. The risk of adverse related to HHD is low, but patients performing HHD fear medical isolation and difficulty with troubleshooting issues. Access to telehealth can alleviate some of these concerns for patient and care partner.

Technology

RPM involves collecting patient data and transmitting to observer at a remote location. The transmission of data can be in real time or stored and forwarded. The RPM is utilized since 1970, although not in the current form. The data and alarms were transmitted in real time to a central observer. The observer called the patient to address the alarms or concerns. The previous RPM technology lacked actionability by the observer as they were not medical professionals. In early 2000, Fresenius developed iCare monitoring system that prioritized the alarms. iCare had limitation as it could be only used with Fresenius machines [26]. The real-time monitoring fell out of favor due to overall resource and cost-effectiveness as the treatments were overall safe.

The RPM is asynchronous with NxStage machines and real-time with Tablo and Quanta SC+ (not approved for HHD in the United States). The NxStage telemedicine platform called Nx2me Connected Health transmits data after the patient's treatment is completed through a secure server for the clinical team to access [27]. The records include vitals, access pressure, ultrafiltration, alarms, and medications, and a patient can enter comments. Weinhandl and Collin's retrospective analysis indicated that usage of Nx2me helps reduce attrition rates and technique failure [28]. In addition, both Tablo and Quanta SC+ machines connected health platforms that allow real-time access to data on-demand [29, 30].

Utility of Remote Patient Monitoring

The COVID-19 pandemic revolutionized telehealth services' adoption and utility, mainly by removing the regulatory barriers. Prior to the COVID-19 pandemic, the 2018 Bipartisan Budget Act enabled telehealth access to home dialysis patients using the home as the originating site beginning in 2019. Under the act, two out of every three monthly visits can occur via telehealth. Although the home dialysis patients do not travel three times, reducing the monthly clinic visits does significantly reduce the burden of therapy [31]. Most HHD patients draw laboratories at home, which takes care of monthly visits for laboratory draws. These clinic visits are not only for physician encounters but also for the interdisciplinary team for emotional check-in by a social worker and dietary counseling.

RPM helps the patient feel connected to the medical team as they are being monitored. It also allows the team to monitor patients whom we think may not do well on home dialysis, thus offering HDD to more patients. With the data from the platform, we can educate the patients on alarms and maybe avoid hospitalization or ER visits. In-home hemodialysis monitoring provides reassurance to the care partner and the patient, especially in the initial stages. Many patients expect some monitoring as part of clinical care while performing treatments. The patient and care partner performing nocturnal HHD perceived RPM as surrogate support of care partners [7].

The treatment details can be helpful for routine clinical care, especially in HHD, as patients' treatments are not directly monitored. For example, if the nurses notice increased arterial pressures, they inquire about increased post-treatment bleeding and possibly intervene before permanent access dysfunction. Similarly, post-weights, blood pressure, and vitals point help adjust the dry weight. The nurses can monitor the compliance with treatment via the connected health portals. In our clinic, the nurses routinely perform surveillance of the treatment records and discuss with patients if any discrepancy is noted. The surveillance of RPM data and intervening depending on the data enhances routine clinical care and reduces hospitalization/ ER visits. However, the impact of RPM on cardiovascular (CV) outcomes needs to be further explored.

Discontinuation of Therapy

Discontinuation of HHD contributes to the low prevalence of modality. According to USRDS, for the patients who initiated HHD in 2017–2018, the conversion from HHD to in-center hemodialysis was 25%. The cumulative incidence of conversion was higher for older patients (>80) and blacks. Other factors contributing to technique failure are small facilities, rural settings, obesity, and smoking. Although data suggests the risk of hospitalization during the 6 months preceding HHD technique failure is from 278.7 admissions per 100 person-years in 2009 to 239.2 admissions per 100 person-years in 2019, the transition period to in-center attributed to emotional and physical distress of patient and care partner. In 2019, 31% of HHD patients accumulated between 1 and 12 sessions, suggesting these may even have discontinued training before transitioning to home [32] (Table 9.1). Unfortunately, there is not much data on factors impacting the completion of training. The complexity and initial fear of the therapy may contribute to non-completion of training. The retention strategies for identifying high-risk patients at the beginning of training and supporting them from the beginning may reduce

Table 9.1 Summary of factors associated with technique survival

1.	Patient training	
	(a)	Learning difficulties
	(b)	Grief/stress
	(c)	Home remodeling
	(d)	Lifestyle adjustments
	(e)	Financial loss
2.	Machine-related	
	(a)	Water system
	(b)	Machine setup
	(c)	Machine repairs/breakdown
	(d)	Blood loss
	(e)	Air embolism
	(f)	Supplies and medication stocking
	(g)	Blood draws
3.	Vascular access	
	(a)	Cannulation
	(b)	Needle dislodgement/ disconnection
	(c)	Infections
	(d)	Interventions
4.	Psychological	
	(a)	Caregiver burnout
	(b)	Depression/anxiety

technique failure. Assisted HHD may be another strategy to support these patients. Initial data reported by Hussein et al. from assisted peritoneal dialysis (PD) in the United States is promising, although exploring the options for assisted HHD needs further studies [33].

The technology and training for HHD have undergone many changes over decades. Although the technique survival varies from center to center, standardization is needed. The new technologies are promising to improve patient experience and reduce burnout. However, health policy changes are required to revolutionize HHD training in the current era of nursing shortage.

References

1. Advancing American Kidney Health. https://aspe.hhs.gov/pdf-report/advancing-american-kidney-health. Accessed 21 May 2020.
2. Perl J, Na Y, Tennankore KK, Chan CT. Temporal trends and factors associated with home hemodialysis technique survival in Canada. Clin J Am Soc Nephrol. 2017;12:1248.
3. United States Renal Data Report. https://adr.usrds.org/2021/end-stage-renal-disease/2-home-dialysis. Accessed 15April 2022.
4. Blake PG. Global dialysis perspective: Canada. Kidney360. 2020;1(2):115–8.
5. Seshasai RK, Mitra N, Chaknos CM, et al. Factors associated with discontinuation of home hemodialysis. Am J Kidney Dis. 2016;67(4):629–37.
6. Clarke AL, Yates T, Smith AC, Chilcot J. Patient's perceptions of chronic kidney disease and their association with psychosocial and clinical outcomes: a narrative review. Clin Kidney J. 2016;9(3):494–502.
7. Cafazzo JA, Leonard K, Easty AC, Rossos PG, Chan CT. Patient perceptions of remote monitoring for nocturnal home hemodialysis. Hemodial Int. 2010;14(4):471–7.
8. Shafi T, Jaar BG. Maintaining patients on home hemodialysis: the journey matters as does the destination. Clin J Am Soc Nephrol. 2017;12:1209.

9. Courts NF. Psychosocial adjustment of patients on home hemodialysis and their dialysis partners. Clin Nurs Res. 2000;9(2):177–90.
10. Wong B, Zimmerman D, Reintjes F, et al. Procedure-related serious adverse events among home hemodialysis patients: a quality assurance perspective. Am J Kidney Dis. 2014;63(2):251–8.
11. Suri RS, Larive B, Sherer S, et al. Risk of vascular access complications with frequent hemodialysis. J Am Soc Nephrol. 2013;24(3):498–505.
12. Rivara MB, Soohoo M, Streja E, et al. Association of vascular access type with mortality, hospitalization, and transfer to in-center hemodialysis in patients undergoing home hemodialysis. Clin J Am Soc Nephrol. 2016;11(2):298–307.
13. Lok CE, Sontrop JM, Faratro R, Chan CT, Zimmerman DL. Frequent hemodialysis fistula infectious complications. Nephron Extra. 2014;4(3):159–67.
14. Muir CA, Kotwal SS, Hawley CM, et al. Buttonhole cannulation and clinical outcomes in a home hemodialysis cohort and systematic review. Clin J Am Soc Nephrol. 2014;9(1):110–9.
15. Vachharajani TJ, Wong L, Niyyar VD, Abreo KD, Mokrzycki MH. Buttonhole cannulation of arteriovenous fistulas in the United States. Kidney360. 2020;1(4):306–13.
16. Schachter ME, Tennankore KK, Chan CT. Determinants of training and technique failure in home hemodialysis. Hemodial Int. 2013;17(3):421–6.
17. National Kidney Foundation PEERS. https://www.kidney.org/peers. Accessed 7 June 2022.
18. Home Dialyzors United. https://www.homedialyzorsunited.org/. Accessed 7 June 2022.
19. Jaber BL, Finkelstein FO, Glickman JD, et al. Scope and design of the Following Rehabilitation, Economics and Everyday-Dialysis Outcome Measurements (FREEDOM) study. Am J Kidney Dis. 2009;53(2):310–20.
20. Unruh ML, Larive B, Chertow GM, et al. Effects of 6-times-weekly versus 3-times-weekly hemodialysis on depressive symptoms and self-reported mental health: Frequent Hemodialysis Network (FHN) trials. Am J Kidney Dis. 2013;61(5):748–58.
21. Suri RS, Larive B, Garg AX, et al. Burden on caregivers as perceived by hemodialysis patients in the Frequent Hemodialysis Network (FHN) trials. Nephrol Dial Transplant. 2011;26(7):2316–22.
22. Schatell Dori WB. Measuring dialysis patients' health-related quality of life with the KDQOL-36. https://www.kdqol-complete.org/pdfs/kdqol-36.pdf. Accessed 7 June 2022.
23. Damery S, Brown C, Sein K, Nicholas J, Baharani J, Combes G. The prevalence of mild-to-moderate distress in patients with end-stage renal disease: results from a patient survey using the emotion thermometers in four hospital Trusts in the West Midlands, UK. BMJ Open. 2019;9(5):e027982.
24. Suri RS, Larive B, Hall Y, et al. Effects of frequent hemodialysis on perceived caregiver burden in the Frequent Hemodialysis Network trials. Clin J Am Soc Nephrol. 2014;9(5):936–42.
25. Telehealth: Defining 21st Century Care. https://www.americantelemed.org/resource/why-telemedicine/. Accessed 7 June 2022.
26. Diaz-Buxo JA, Schlaeper C, Vanvalkenburgh D. Evolution of home hemodialysis monitoring systems. Hemodial Int. 2003;7(4):353–5.
27. Nx2me Connected Health https://www.nxstage.com/patients/nx2me. Accessed 8 June 2022.
28. Weinhandl ED, Collins AJ. Relative risk of home hemodialysis attrition in patients using a telehealth platform. Hemodial Int. 2018;22(3):318–27.
29. Tablo systems now equipped with remote patient monitoring through TabloHub. https://www.outsetmedical.com/perspective/tablo-systems-now-equipped-with-remote-patient-monitoring-through-tablohub/. Accessed 8June 2022.
30. Quanta. https://www.quantadt.com/. Accessed 8 June 2022.
31. H.R.1892. Bipartisan Budget Act of 2018, 115th Congress (2017–2018). https://www.congress.gov/bill/115th-congress/house-bill/1892?q=%7B%22search%22%3A%5B%22bipartisan+budget+act+of+2018%22%5D%7D. Accessed 8 June 2022.
32. United States Renal Data System. 2020 USRDS Annual Data Report: epidemiology of kidney disease in the United States. Bethesda: National Institutes of Health, National Institute of Diabetes and Digestive and Kidney Diseases; 2020.
33. Hussein WF, Bennett PN, Anwaar A, et al. Implementation of a staff-assisted peritoneal dialysis program in the United States: a feasibility study. Clin J Am Soc Nephrol. 2022;17(5):703–5.

Home Hemodialysis Program Development

10

Joel D. Glickman

Introduction

The success of a home hemodialysis (HHD) program requires focus on the structure and support of the entire nephrology practice. Practitioners have to do more than just adopt a "home first" attitude. They also need to develop and utilize workflows that encourage the use of HHD. At a minimum, all practitioners should have a thorough, but not necessarily expert, knowledge of quality-of-life advantages, medical benefits, and burdens of HHD. More importantly, they must also have a positive "can do" attitude as opposed to a negative "I don't think it will work" approach. Patients need encouragement to do home dialysis, and the home team must be innovative with "out of the box" attitudes and solutions that will enable patients with the most challenging situations to succeed at home. When patients express interest in HHD, the initial answer should either be "yes we can" or "let's talk to the home dialysis team before we make any decisions"; it rarely should be "no." Ideally, the practice should designate one "HHD expert" and medical director for the home program who will be a much needed resource for all staff regarding questions related to HHD. This "expert" will be a liaison to help identify patients from every venue in the nephrology practice who are interested in HHD and will develop programs such as chronic kidney disease (CKD) education, transitional care units, and modality education for patients on dialysis. The lead HHD physician should also develop relations with other HHD advocates in other locales and academic institutions that will help problem-solve difficult patient and facility problems, as well as offer opportunities to collaborate on clinical and research projects.

A HHD program should be part of a home dialysis program that includes peritoneal dialysis (PD). The synergy between these two modalities complements and enhances each other. Intentionally and functionally, we describe how to build a

J. D. Glickman (✉)
Perelman School of Medicine, University of Pennsylvania, Philadelphia, PA, USA
e-mail: joel.glickman@pennmedicine.upenn.edu

A. Shah et al. (eds.), *Applied Home Hemodialysis*,
https://doi.org/10.1007/978-3-031-77244-3_10

successful home dialysis program as opposed to just an HHD program because the many similarities between HHD and PD logically dictate that these two programs live under one roof. Strategies to increase utilization of HHD will also increase utilization of PD [1]. Teaching methods to improve training and retraining of patients are similar for HHD and PD. Programs to develop QA and continuous quality improvement (CQI) initiatives overlap for these two modalities. Finally, the goals, philosophy, and mission of PD and HHD programs are the same and should be clearly stated and practiced.

Program Goals

Creating a culture that encourages home dialysis and patient success will develop over time with the right leadership driving the process. Implementing a culture change should start with a mission statement. It will help keep the home dialysis team focus on goals and can help them navigate challenging problems that require difficult decisions. The patient's success is the ultimate goal, and therefore, a "patient-centric" mentality is paramount. A recurring scenario of the difficult patient situation is easier to resolve when the staff can set aside their own feelings and focus on the patient's situation. For example: why should the staff feel angry with a non-adherent patient when the correct response should be "what are the barriers that prevent this patient from succeeding" or "what can we do to ease the burden and maximize the benefit for the patient." Some other important ideas for the mission statement could include: offering all patients the opportunity to do home dialysis without bias or prejudice, helping patients achieve their life goals, providing patients a safe environment to voice their concerns, guaranteeing patients receive the best care possible, and incorporating innovative thinking and solutions to enhance the lives of home dialysis patients.

Eventually, as the program's experience develops, the team will gain confidence and will be able to take care of more difficult patient situations. Problem solving with "out of the box" solutions will empower the team to take care of very complicated patients that many programs cannot or will not. Program success occurs when the home team is presented with a challenging patient that no other program would accept, and they say with confidence "Someone has to take care of this patient. It should be our team because we have the experience to enable this patient to succeed."

Nevertheless, the most important goal is the patient's personal perception of success. Dialysis is associated with burdens regardless of the modality, but the burden of HHD is much more than that of in-center hemodialysis (ICHD). The patient-perceived benefit of HHD must significantly exceed the inevitable burden of therapy, or else, the patient will likely "burn out." The benefit/ burden ratio is modifiable. For example: we typically present patients with several options for initial prescriptions and changes to therapy in order to make sure our plans are compatible with their lifestyle. We organize comprehensive, multidisciplinary monthly clinic visits that minimize patient visits and allow us to address all of their needs at one time.

To understand the patient's perception of benefit, the home team needs to explore the patient's goals, aspirations, social setting, work, and personal obligations that the patient values. In contradistinction to ICHD which has limited options to adjust schedule and treatment duration, HHD has multiple modifiable treatment options: treatments per week, days of treatment that can vary from week to week, and duration of treatment depending on the patient's schedule. A progressive example of a unique prescription allows a patient to choose either a short daily or nocturnal treatment on different days depending on the patient's schedule and how they feel. Though flexibility is certainly a benefit of home dialysis, too much flexibility may paradoxically be stressful for patients [2]. Though there are no guidelines for HHD prescriptions that focus on patient goals, we can learn from guidelines for PD prescriptions [3]. One way to assess patient benefit is to longitudinally quantitate patient-reported outcome measurements.

A crucial and measurable goal is the degree of patient utilization of home therapies. Predicting program size is difficult, but with a robust CKD education program, about 35–40% of office patients will start dialysis on a home modality with HHD comprising about 8–10% of the new dialysis start. A reasonable target for the prevalence of home dialysis patients in a practice should be 25–35% of which about 5–8% are on HHD. A more experienced and committed home team, with appropriate clinical and patient social support, should have higher utilization of home dialysis. Program size will influence plans for physical space for the program and targets for staffing. During the initial years of a new HHD program, nurses will likely spend more of their time training patients, but in a mature program, the nurses will focus on clinics and daily patient-related problems. The growth of the program is related not only to new patients but also to the number of patients who exit the program due to modality switch (to PD or in-center HD), transplant, or death. Unfortunately, there is a high early dropout rate from HHD, in the order of 25% in the first year [4]. The number of patients who exit the program is a measure of the program quality. It is reasonable to assume that larger program size, and therefore more clinical experience, may associate with improved outcomes as is true in PD. Every project, miscue, and opportunity for improvement in the process of setting up a home program will turn into a success if the entire home dialysis team focuses on the patient's needs (and not necessarily ours).

The success of the program must include financial matters too. A dialysis provider may limit access to dialysis products or medications if cheaper, equivalent options are available. The staff should advocate for patients if they feel the extra costs are warranted. At the same time, the home team should be careful how they spend "other people's money." If the program is financially successful, chances are the dialysis provider will be more willing to accommodate the home team's request for more expensive options in special circumstances.

Patient Recruitment

Consistent with a patient-centric attitude, the term "patient recruitment" should replace the physician-centric term "patient selection."

Every patient encounter in any setting (office practice, hospital, and dialysis unit) is an opportunity to educate and encourage patients about the benefits of HHD. Education should include the medical benefits of HHD and quality-of-life considerations. It is imperative to explore in detail the goals, preferences, and priorities of the patient and the healthcare partner to enable the practitioner to appropriately counsel the patient. The best home dialysis patient is the patient who is highly motivated and not the patient who decided to do HHD because "my doctor thought it would be a good idea." Ongoing modality education for HHD patients and ICHD patients reminds them that other options are available if circumstances dictate that they need a change. Maintaining relationships with referring physicians and especially transplant services will positively impact patient care and will likely increase referrals to the home program.

CKD education, ideally as part of a CKD management program, helps patients understand their disease, as well as dietary interventions and treatment options that may slow the progression of renal disease. Modality education when done correctly will increase patient utilization of home modalities. Classes and written materials are helpful for most patients, but patients need more than just one educational session to make the right choice for themselves. Patients interested in HHD should visit the home program to see the equipment they will need at home. The best promoters of HHD are HHD patients. The home program should generate a list of current and former HHD patients who are willing to speak to prospective HHD patients.

The transition from the CKD clinic to dialysis can be complicated for many patients and often leads to preventable hospital admissions for initiation of dialysis that are associated with higher mortality and morbidity. Often, these patients are sent to an outpatient HD center and never have the opportunity to do HHD even if they were interested in it prior to hospitalization. The CKD management team can develop relationships with home programs to facilitate a successful transition to home dialysis without hospitalizations and complications.

Unfortunately, an unacceptably high percentage of dialysis patients start dialysis without sufficient CKD education. Though these patients often start dialysis on hemodialysis with a central venous catheter, they should all be considered to be potential home dialysis patients. An in-patient modality education program with follow-up can increase utilization of home dialysis [5]. For those patients who have not had the benefit of education prior to the initiation of dialysis, transitional care units may improve utilization of home therapies [6]. Typically, a transitional care unit will offer more frequent short daily hemodialysis treatments and personalized education about home dialysis therapies, and help patient acclimate to dialysis in a calm and supportive environment.

Infrastructure

A HHD program should be in the same space as a PD program because the requirements for training rooms, exam rooms, storage, and staff are very similar. It can be in the same structure as an existing ICHD program, as an addition to an existing PD program or as a new stand-alone home dialysis facility. Retrofitting an existing space is more challenging compared to building a new facility because it may not have the ideal amount of space to present an aesthetically pleasing place for patients and to develop efficient workflows for the staff. Ideally, the space needs to accommodate enough training rooms and exam rooms to support the targeted census of the program. Training rooms can double as clinic rooms though standard exam rooms should also be built because they require less space and less plumbing. The training rooms must be large enough to accommodate a dialysis machine, water and dialysate equipment, clean and waste sinks, cabinets for supplies, comfortable chairs for patients and their care partners, and workspace for the nurse. The space should not be claustrophobic and should attempt to mimic the comfort of home. Windows to the outside or facing the clinic make the patient rooms feel more open and brighter. There are regulations that vary from state to state with regard to space and equipment requirements. Training rooms do not need central delivery of treated water or dialysate because patients will need to learn how to use equipment to produce dialysate for use at home. The training rooms require a municipal water source, and the faucet should be prominently and appropriately labeled. Of course, the rooms are constructed with drains for spent dialysate. Ideally, the rooms are set up identically, so staff can easily locate any supplies they need. Patients need to be organized at home, and therefore the clinic should be a perfect model for them.

Staff

The Home Team

The home team staff includes physicians, nurses (potentially both R.N. and L.P.N), patient care technicians, dieticians, social workers, administrative assistants, biomedical technicians, and a facility administrator. Ideally, the medical director and facility administrator are involved in the interview process of hiring home dialysis staff. The applicant should also have the opportunity to tour the facility and meet other staff members. A highly qualified ICHD nurse may not necessarily be the ideal HHD nurse because the skill set requirement for these two positions is very different. The HHD nurse needs to be a great communicator with patience to teach patients of varied backgrounds and learning styles. The home dialysis nurse also needs to be confident, independent, and capable to manage patients without the constant presence of other support staff. Finally, often the work hours may be very different than ICHD and there usually is a need for off-hours on-call duties. Similarly, the skill set and knowledge base for dieticians, social workers, and biomedical technicians may also be different compared to ICHD.

Staff Training

Dialysis organizations have formal training programs for new HHD nurses. In addition to lectures, a significant portion of the training involves working with a trained HHD nurse for several months. The training criteria required for a HHD nurse to work independently vary by state regulations. Though the nurse is "adequately" trained, the physicians need to provide clinical support that will improve the clinical skills of the nurse. Compared to ICHD nurses, HHD nurses need more experience with patient assessment and management. In fact, physicians and HHD nurses learn from each other. Typically, the nurse knows more about the dialysis equipment and has more current information regarding the status of the patients. In reality, differences in management of the home dialysis patient are present for all members of the team. Investing time educating the staff will improve the care of home dialysis patients, help create a safer environment, build team cohesiveness, enhance job satisfaction for the staff, and inevitably make the job of physicians much easier.

Staffing Models

It may be hard to recruit a HHD nurse. One reason is the work schedule. ICHD nurses often work 10- to 12-h shifts 3–4 days a week. HHD nurses often work 5 days per week because most short daily hemodialysis patients receive five treatments per week and patient problems can occur daily. To ensure patients get adequate HD treatment during training, acute patient problems are appropriately addressed promptly, and improved work schedules for HHD nurses are developed, new staffing models should be developed that permit HHD patients to work 4 days per week or have variable work hours when needed. For example: patients could train 4 days per week (especially if they have residual renal function) and if necessary have an occasional ICHD treatment. A patient care technician can be trained to assist the HHD nurse. HHD nurses from different facilities can cross-cover each other. If the nurse is not actively training a patient, she may be able to work from home periodically. The facility administrator should make sure that nurses spend their time on "home dialysis nursing" and designate other tasks that require less training to other staff members. For example, patient care technicians can draw laboratories, process specimens, give patients supplies they need for blood and urine collections, and set up dialysis equipment. An administrative assistant should be able to make sure all regulatory documents are completed on time, make appointments for next home clinics, and answer phone calls that can be disruptive to the nurse.

Professional Development

To improve the quality of the program, retain staff, and keep the home team engaged, programs to promote professional development are indispensable. All HHD staff should attend monthly quality assurance meetings. These meetings ought to prompt new CQI projects that can be managed by different staff members depending on the subject matter of the project. Professional dialysis meetings keep the HHD team up to date and can promote relationships with other HHD programs. Inevitably, CQI projects, interesting cases, and new approaches to patient care create opportunity for writing papers and abstracts, as well as oral presentations at meetings. These types of projects will create a sense of professional satisfaction for the staff that will lead to improved patient care and dedication to the HHD program.

Role of the Medical Director

The fundamental responsibilities of the medical director are outlined in the CMS conditions of coverage [7]. However, to develop a successful program, the medical director also needs to be the expert on home dialysis therapies, the chief educator for the home team, and the enthusiastic cheerleader for patients and staff. If nephrology fellowships don't provide high level education on HHD (which is typical), the medical director will need to attend a comprehensive home dialysis course, read pertinent medical literature, and develop relationships with other HHD physicians who can provide advice regarding program function and patient care. It is unrealistic for the medical director to have a detailed knowledge of all the technical aspects of the dialysis equipment, as well as how to train patients, but they should have a strong background and interest in these subjects. The nurse will be the expert on training and will know more about the dialysis equipment as will the biomedical technician.

The medical director needs to make sure that the patient can dialyze safely at home. One of the challenges of a HHD program is that each patient at home essentially runs their own dialysis facility. These multiple "home dialysis facilities" have to generate quality dialysate (e.g., routine cultures), manage equipment failures, provide preventive maintenance and monitoring of equipment, and avoid potential supply problems, and are subject to power and water supply outages. The medical director needs a system to make sure all these issues are monitored at a predetermined schedule and policies are in place to address potential problems. The medical director needs to make sure that the patient and potential care partner are competent to perform dialysis at home with the same standards that certify HHD staff to be competent in HHD.

Patient Clinic Visits

Monthly physician and nursing visits are mandated by CMS conditions of coverage that can be achieved by several different models. Multidisciplinary (physician, nurse, social worker, dietician) visits in the same venue promote a better team approach to clinical care, and facilitate communication between team members and the patient. Often, patients develop different relationships with different members of the team and may feel more comfortable discussing personal problems with a particular staff member regardless of their role. As an example, a patient might feel closer to the dietician and confide in that person rather than the nurse or physician. Some physicians prefer to see patients in their office, but the patient is still required to have a second visit with the nurses in the dialysis facility. This added visit to the physician is a burden for the patient and does not improve patient care. If anything, it might compromise care because the communication between the physician and the rest of the home team may become fragmented. Fortunately, telemedicine visits are permitted by Medicare. The first 3 months after training must be in-person visits, but after that, only one visit every 3 months needs to be in-person. The team needs to develop a plan for effective telemedicine visits [8]. For urgent issues, additional visits may be necessary.

Blood tests are required monthly and include *Kt/V* that is derived from pre- and post-treatment serum BUN measurements. Obviously, it is difficult to obtain post-treatment BUN levels during a clinic visit. Therefore, patients are taught how to draw laboratories at home and mail them to a central laboratory.

HHD patients can self-administer intravenous erythropoietin-stimulating agents and vitamin D analogues. Depending on the dialysis provider, patients can also self-administer intravenous iron and some antibiotics. At times, patients are treated with intravenous antibiotics that cannot be administered during dialysis at home. Alternative options include going to the clinic for antibiotic infusion several days per week, short-term conversion to ICHD, or home infusion service that administers antibiotic by a non-dialysis venous access.

Respite Care

The HHD team should never underestimate the burdens that HHD patients and their caregivers experience. They must also realize that patients are not always forthcoming with personal problems and at times may not even recognize the personal impact of all the responsibilities they have. Primarily, the social work tries to discover these problems but they manifest as emergencies, but other staff need to be vigilant in detecting difficulties that occur for the patient. Respite HHD care, providing patients dialysis treatments in the home clinic or ICHD facility, can temporarily relieve some of the burden patients experience until the problems they face can be corrected. Patients must be told often that respite care is available should they need it, so it can be utilized before a crisis occurs.

References

1. Rioux JP, Bargman JM, Chan CT. Systematic differences among patients initiated on home haemodialysis and peritoneal dialysis: the fallacy of potential competition. Nephrol Dial Transplant. 2010;25:2364–7.

2. Seshasai RK, Wong Y, Glickman J, Shea JA, Dember LM. The home hemodialysis patient experience: a qualitative assessment of modality use and discontinuation. Hemodial Int. 2019;23(2):139–50.
3. Brown EA, Blake G, Boudville N, Davies S, De Arteaga J, Dong J, et al. International Society for Peritoneal Dialysis practice recommendations: prescribing high-quality goal-directed peritoneal dialysis. Perit Dial Int. 2020;40(3):244–53.
4. Seshasai RK, Mitra N, Chaknos CM, Li J, Wirtalla C, Negoianu D, et al. Factors associated with discontinuation of home hemodialysis. Am J Kidney Dis. 2016;67(4):629–37.
5. Rioux JP, Cheema H, Bargman JM, Watson D, Chan C. Effect of an in-hospital chronic kidney disease education program among patients with unplanned urgent-start dialysis. Clin J Am Soc Nephrol. 2011;6:799–804.
6. Hussein WF, Bennett PN, Schiller B. Innovations to increase home hemodialysis utilization: the transitional care unit. Adv Chronic Kidney Dis. 2021;28(2):178–83.
7. http://www.cms.gov/Medicare/Provider-Enrollment-and-certification/GuidanceforLawsAndRegulations/Downloads/esrdpgmguidance.pdf. Accessed 7 Nov 2022.
8. Lew SQ, Wallace EL, Srivatana V, Warady BA, Watnick S, Hood J, et al. Telehealth for home dialysis in COVID-19 and beyond: a perspective from the American Society of Nephrology COVID-19 Home Dialysis Subcommittee. Am J Kidney Dis. 2021;77(1):142–8.

Water Treatment and Dialysate Production in the Home

11

Hannah Webb and Brent Miller

History of Water Purification and Dialysate Production in Home Hemodialysis

Home hemodialysis requires a consistent and large-volume water supply in the home. Based on water rejection from the purification system, and the ultimate dialysate flow rate, water consumption during home hemodialysis can range between 500 and 1500 mL/min to produce a final dialysate flow of 100–800 mL/min. Further, a hemodialysis patient is often exposed to more water in 1 week than most seen in a lifetime, and many home hemodialysis patients typically see even more water than conventional hemodialysis given longer and more frequent sessions that are currently prescribed. Given only a thin, semipermeable membrane separating the patient's blood from water (dialysate), it is crucial for this water to be reliably purified to the appropriate standards. The dangers of water purification and dialysate production mishaps are significant, and they have been shown throughout the history of dialysis.

The extracorporeal circuit can also cause problems during hemodialysis. Human error, faulty equipment, and environmental factors can all have disastrous consequences for patients performing hemodialysis in their home. For example, a misconnection of tubing between water purification systems and hemodialysis machines can lead to dialysate production with wastewater, infusing toxic amounts of calcium into patients' blood [1]. As first described in the 1980s, dialysis tubing can release silicone particles up to 5 μm, called spallation, as well as volatile hydrocarbons into the blood. These events can be markedly reduced by rinsing components with 500 mL of saline prior to each session [2, 3]. While air in the circuit is reliably monitored during hemodialysis, microbubbles up to 10 μm can enter the body. Most of these are dissolved in the pulmonary circulation, although they have been found

H. Webb · B. Miller (✉)
Division of Nephrology, Indiana University School of Medicine, Indianapolis, IN, USA
e-mail: htwebb@iu.edu; bwm1@iu.edu

A. Shah et al. (eds.), *Applied Home Hemodialysis*,
https://doi.org/10.1007/978-3-031-77244-3_11

in the carotid artery even in the absence of a patent foramen ovale, potentially due to pulmonary edema and shunting [4]. Other considerations within the dialysis circuit include the membrane composition, which could contribute to both platelet and neutrophil or complement activation, as well as chronic exposure to anticoagulants and the effects of this over many years.

Water Sources

Water for home hemodialysis is generally supplied from the municipal water system, although patients living in rural or remote areas may rely on feed sources such as wells, tanks, reservoirs, and lakes. Batch supply water is less frequently used but can be an option in the absence of water purification systems. The municipal water supply is fairly standardized in terms of contaminant removal, and often provides a reliable source for home hemodialysis. Feed sources require an initial biochemical analysis to determine necessary filters prior to reverse osmosis (RO) or deionization installation in the home (Fig. 11.1).

History of Water Contaminants in Home Hemodialysis

The water purification system plays a critical role in safe hemodialysis, eliminating harmful contaminants from any water supply source. Historical examples have taught lessons about water sanitization and ultimately lead to modern purification systems commonly used today in hemodialysis centers and at home (Table 11.1).

The municipal water supply can be contaminated by industrial waste products that can enter the dialysate and are difficult to test for routinely, such as in a 2014

Sample reeived in acceptable condition unless otherwise noted. Results reflect the sample as received in the laboratory. Low reportable limits are set based on AAMI requirements and not intended for drinking water quality.

Assay Date/Time: 11/08/17 13:00

Aluminum, Water[1]	**0.055**	**H**		0.000–0.010	mg/L
Antimony, Water			<0.005	0.000–0.006	mg/L
Arsenic, Water			<0.002	0.000–0.005	mg/L
Barium, Water			0.022	0.000–0.100	mg/L
Beryllium, Water			<0.0004	0.0000–0.0004	mg/L
Cadmium, Water			<0.0010	0.0000–0.0010	mg/L
Calcium, Water	**14.761**	**H**		0.000–2.000	mg/L
Chromium, Water			<0.005	0.000–0.014	mg/L
Copper, Water			<0.005	0.000–0.100	mg/L
Fluoride, Water	**0.82**	**H**		0.00–0.20	mg/L
Lead, Water			<0.002	0.000–0.005	mg/L
Magnesium, Water			3.757	0.000–4.000	mg/L
Mercury, Water			<0.0002	0.0000–0.0002	mg/L
Nitrate, Water			0.36	0.0–2.0	mg/L
Potassium, Water			2.388	0.000–8.000	mg/L
Selenium, Water			<0.005	0.000–0.090	mg/L
Silver, Water			<0.003	0.000–0.005	mg/L
Sodium, Water			27.079	0.000–70.000	mg/L
Sulfate, Water			36.1	0.0–100.0	mg/L

Fig. 11.1 Example of home water analysis

Table 11.1 Common water contaminants and their source

Contaminant	Source
Aluminum	Drinking water additive
Cadmium	Industrial waste
Calcium/magnesium	Naturally occurring
Chlorine/chloramines	Drinking water additive
Chromium	Steel mills and wood preserving
Copper	Pipes/infrastructure
Fluoride	Drinking water additive
Lead	Pipes/infrastructure
Nitrates	Fertilizer runoff
Bleach (sodium hypochlorite)	Dialyzer sterilization
Sulfate	Naturally occurring or industrial waste
Zinc	Infrastructure or feedwater sources

incident in West Virginia in which drinking water was exposed to 4-methylcyclohexane methanol that leaked from a storage tank [5]. Well water can pose specific threats such as methemoglobinemia given the higher prevalence of nitrates in groundwater [6]. The equipment used to deliver the dialysate can also be a source of dangerous contaminants, as seen in 1991 at a dialysis center in Pennsylvania that installed electric pumps with aluminum housing to add bicarbonate to dialysate were soon after found to have dangerously high levels of aluminum in the blood of patients who required more bicarbonate with dialysis [7].

Water purification equipment that is not properly maintained can lead to dangerous contaminants in dialysate. In 1970, a phenomenon was first described in which patients suffered from hemolytic anemia related to copper toxicity that occurred when a deionizing system was exhausted allow copper from tubing to leach into dialysate [8]. Similarly, continuing use of a deionization system after the ion binding resin is depleted can lead to fluoride contamination in dialysate from the municipal water supply due to displacement of low-affinity ions (i.e., fluoride) from the resin, as occurred in a dialysis center in Chicago in 1994 [9].

How Potable Water Is Produced

Municipal water undergoes multiple steps of purification prior to release into the local water supply. These steps ensure a potable water source for all residents of a community. First, a gross screening allows for the removal of large debris. The addition of aluminum sulfate and calcium hydroxide allows for purification. Water is then filtered for the removal of smaller particles. Chlorine and chloramine are added for their disinfectant properties, and calcium hydroxide is used to adjust pH. However, many of the additives to make water safe for drinking are potentially harmful in the circulation in larger concentrations.

AAMI Standards

Since 1981, the Association for the Advancement of Medical Instrumentation (AAMI) has published minimum standards for both in-center and home hemodialysis water purification. Water must undergo yearly biochemical analysis to ensure safety and purity as defined by the AAMI. In addition, monthly testing for colony count and endotoxin can detect bacterial contamination. Finally, chlorine testing is required on every dialysate.

AAMI has also defined standard and ultrapure dialysate, determined by the number of colony-forming units (maximum 100 versus 0.1, respectively) and endotoxin (<0.5 versus <0.003 EU/mL) [10]. Ultrapure dialysate ensures that when backfiltration occurs—movement of dialysate water into the blood due to the pressure differential between the two compartments—there is less risk of contamination. Backfiltration that occurs after convection in an ultrapure dialysate can enhance large molecule clearance from the blood although clinical studies have not shown consistent long-term clinical benefits of ultrapure water for dialysate production.

Methods of Producing Dialysate Water

Water for dialysate must go through sophisticated water purification systems prior to use in hemodialysis to prevent complications such as those previously described. Similar concepts are utilized in both in-center and home dialysate production, so we will start with a review on the former to explain the adaptations needed for the latter.

Multimedia Filtering Tank

The first step in a water purification system generally involves a multimedia filtering tank. The role of this process is to remove large particulate matter from the water including mud, clay, silica, and other large sediments.

Carbon Tanks

Carbon tanks are used in the absorption of organic materials, chlorine and especially chloramines, which are added to the municipal water supply for antimicrobial properties. These compounds are oxidative agents that kill bacteria but can rapidly enter the blood and cause hemolysis. Carbon in the carbon bed reacts with chlorines and chloramines to produce chloride and carbon dioxide, and also to remove organics and sediment from the water. Monitoring should focus on detection of bacterial growth, release of fine particles, and release of chloramines into water when the carbon is exhausted. Two carbon tanks are commonly installed in sequence to ensure effective removal of chlorines from the water supply.

Water Softener

The water softener acts to remove calcium and magnesium from the water supply, in effect exchanging calcium, magnesium, iron, and manganese, among other cations from the source water, for sodium in the product water. This protects the downstream RO or deionizing system from exhaustion, thereby extending the life of more costly equipment and supplies. The water softener needs to be monitored for bacterial growth and exhaustion on a regular basis.

Micron Filters

Micron filters remove smaller particles, particularly bacteria and endotoxin, and act as a final safeguard against microbials that may have contaminated the water from within the purification system. Micron filters are particularly important in sequence after deionizing systems given their propensity for internal bacterial proliferation.

Ultraviolet Light

Ultraviolet light works as an antibacterial by altering bacteria's DNA, preventing replication. These devices are used in several home hemodialysis water purification systems, but do not reduce endotoxin and are not effective if a biofilm is present.

Reverse Osmosis

RO systems remove dissolved particles by using a high-pressure force to push water through a semipermeable membrane that is not permeable to dissolved solutes in the water. Water pressure pre- and post-RO and solute concentration of water can be used to assess the efficacy of the system. In home hemodialysis, these machines are portable and connect directly to the dialysis system, but have a high rate of water waste, leading to more utility costs in both water and sewage expenses, as well as environmental considerations related to water usage. RO systems also require membrane disinfection and changing. Online systems track both water flow and membrane pressure of the RO system and alert the user when the membrane has been depleted.

Deionization

Deionization (DI) machines work to remove cations and anions using resin beads, and replace them with hydrogen and hydroxyl molecules, respectively, to form pure water. Like RO, DI systems are portable in the home hemodialysis setup and are connected directly to the hemodialysis machine to supply pure water. DI machines tend to be a less expensive option in home hemodialysis as compared to RO and produce less water waste with nearly 100% water use as compared to a 50–90% rejection rate in RO systems. These systems are generally quieter options than RO setups. Internal monitors continuously measure resistivity, that is, the inverse of conductivity, of the water to assess the efficacy of the DI water purification. When the resistivity increases above a certain level, the machine will indicate that the resin beads are depleted [11].

Sorbent

Due to the financial and economic impacts of high water usage with single-pass water purification systems, there has been prior interest in sorbent technology, or adsorption of impurities from "used" dialysate to produce ultrapure water and eventually new dialysate. Adsorption occurs in sequence by passing impure dialysate through a column containing first activated charcoal, then zirconium phosphate, urease, and lastly zirconium oxide and zirconium sulfate.

Sorbent systems require less water usage because of their ability to recycle dialysate, making the system more portable and eco-friendly. In the past, systems such as the Baxter Redy, Fresenius PAK, and Renal Solutions Allient were available and used frequently in home hemodialysis. Currently, no machines in the United States use sorbent systems, although the technology could come back into favor as home hemodialysis becomes more prevalent.

Ensuring Home Dialysis Water Quality

To ensure safe contaminant-free water for home hemodialysis, source water must be tested and treated appropriately prior to purification, especially if the water is from a feed source such as a well or reservoir. Water, described as "product water," should also be tested after purification to confirm efficacy of the system in place.

Installation of Water Treatment in the Home

Cost/Supplies/Delivery

Several different methods incorporating the above principles are available to produce water for dialysate production in the home. In current practice, those methods can be divided into a "batched" production method and an "on-demand" production method. A batched production method requires that the water and dialysate be prepared ahead of the planned hemodialysis treatment. The volume of the batch will limit the amount of dialysate that can be utilized and hence the dose and/or time of dialysis delivered.

One more costly alternative to water purification and dialysate production in the home is bagged, premade dialysate, which is utilized by the Physidia® home dialysis system. This system avoids the time and space restraints of installing a water purification system in the home and making dialysate for each session by shipping 5-L bags of sterile dialysate in various formulations to the patient. The added benefit of this system also lies in the guarantee of sterility and endotoxin-free dialysate without as much reliance on individual patients to maintain and test personal water purification systems.

The only batched dialysate water system currently approved by the United States Food and Drug Administration is the NxStage Pureflow Water Treatment System®

(Fig. 11.2a). Designed for home hemodialysis and utilizing DI technology, the system includes a pre-DI sediment filter, ultraviolet light for decontamination, and carbon tank in one unit to produce a bag of 60 liters of ultrapure water from tap water. Dialysate is produced by directly mixing the ultrapure water product into a bag with liquid solutes. Water purification and subsequent dialysate mixing take about 8 h and are available for 96 h.

The other home dialysis machine currently approved for use in the United States, the Tablo by Outset Medical, utilizes an inline RO system that produces dialysate water proportioned with dialysate acid and base concentrates at the time of use, as illustrated in Fig. 11.2b.

Production of Dialysate

Components of Dialysate (Table 11.2)

- Base
- Historically, three bases have been utilized in hemodialysis: acetate, lactate, and bicarbonate (Table 11.3). Acetate is no longer utilized as the primary base due to the symptoms it produces in the patient prior to conversion in the body to bicarbonate. Lactate has the advantage of being both less prone to microbiological contamination and biochemically stable, as well as not causing precipitation of calcium. Bicarbonate is generally very well tolerated by the patient, but care must be taken to prevent microbiological contamination and precipitation of calcium. Thus, the design of a bagged or batched system would favor lactate and an on-demand system would favor bicarbonate.
- Lactate and acetate present the biochemical issue of needing conversion to bicarbonate by the body. The human body is capable of metabolizing about 1500 mmol of lactate daily from any source, but total capacity is 1400 mL/min of plasma. This capacity generally does not decrease until liver blood flow decreases to about 25% of normal. On average, a home dialysis treatment would diffuse between 800 and 1350 mmol lactate into the circulation. The plasma level of lactate rises slightly during the treatment and promptly returns to normal after the treatment.
- When lactate is used as the base for dialysate in home hemodialysis, there is a temporary measurable increase in serum lactate concentrations up to 3.48 mEq/L on average immediately post-treatment, decreasing back to normal levels within 1 h following a session [12]. At these levels—which may be due to the lower dialysate flow and generally short dialysis time utilized in home hemodialysis—no significant difference in symptoms such as headache, fatigue, or nausea/vomiting has been shown between patients using lactate- or bicarbonate-based dialysate.
- Potassium
- Potassium concentration is one of the most important components of dialysate as both hypokalemia and hyperkalemia in hemodialysis patients have significant

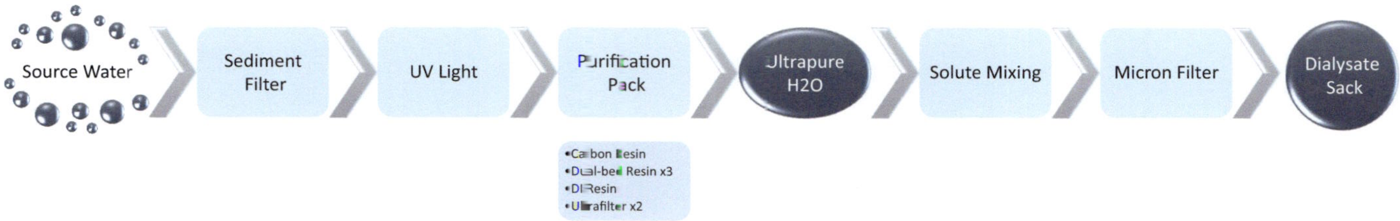

Fig. 11.2a NxStage Pureflow® water treatment system

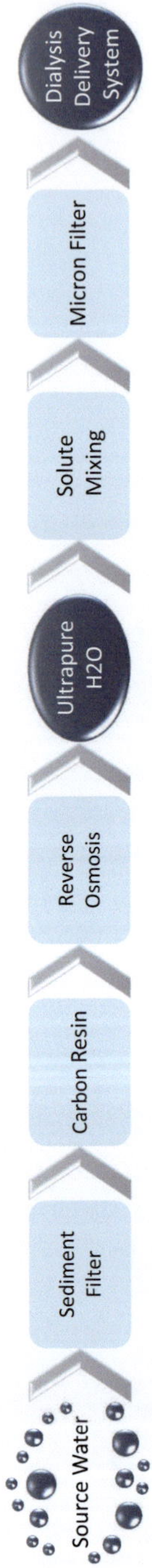

Fig. 11.2b Tablo® by Outset Medical

Table 11.2 Available dialysate compositions in NxStage Pureflow® and Tablo® systems

Constituent	Nxstage Pureflow®	Tablo®
Base	40–45 mEq/L (lactate)	30–40 mEq/L (bicarbonate and acetate)
Potassium	1, 2, 3 mEq/L	0, 1, 2, 3 mEq/L
Sodium	140 mEq/L	130–145 mEq/L
Calcium	3–3.5	0–3.5

Table 11.3 Comparing base/buffer in home dialysate

	Bicarbonate	Lactate	Acetate
Conversion	None	To bicarbonate	To bicarbonate
Symptoms[a]	Minimal	Minimal	Significant
Calcium precipitation	Yes	None	None
Microbial contamination risk	Significant	Less	Less
Lactate elevation	None	Average 3.48 mEq/L	None

[a]Headache, nausea/vomiting, weakness, hypotension, cramping

morbidities. 95% of potassium removal from the body in normal kidney function is performed by the kidneys. In the end-stage renal disease, the gastrointestinal (GI) tract increases potassium excretion from 5% to approximately 35% of the total to make up for the lack of kidney function. However, this still requires dialysis to remove 40–70 mEq per day (or 80–140 mEq per session if dialysis is performed three times weekly), assuming an average potassium intake of 0.75–1 mEq/kg/day [13].

- Potassium removal during dialysis is dependent on both the dialysate potassium concentration gradient between plasma and dialysate and the rate of efflux of potassium from the intracellular space as dialysis ensues. The first quarter of a treatment removes potassium from the intravascular and extracellular space, while the last three quarters of any dialysis session extract potassium from the intracellular compartment. There is a redistribution of potassium within the 6 h following a dialysis session of potassium from the intracellular compartment to the intravascular and extracellular space [13].
- In low-flow hemodialysis, as is commonly performed at home, the dialysate flow rate is reduced from 600–800 mL/min in conventional dialysis to 100–200 mL/min and the total dialysate utilized is 20–60 L. Thus, the gradient in the dialysate is not maintained, and an increased gradient is required to ensure adequate potassium removal. For example, a patient with a serum potassium concentration of 4 mEq/L who dialyzes with a Qd of 150 mL/min for a total of 30 L of dialysate with a potassium concentration of 1 mEq/L and 2 L ultrafiltration removes 96 mEq of potassium during a session (32 L × (4–1 mEq/L)), assuming a 100% dialysate saturation. In this way, performing hemodialysis six times weekly with low-flow dialysate can easily meet potassium removal needs of most patients, and reduces much of the variability in serum potassium levels seen in in-center hemodialysis patients receiving treatments three times weekly (Fig. 11.3).
- Sodium

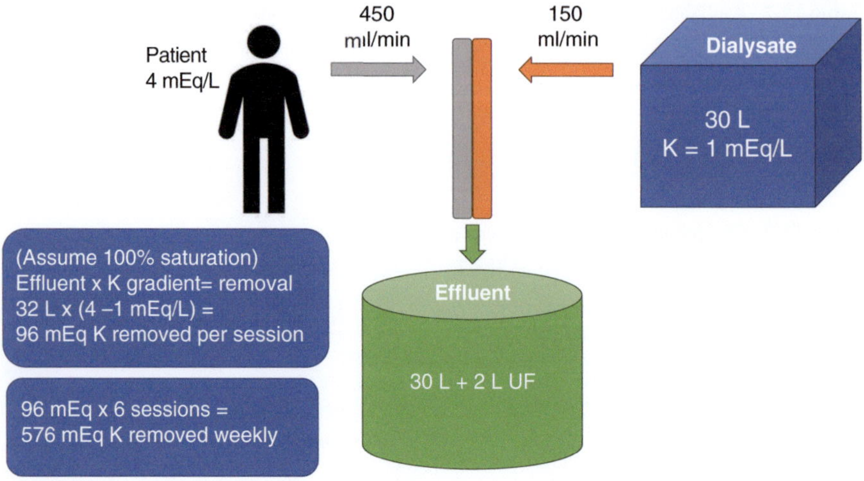

Fig. 11.3 Potassium removal in home hemodialysis

- Most of the sodium removal in a hemodialysis treatment occurs with ultrafiltration; thus, the most important decision is the target weight. The dialysate sodium concentration and the subsequent gradient between the plasma and dialysate will allow for sodium removal via diffusion. Notably, there is a theoretical phenomenon, the Gibbs-Donnan effect, which postulates a breakdown in the sodium gradient as a driving force and therefore less sodium removal during dialysis because of the impermeability of the dialysis membrane to albumin, which is an anion. As albumin becomes more concentrated in the blood (i.e., with more ultrafiltration), less sodium moves into the dialysate due to electronegative forces [14].
- Magnesium
- Magnesium retention tends to occur in patients undergoing hemodialysis, so the dialysate bath utilized encourages magnesium removal. However, observational studies suggest that lower magnesium baths also have adverse cardiac complications, so hemodialysis magnesium baths have been more recently increased to 1 mEq/L. This is also true for home hemodialysis [15].
- Calcium
- Calcium mass balance during hemodialysis is highly variable compared to potassium because of calcium binding to protein, its divalent status, the effect of phosphorous levels on calcium diffusion across the dialysis membrane, and Gibbs-Donnan equilibrium effects. Opinion has also shifted over the last 40 years on whether calcium balance during hemodialysis should be positive, negative, or neutral. Although urinary calcium is a significant source of excretion with lower amounts of calcium intake and normal kidney function, the GI tract has been shown to quickly decrease calcium absorption at higher levels of intake, minimizing any positive calcium balance that could occur [16]. This would imply that even patients with end-stage renal disease who have no urinary calcium excretion will not automatically accumulate calcium significantly between dialysis

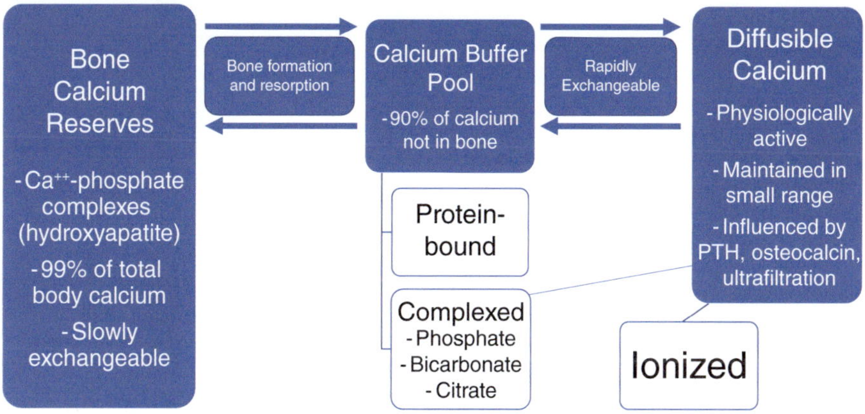

Fig. 11.4 Modeling calcium balance during dialysis

sessions. Thus, it is often necessary to remove only small amounts of calcium during dialysis. This is even less of a concern in nocturnal home dialysis, which is performed more frequently, due to less prevalence of hyperphosphatemia and almost no requirement for calcium-based phosphorous binders.

- Calcium removal on dialysis is based on serum concentration, dialysate concentrate, blood flow rate, and dialysate flow rate. Serum concentration will not change significantly even with varying dialysate concentrations due to a large pool of calcium that can quickly be mobilized or sequestered based on increases or decreases in serum calcium levels [17]. Calcium balance during dialysis is also dependent on ultrafiltration, PTH levels, and osteocalcin [18]. In the setting of using lower total dialysate volumes as is often done in home hemodialysis, even under optimum diffusion circumstances, only a small amount of calcium could be either removed from or added to the patient (Fig. 11.4).
- Glucose
- In the 1970s, the common glucose concentration in hemodialysis was 200 mg/dl with the concept that this would both prevent hypoglycemia and improve the nutritional status of the patients. However, as the adverse metabolic consequences of hyperglycemia became apparent, the standard glucose concentration for hemodialysis changed to 100 mg/dL in the 1990s and this remains the typical concentration in home hemodialysis.

How Much Dialysate Is Necessary to Achieve Clearance?

Solute clearance in dialysis is dependent on both dialysate flow rate and time on dialysis. Home hemodialysis prescriptions tend to use lower flow rates with longer and more frequent sessions, oftentimes nocturnal. This structure allows for adequate solute clearance by taking advantage of the time variable, while decreasing the amount of dialysate (and water) required for treatment. Time on dialysis,

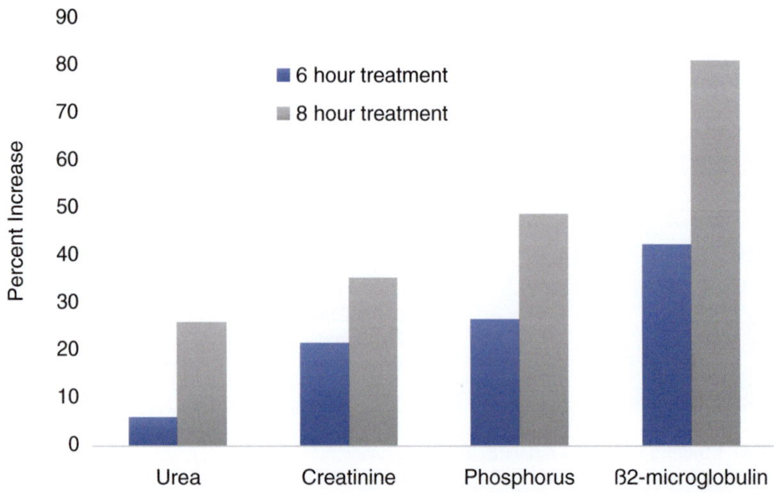

Fig. 11.5a Effects of treatment duration on solute clearance. (Adapted from Ref. [18])

independent of volume of dialysate utilized, significantly increases solute clearance, as illustrated in Fig. 11.5a [19].

Prior studies have shown only small benefits to higher dialysate flow rates (Q_D) (800 mL/min instead of 500 mL/min) even when the length of dialysis treatment is held constant. For example, as seen in Fig. 11.5b, decreasing Q_D from 800 to 500 mL/min would decrease urea clearance by 7%, decrease phosphorous clearance by 4%, and have no effect on $ß_2$-microglobulin clearance (a surrogate for middle molecular weight molecule clearance) [20]. None of these benefits are likely to be clinically significant in increasing efficacy of dialysis treatment. In addition, the proportion of solute removed compared to dialysate use was constant regardless of dialysate flow rate.

Summary and Future Directions

Water and dialysate production is critical to the success of home hemodialysis and if done incorrectly or not monitored carefully can harm the patient. The supplies and equipment utilized can often add significant cost to the therapy and even add to the patient's own water bill. Although progress continues to be made to simplify this portion of home hemodialysis, several advancements are needed:

- Technologies that utilize less water to produce dialysate
- Further refinement in the optimum amount of dialysate to be utilized in a hemodialysis treatment
- Further ability to individualize components of the dialysate bath at the point of care

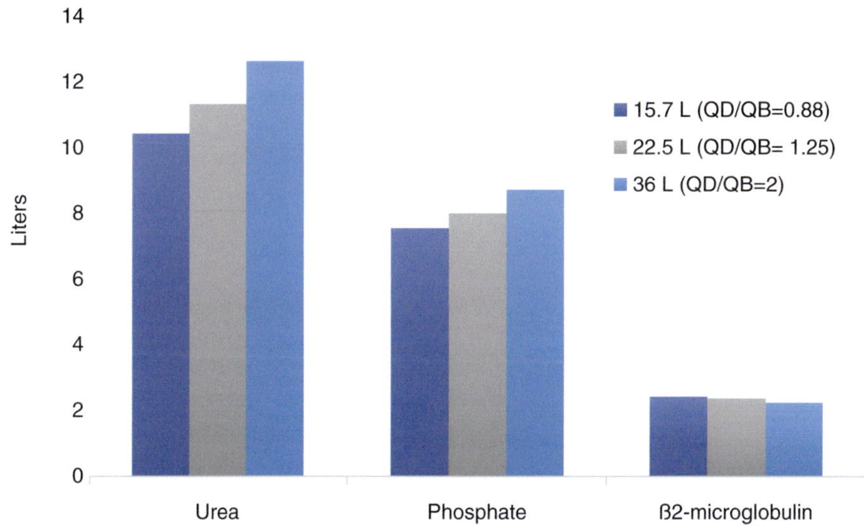

Fig. 11.5b Effects of dialysate flow rate on solute clearance. (Adapted from Ref. 19)

- Development of other technologies such as sorbent or cellular membranes that don't rely on convective and diffusive clearance

References

1. Murlidharan P, Chan CT, Bargman JM. Catastrophic hypercalcemia as a technical complication in home hemodialysis. NDT Plus. 2011;4:251–2.
2. Bommer J, Pernicka E, Kessler ER, Ritz E. University of Heidelberg,* Max-Planck-Institut für Kernphysik, Heidelberg, FRC. Proc EDTA—ERA; 1984.
3. Lee HJ, Meinardi S, Pahl MV, Vaziri ND, Blake DR. Exposure to potentially toxic hydrocarbons and halocarbons released from the dialyzer and tubing set during hemodialysis. Am J Kidney Dis. 2012;60:609–16.
4. Stegmayr B, Brännström T, Forsberg U, Jonson P, Stegmayr C, Hultdin J. Microbubbles of air may occur in the organs of hemodialysis patients. ASAIO J. 2012;58:177–9.
5. Unger D. West Virginia chemical spill: what's 4-methylcyclohexane methanol? Christ Sci Monit. 2014;
6. Carlson DJ, Shapiro FL. Methemoglobinemia from well water nitrates: a complication of home dialysis. Ann Intern Med. 1970;73:757–9.
7. Burwen DR, Olsen SM, Bland LA, Arduino MJ, Reid MH, Jarvis WR. Epidemic aluminum intoxication in hemodialysis patients traced to use of an aluminum pump. Kidney Int. 1995;48:469–74.
8. Manzler AD, Schreiner AW. Copper-induced acute hemolytic anemia. A new complication of hemodialysis. Ann Intern Med. 1970;73:409–12.
9. Arnow PM, Bland LA, Garcia-Houchins S, Fridkin S, Fellner SK. An outbreak of fatal fluoride intoxication in a long-term hemodialysis unit. Ann Intern Med. 1994;121:339–44.
10. Association for the Advancement of Medical Instrumentation: American National Standard. ANSI/AAMI/ISO2009.

11. Network NR. Monitoring your dialysis water treatment system. Seattle: Northwest Renal Network; 2005.
12. Dalal S, Yu AW, Gupta DK, Kar PM, Ing TS, Daugirdas JT. L-lactate high-efficiency hemodialysis: hemodynamics, blood gas changes, potassium/phosphorus, and symptoms. Kidney Int. 1990;38:896–903.
13. Rachoin JS, Weisberg LS. How should dialysis fluid be individualized for the chronic hemodialysis patient? Potassium Semin Dial. 2008;21:223–5.
14. Kawanishi H. Is there enough evidence to prove that hemodiafiltration is superior? Blood Purif. 2018;46:3–6.
15. Pun PH, Middleton JP. Dialysate potassium, dialysate magnesium, and hemodialysis risk. J Am Soc Nephrol. 2017;28:3441–51.
16. Spencer H, Kramer L, Rubio N, Osis D. The effect of phosphorus on endogenous fecal calcium excretion in man. Am J Clin Nutr. 1986;43:844–51.
17. Gotch F, Kotanko P, Handelman G, Levin N. A kinetic model of calcium mass balance during dialysis therapy. Blood Purif. 2007;25:139–49.
18. Karohl C, de Paiva PJ, de Castro MC, et al. Effects of bone remodelling on calcium mass transfer during haemodialysis. Nephrol Dial Transplant. 2010;25:1244–51.
19. Eloot S, Van Biesen W, Dhondt A, et al. Impact of hemodialysis duration on the removal of uremic retention solutes. Kidney Int. 2008;73:765–70.
20. Bhimani JP, Ouseph R, Ward RA. Effect of increasing dialysate flow rate on diffusive mass transfer of urea, phosphate and beta2-microglobulin during clinical haemodialysis. Nephrol Dial Transplant. 2010;25:3990–5.

Pediatric Applications of Home Hemodialysis

12

Iona Madden, Bradley A. Warady, and Daljit K. Hothi

Introduction

Chronic kidney disease (CKD) is a rare condition in children and adolescents. Kidney transplantation is well recognized to be the optimal treatment for the majority of children with end-stage kidney disease (ESKD) [1–3]. However, pre-emptive kidney transplantation is not possible for all children, and thus dialysis is frequently required either before transplantation or after a failed transplant. Whereas dialysis is considered a bridge to transplantation, it ideally is also an important component of a clinical strategy intended to successfully address the disadvantages and comorbidities associated with ESKD.

Children make up a unique ESKD population, differing from adults in several ways. Comorbidities that are often taken into account in adults such as diabetes, smoking, cerebrovascular disease, and gout are rarely relevant to children, while special attention is required regarding neurocognitive and behavioral disorders (developmental delay, seizure disorders), congenital anomalies (gastrointestinal disorders and need for colostomies), metabolic disorders, as well as education and family dynamics [4].

Pediatric home hemodialysis (HHD) is infrequently and inconsistently used as a kidney replacement therapy for children with ESKD, despite the availability of promising data describing the benefits of the therapy when compared with hospital-based hemodialysis (HD) [5–9]. There is increasing evidence, particularly in adults, of the benefits of intensified HD schedules in terms of both patient outcome and health-related quality of life; however, providing augmented schedules, especially

I. Madden · D. K. Hothi (✉)
Department of Pediatric Nephrology, Great Ormond Street Hospital, London, UK
e-mail: Iona.Madden@gosh.nhs.uk; daljit.hothi@gosh.nhs.uk

B. A. Warady
Children's Mercy Kansas City, Kansas City, MO, USA
e-mail: bwarady@cmh.edu

A. Shah et al. (eds.), *Applied Home Hemodialysis*,
https://doi.org/10.1007/978-3-031-77244-3_12

in children, remains a challenge [10–15]. It is, of course, recognized that the provision of an augmented schedule is often easiest in the home setting, which can be accompanied by a level of convenience and flexibility not achievable in-center. The literature on HHD and augmented home dialysis schedules therefore overlaps substantially. The successful application of HHD has resulted in recently published HD guidelines in the UK to include the recommendation that HHD should be available in all dialysis programs as part of a comprehensive kidney replacement therapy program. Most importantly, it was noted that HHD has many advantages for children, allowing an augmented schedule without institutionalization and providing dialysis management flexibility, which can reduce the negative impact that dialysis can have on social development [16].

This chapter dedicated to pediatric HHD outlines the epidemiology and the availability of HHD for children, the potential benefits and outcomes of pediatric HHD, the process of patient selection and training, as well as the infrastructure, economics, and technology necessary for a successful pediatric HHD program. Also discussed is the HHD prescription, HHD complications, and potential barriers to HHD implementation in children, in addition to unique pediatric aspects of dialysis, specifically the transition from pediatric to adult nephrology care.

Epidemiology

The incidence, prevalence, and treatment modality data pertaining to pediatric ESKD worldwide are only partially known because of differences in pediatric patient definitions, disease classification, and lack of national registries and health information systems, especially in low- and middle-income countries. Most of the epidemiological data on pediatric ESKD patients requiring kidney replacement therapy (dialysis or kidney transplantation) is derived from high-income countries due to the availability of robust national or international registries primarily in Europe, Australia, and New Zealand, and the United States. Based on this registry data, the incidence of ESKD in children varies widely across different countries but ranges from 5 to 15 cases per million children per year among patients under 20 years [17, 18]. The prevalence of ESKD in children (<21 years of age) is 20-fold less than in adults, while pediatric patients account for only 1% of the prevalent population receiving kidney replacement therapy [18–21]. In Europe and the United States, approximately 20–25% of children with ESKD receive a pre-emptive kidney transplant as their initial kidney replacement therapy [17, 18]. Children who do not receive pre-emptive kidney transplantation typically receive peritoneal dialysis (PD) or HD, but the percentage of children who initiate dialysis and use each of these modalities varies substantially depending on the patient's age, center expertise and resources, country, reimbursement system for ESKD care, and public policies (Fig. 12.1).

HHD is offered to a very small number of selected children by a few centers [5]. In turn, very limited data exists regarding the incidence and prevalence of HHD in children. The US Renal Data System (USRDS) 2021 Annual Data Report states that

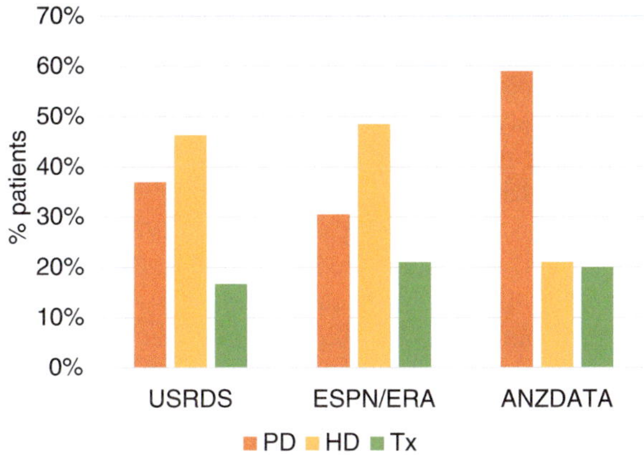

Fig. 12.1 Treatment modality at initiation of kidney replacement therapy in Europe, the United States, New Zealand and Australia in 2020–2021. Data was collected from the European Registry for Children on Renal Replacement Therapy (ESPN/ERA-EDTA Registry, annual report 2021 https://www.era-online.org/research-education/era-registry/annual-reports/), the United States Renal Data from 2021, published in the 2023 USRDS annual data report (https://www.usrds.org/) and the Australia and New Zealand Dialysis and Transplant (ANZDATA) Registry (https://www.anzdata.org.au/anzdata/). HD, haemodialysis; PD, peritoneal dialysis; Tx, transplantation

among all incident HHD patients in 2019, only 0.5% of patients were aged between 0 and 17 years [22]. In a survey conducted for this chapter aiming to provide information regarding the number of centers providing pediatric HHD worldwide, only 4 (all in Europe) out of the 21 centers who replied offer HHD. Two of these centers currently have between 6 and 10 patients on HHD; 1 center is currently providing HHD to 1–5 children, and the last center offers HHD but does not have any children on this modality currently.

Rationale, Potential Benefits and Outcomes

Case

An 8-year-old boy with a history of inflammatory bowel disease treated with tacrolimus presented to the renal team with a history of increasing edema, proteinuria, and hypoalbuminemia. Diagnosed with nephrotic syndrome, he was treated with a course of prednisolone but was found to be steroid resistant. A subsequent kidney biopsy confirmed a collapsing variant of focal segmental glomerulosclerosis (FSGS). Genetic screening was negative. Despite trials with a number of immunosuppressants and liposorber apheresis treatment, his kidney function deteriorated and he became increasingly hypertensive. As a result, he started 4 h of in-center HD, 3 times per week. Hypertension continued, triggering two episodes of Posterior Reversible Encephalopathy Syndrome (PRES) manifesting as tonic-clonic seizures. He then underwent bilateral nephrectomies in an attempt to correct the hypertension. Thereafter, he became increasingly hypotensive with volume overload necessitating additional weekly dialysis sessions and high UF rates. Eight months later, he experienced acute deterioration with pulmonary edema and worsening hypotension. An echocardiogram confirmed severe dilated cardiomyopathy. He was fluid restricted to 400 mL per day and his dialysis time was increased to 3–4 h, 5–6 times per week. Despite this treatment, his cardiac function continued to deteriorate, and he was referred to the HHD program.

Children on dialysis are at a heightened risk of mortality and life-threatening comorbidities [3, 23, 24] when compared to healthy children, and their lives and quality of life are often dictated by frequent clinic appointments, hospital admissions, invasive interventions, numerous medications, infections and lifestyle restrictions. They frequently experience pain, sleep difficulties, changes in their appearance, growth restrictions, and fatigue, all of which can be debilitating in day-to-day life. Many of these symptoms may in fact be improved by HHD (Fig. 12.2). Whereas the available literature on the benefits of HHD in children is limited and mainly based on single-center experiences in cohorts of fewer than ten patients (Table 12.1), the pediatric experience seems to reflect similar benefits to those described in adults [5–7, 27, 28].

Impact on Cardiovascular Disease (CVD)

Cardiovascular disease (CVD) is the leading cause of death in children with CKD. According to the USRDS 2021 Annual Data Report, CVD accounted for 28% and 33.5% of deaths in children (0–17 years) on HD and peritoneal dialysis, respectively, in 2010–2019 [22]. While conventional thrice-weekly HD provides adequate dialysis to prevent mortality, CVD-related morbidity is prevalent in the pediatric

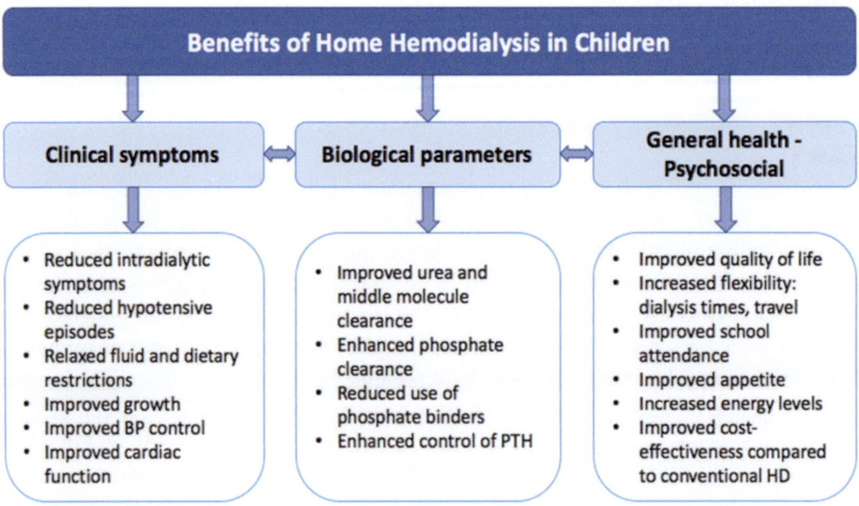

Fig. 12.2 Potential benefits of HHD in children. HD, hemodialysis

Table 12.1 Summary of studies on intensified HD in children

Author	Number of patients (*n*)	Age (years)	Intensified dialysis modality	Results
Geary et al. [6]	2	12–16	Conventional HD or PD to nocturnal HHD	– Discontinuation of phosphate binders – No fluid and dietary restrictions – Improved appetite – Improved school attendance – Improved physical and psychological HRQoL scores
Hothi et al. [47]	4	12–16	Nocturnal HHD	– Discontinuation of phosphate binders – No dietary restrictions – Reductions in intact PTH levels – Net positive calcium balance
Fischbach et al. [46, 48]	12	2–16	In-center daily online hemodiafiltration in 3-h sessions, 5–6 times per week	– No dietary restrictions – Reduced amount of medications: antihypertensive drugs, potassium and phosphate binders – Improved growth
Goldstein et al. [7]	4	Weight range 38–61.4 kg	Conventional in-center program to home HD for 2–3 h, 6 times per week	– Improved blood pressure control – Fewer medications – Improvement in serum phosphate without change in dose of phosphate binders – Improved parent-reported HRQoL scores
Müller et al. [25]	1	16	Nocturnal in-center HD	– Fewer medications – Improved well-being

(continued)

Table 12.1 (continued)

Author	Number of patients (*n*)	Age (years)	Intensified dialysis modality	Results
Hoppe et al. [43]	16	0.5–17	Nocturnal in-center HD	– Decreased serum phosphate and PTH levels – Improved urea clearance – Improved blood pressure control – Reduced amount of medications: antihypertensive drugs, potassium and phosphate binders – Improved hemoglobin levels – No dietary and fluid restrictions – Improved appetite – Improved general and psychosocial well-being – Improved school attendance
de Camargo et al. [26]	24	0.25–16	Daily HHD with 90–120 min sessions, 6 days per week	– Improved growth – Improved appetite
Melhem et al. [34]	1	13	Daily HHD with 5-h sessions, 5 times a week Then nocturnal HHD	– Improved exercise tolerance – Improved appetite and energy levels – Improved school attendance – No dietary restrictions and reduced fluid restriction – Improved urea clearance – Improved blood pressure control – Normalization of biventricular function and reduction in left ventricular volumes

(continued)

Table 12.1 (continued)

Author	Number of patients (*n*)	Age (years)	Intensified dialysis modality	Results
Thumfart et al. [28]	7	13.4–16.3	Conventional HD to intermittent nocturnal HD and intermittent nocturnal online HD (NHD) for 3 months, then Hemodiafiltration (HDF) for 3 months, and then changed back to NHD for 3 months (each 8 h, 3 times per week)	– Increased urea clearance – Improved blood pressure control – Reduced PTH and serum phosphate levels – No dietary restrictions – Decreased intradialytic hypotensive episodes
Laskin et al. [71]	6	15.9–18	Prospective, open-label, randomized, cross-over pilot trial over two successive 12-week (3-month) study periods: either conventional HD treatment 3 days per week for 4 h, then in-center HD 5 days per week For 2 h 25 min	– Improved blood pressure control
Hothi and Fenton [33]	3	0.6–13	Daily and nocturnal HHD	– Normalization of cardiac function in patients with a history of moderate-to-severe cardiac failure – Fewer medications

HD hemodialysis, *HHD* home hemodialysis, *HRQoL* health-related quality of life, *PD* peritoneal dialysis

population [29, 30]. Conventional HD sessions are often complicated by inadequate fluid control between sessions, intradialytic hypotensive episodes, and myocardial ischemia associated with aggressive fluid removal, along with poor control of serum phosphorus, all of which contribute to an increased risk of CVD. Moreover, a non-negligible proportion of children on dialysis present with other cardiac comorbidities, often in the context of congenital, genetic, and metabolic disorders.

With a goal of decreasing the prevalence of CVD, risk factors in dialysis patients such as hypertension, dyslipidemia, abnormal mineral metabolism, inflammation, anemia, vascular calcification, and metabolic syndrome should be identified and treated, and the use of HHD has proven to be a beneficial therapeutic strategy.

Left ventricular hypertrophy (LVH) and left ventricular dysfunction are both well-described independent predictors of cardiovascular morbidity and mortality in adults on dialysis that likely influence the outcome of children on dialysis as well [31]. Most importantly, hypertension and fluid overload are modifiable risk factors for LVH. However, LVH reversal is difficult to achieve in children on conventional

HD and PD due to poor volume and BP control [32]. In contrast, HHD has resulted in improved BP control and relaxed fluid restrictions in children [5–7, 33]. Promisingly, several small, single-center studies in pediatric patients on intensified dialysis regimens have shown a reduced percentage of patients with an elevated LV mass index and LVH. Two studies have even provided evidence of cardiac recovery in a small number of children on HHD with a history of severe cardiac failure [33, 34]. The reasons for the improved outcomes are speculative and multiple and include the capacity to increase the frequency and duration of dialysis with HHD, both of which result in superior purification of the uremic milieu and allowance for a lower ultrafiltration (UF) rate and a decreased risk for intradialytic hypotension. Movilli et al. previously demonstrated a critical safe point, with better patient survival associated with HD UF rates of less than 12.37 mL/kg/h [35]. In a recent study, adult HD patients who did not experience frequent episodes of UF rates above 13 mL/kg/h during the first 3 months of their dialysis tenure had a significantly lower risk of death compared to patients with frequent HD sessions associated with higher UF rates [36]. In pediatric HHD patients, UF rates have been able to be effectively lowered, individually set at rates associated with symptom-free treatments and minimal intradialytic BP and heart rate changes, thus attenuating the risk of repeated myocardial stunning [37, 38]. Thumfart et al. reported only one intradialytic hypotensive episode in their 7 pediatric patients undergoing nocturnal HD and nocturnal hemodiafiltration, as compared to 13 episodes in patients on conventional HD [28].

Transitioning patients home on HD has also created the potential for a more consistent approach to the dialysis treatments directed by a single provider, the nephrologist, in contrast to a number of different expert voices that may direct management within a single dialysis program. This has permitted the determination of clinical patterns that have regularly emerged in children who receive HHD and a structured analysis of what does and does not work well. Cardio-protective interventions have subsequently been integrated within the pediatric HHD prescription, such as the use of higher calcium dialysate solutions and not allowing more than a 24 h interval between dialysis sessions. Improved nutrition, thanks to relaxed dietary restrictions, has also probably contributed to cardiac recovery in some patients [39].

Impact on CKD Mineral and Bone Disorder

Optimal control of phosphate, calcium, and Parathyroid hormone (PTH) is particularly relevant for children because of the influence of metabolic control on bone integrity and statural growth and the prevention of skeletal abnormalities and vascular calcification. Unfortunately, complications of mineral bone disease are common and contribute to the high morbidity and mortality in children on dialysis [30, 40]. Management in dialysis patients includes dietary adjustments (calcium and phosphate intake), use of phosphate binders, calcium, vitamin D, calcitriol, and calcimimetic supplementation, accompanied by modifications of the dialysis prescription. Existing studies demonstrate that dialysis time is the most significant determinant of phosphate clearance [41, 42]. In turn, there is good evidence that, compared with conventional HD, children prescribed all forms of intensified dialysis, including HHD, have a reduced need for dietary phosphate restriction and the use of phosphate binders [5–7, 28, 43]. Close monitoring of trends in serum calcium (or ideally ionized calcium, if available), phosphate, PTH, alkaline phosphatase, and 25-vitamin D levels is necessary, as some patients on HHD may require phosphate and calcium supplementations or dialysate adjustments [40]. Calcium and phosphate levels should be within the normal range according to the patient's age, and vitamin D and PTH levels should be targeted in accordance with published guidelines [40].

Impact on Growth

Growth failure is a major complication of CKD in children and is a marker of disease severity. Approximately 40% of children with ESKD have a reduced final height (below the third percentile) compared with that of healthy age-matched and sex-matched controls [44, 45]. Growth failure is associated with poor health and social outcomes, including reduced quality of life, poorer graft function, an increased number of hospital admissions, and an increased mortality risk [45]. Given the strong association between growth, clinical outcomes, and quality of life in children receiving dialysis, adequate growth becomes a marker of "optimal dialysis." The 2011 annual dialysis report from the North American Pediatric Renal Trials and Collaborative Studies (NAPRTCS) registry showed that children on conventional HD had worse height deficits compared with children who received PD, highlighting the importance of finding solutions for better growth for children receiving HD. Several small studies have provided promising data regarding intensified dialysis and improved growth. Fischbach et al. reported remarkable catch-up growth in several oligo-anuric patients who received daily online hemodiafiltration [46, 47]. The reasons for improved growth of HHD are most likely multifactorial: a free diet with a better appetite leading to reduced rates of malnutrition, improved response to growth hormone treatment, and less uremic protein wasting likely all contribute [45, 46, 48].

Impact on General Health and Quality of Life

Dialysis has an immense impact on the quality of life of the child and their caregivers as a result of invasive interventions, appointments, hospitalizations, infections, complex treatment regimens, lifestyle restrictions, poor school attendance, pain, fatigue, sleep problems, growth restrictions, and changes in appearance. Tjaden et al. conducted a systematic review of qualitative studies exploring the experiences of children on dialysis. Five major themes were identified: (1) loss of control (high reliance on caregivers, parental overprotectiveness, unrelenting dependence on a machine, impaired body integrity), (2) restricted life (limited socialization opportunities, struggle to perform academically), (3) managing treatment (ownership, proactive involvement, adherence to fluid and diet restrictions), (4) feeling different (abnormal physical appearance, injustice, being a burden), and (5) coping strategies (hope for a kidney transplant and medical advances, social support, positive determination and self-awareness, engaging in activities, denial) [49]. In addition, adults diagnosed with CKD during childhood have worse educational, vocational, and social outcomes than the general population [50].

Consequently, life participation and quality of life are considered core outcomes for children with CKD, especially for children receiving dialysis. The Standardized Outcomes in Nephrology—Children and Adolescents (SONG-Kids) initiative included life participation as one of their high-priority goals for future studies of children with CKD and highlighted the importance of capturing the quality of life of the child and entire family in these studies [51].

A number of randomized clinical trials/meta-analysis/large prospective studies in adults have shown a significant improvement of both physical and mental health-related quality of life in patients on HHD relative to conventional HD, with reduced rates of clinical depression, better sleep quality, shorter recovery time, improved social lives, and more flexibility [52–56]. However, there is limited pediatric data on the subject. Goldstein et al. noted improvement in parent-reported physical, emotional, and psychological health-related quality of life scores in children undergoing HHD [7]. Geary et al. described improved school attendance in three of four adolescent patients who switched to a nocturnal hemodialysis (NHD) program, with better school performance and improved energy levels [6]. In a survey of 15 patients receiving HHD conducted prior to the writing of this chapter, 75% of respondents rated their quality of life on HHD as "good" or "very good." In the same survey, all patients who had received in-center HD and HHD reported that their overall quality of life on HHD was "better" or "much better" and that their social lives, school attendance, and treatment flexibility were "much better." None of the patients who had received treatment with several dialysis modalities replied that their quality of life, social lives, school attendance, treatment flexibility, or body appearance were "worse" or "much worse" on HHD compared with either PD or in-center HD.

Outcomes of HHD Versus Other Dialysis Modalities

In a systematic review of adults conducted to compare survival, hospitalization, CVD, nutrition, and quality of life in patients who had received HHD compared to in-center HD, 66% of the publications reviewed demonstrated improved clinical outcomes in patients who chose HHD. HHD was associated with appreciably better survival and lower risks of mortality and treatment failure compared to PD in adults [14, 57, 58]. Thus, even though HHD may not be the preferred dialysis modality for all patients, this review of the literature suggested that HHD should ideally be provided as a modality choice for substantially more than the small proportion of patients that currently benefit from it [59].

Unfortunately, no studies comparing patient survival between HHD, PD, or in-center HHD have been conducted in children. This may in part relate to the fact that mortality is not the most meaningful outcome in pediatrics, and pediatric studies would likely be open to criticism resulting from small patient numbers, bias pertaining to patient selection, and numerous confounders. In pediatrics, outcome studies in which dialysis modalities are being compared should instead emphasize outcomes such as symptom control and quality of life. Of course, any presumed advantages of HHD in children require validation in large cohorts of patients such as NAPRTCS or the International Pediatric Dialysis Network (IPDN) if HHD and intensified dialysis programs are to achieve more wide-spread acceptance and application.

Patient Selection and Training

Patient Criteria

The decision to pursue HHD can be triggered by medical, social, and school-related issues, or simply by families exercising their right to choose the dialysis modality for their child, dependent on the maturity and confidence of the service. In consideration of safety, efficacy, and equity in the selection process, the establishment of possible clinical indications for HHD is recommended (Table 12.2).

In the initial stages of setting up an HHD program, it is also advisable to set relatively conservative patient selection criteria that take into consideration a number of factors that include the team's availability and expertise; the infrastructure constraints, available technology, and out-of-hours support; and the local patient demographics and requirements for dialysis therapy. Patient safety should be at the heart of any patient-specific decision that is made, with the perspectives of a multidisciplinary team that includes the patient and family as important components of the decision process. In all cases, the following issues need to be addressed as part of the evaluation of a potential pediatric HHD candidate:

- In order to undertake HHD, an established, well-functioning dialysis access is necessary. The dialysis system and the size of the extracorporeal volume will determine the minimal weight cut-off for patients to be accepted into the HHD program. In certain centers, children weighing as little as 10 kg receive HHD safely and successfully.

Table 12.2 Clinical indications for HHD in children

Patient preference and motivation
Remote residence
Difficult to control hypertension
Patients with cardiac failure
Frequent intradialytic symptoms on conventional HD
Prolonged recovery time
Inadequate urea clearance
Refractory fluid overload
Hyperoxaluria
Chemotherapy

- The medical history is one of the principal considerations and must provide evidence of the overall clinical stability of the patient during in-center HD.
- Suitable housing with sufficient room to accommodate dialysis equipment and consumables is essential. In addition, it is important that families do not live in areas with frequent and prolonged electricity supply disruptions or where an emergency source of power is not available at all times. For some dialysis systems, a reverse osmosis system is required, and thus specific conversations regarding home equipment availability and function are a pre-requisite.
- Social considerations, particularly a family's household hygiene, are an important factor for minimizing the patient's risk of infection with HHD. The capacity to pay water and electricity bills as a direct consequence of patients dialyzing at home should be discussed in advance, and where possible, options for reimbursements should be sought if not currently available and required.
- HHD is burdensome for the patient and those undertaking dialysis at home. It requires a relentless commitment, it demands family time, and it can provoke anxiety and be mentally challenging. In view of the family burden, it is important to assess the caregiver's mental health history and ensure that they have access to adequate support within the family and community.

It is also most important to recognize that failed home PD does not necessarily preclude the possibility of HHD. The reasons for the prior failed experience should, of course, be investigated and taken into consideration if HHD is to be considered. Likewise, for those patients and families that lack immediate confidence to transition home, investing in a slower training process that incrementally supports patients and/or their caregivers from a point of delivering minimal medical care at home to delivering the dialysis treatment in a totally independent manner can be extremely effective.

Training

A robust training program is key to a safe, high-quality pediatric HHD program. The specific design can vary from patient to patient and from unit to unit, but to ensure a high recruitment-to-retention ratio, it is essential to set clear expectations on the likely time commitment and the minimum number of caregivers to be trained. Ideally, it is advisable to train two people from the outset and encourage the young "patient" to learn about the machine set-up, access care, and dialysis prescription. All families should be offered repeated opportunities to enhance their knowledge and skills once they are conducting HHD, and it is specifically recommended following an adverse event, switching from daytime to nocturnal treatments, or changes in dialysis access, such as switching from a central line to a fistula.

When possible, at least part of the training should take place outside the HD unit and within a separate training facility to encourage those training to "step-down" from being medically supported to undertake dialysis independently, in a simulated home environment. The final sign-off should be completed when the caregiver has successfully completed their first dialysis session at home.

Companies supplying dialysis equipment will often provide considerable teaching materials and expertise, but for the vast majority, this needs to be adapted for the pediatric population by the center conducting the training. To ensure that caregivers have completely understood the content, the trainee's competency should be formally assessed and signed off both by the trainee and trainer. Finally, prior to discharge home, an adherence contract signed by the patient and their caregivers can be an extremely important step for reinforcing the shared responsibility of the medical team and family to uphold the safety and quality of the home dialysis treatment.

Infrastructure, Technology, and Economics

Infrastructure

The establishment of a pediatric HHD program requires careful planning with patient safety and risk management working closely with nephrology. The service delivery model may vary between units but is largely influenced by:

- The availability and requirement for partnership with neighboring pediatric or adult HHD services to assist with the delivery of the service, especially in smaller programs that do not have access to dedicated HHD staff.
- The intended spectrum of dialysis regimens that will be offered to patients: daytime/nocturnal, daily/frequent.
- The degree to which home modifications will be required or are feasible, which in turn influences the dialysis system that is selected.

Building an expert, multidisciplinary clinical team is key to the success of any program. At a minimum, the team must consist of a dedicated HD nurse, nephrologist, dietician, dialysis technician, pharmacist, and social worker. In addition, partnering with other allied health professionals, such as a psychologist, community nurses, and, on occasion, local pediatricians and general practitioners, can help meet a variety of patient and family needs.

The other essential component of an HHD program is a commitment to establish a robust remote monitoring and support structure to ensure that families feel safe and connected to expert help and advice whenever they require it. Families need to be clear on how to access medical and technical support when they are setting up and preparing for their dialysis session or during the time when dialysis is being conducted at home. Clarity is further enhanced with written guidelines which include normal ranges for dialysis and physiological parameters and clear instructions on how and when to seek help if the dialyzed child's parameters fall outside the normal range. Although remote monitoring is not universally employed or even recommended, its availability can help relieve many family anxieties. In addition to providing reassurance, remote monitoring through telehealth technology also creates opportunities for the HHD medical team to intervene earlier and make adjustments to treatments outside the hospital clinic reviews. Additional technical modifications are now also available to enhance the families' ability to detect blood and dialysate leaks from disconnections within the circuit.

Technology

There are a number of commercially available HD machines that are suitable for HHD; however, only a fraction of these are licensed for use in pediatric patients. The key differences between the machines are their physical size, the circuit and dialyzer sizes, and the way that dialysate is prepared and delivered.

Conventional, pediatric compatible HD machines such as the Fresenius 5008™ that require water treatment systems to generate large volumes of high-quality dialysate can be used for HHD. In this case, home water conversions are necessary which requires the installation of a cold-water outlet and a drain to allow the carbon filter, reverse osmosis unit, and dialysis machine to be fitted. The cost of this conversion can sometimes become a barrier to the transition of a child to HHD, especially when it is being used as a bridging therapy to transplant. In addition, when HHD is being used, families are required to test their water for chloride prior to every session and to bring in a sample of their dialysate fluid to the hospital monthly to be tested for the presence of chemicals, endotoxins, and bacteria. This can sometimes be seen as a burden and a source of anxiety for families.

Low-flow systems such as the NxStage System One™ are portable home dialysis machine that functions without home water modifications and can also be used for HHD in children. Dialysate is prepared in batches of up to 60 L using the NxStage PureFlow SL™ integrated water purification and dialysate production system from ordinary tap water mixed with sterile-filtered concentrate to produce lactate-buffered dialysate. Premixed bagged dialysate is also available for home patients in sterile, 5 L bags with a variety of fluid configurations. The NxStage System One™ is the only low-flow system to date with circuits that are suitable and licensed for pediatric use. CAR-172-C is the standard circuit with a pre-attached polysulfone dialyzer and an extracorporeal circuit volume of 163 mL (Table 12.3). The CAR-124-C and CAR-125B are modified continuous veno-venous hemofiltration circuits that can house any appropriately sized dialyzer with extracorporeal circuit volumes of 97 and 55 mL, respectively (minus the dialyzer) (Table 12.3).

Table 12.3 NxStage Cartridge options

Cartridges	CAR-125-B Infant	CAR-124-C Pediatric/acute	CAR-172-C Adult
Line volume	55 mL	97 mL	72 mL
Pre-attached dialyser	No pre-attached	No pre-attached	91 mL
Total volume			163
Patient weight for cartridge choice	10–20 kg	20–30 kg	≥30 kg

Economics

The financial case for a pediatric HHD program differs from an adult program. In adult units, the HD patient pool can consist of several hundred patients, whereas in comparison, the pediatric cohort rarely exceeds 25 patients. In adult HHD programs, even with a conservative recruitment rate of 5% of the total HD cohort, that fairly large number of patients will accrue a financial saving from transitioning home, making it much easier to offset the financial investment to establish and maintain the HHD program. Within pediatrics, the cost analysis of an individual HD treatment delivered at home compared with conventional in-center treatment can result in savings of up to 27% [6], largely as a result of decreasing the center's staff requirement to deliver HD treatments in the hospital. However, based on the relatively small number of pediatric patients that are cared for in an in-center HD program, proportionately a higher recruitment rate is required to offset the cost of establishing and sustaining a HHD program. Thus, pediatric HHD programs carry a significantly higher financial risk and may sometimes even experience a net financial loss. In some cases, having a pediatric program as part of a larger adult HHD program, with the provision of appropriate pediatric training, can reduce the financial risk.

Dialysis Access and Prescription

Case Continued

Our young patient was commenced on 5 h of dialysis, 5 times/week, with no longer than a 24-h interval between dialysis sessions; the maximum UF rate was 0.18 L/h at a dry weight of 31 kg. Over the next few months, his exercise tolerance progressively rose, his appetite improved, his energy levels increased, and his seizure frequency significantly dropped.

After 7 months on HHD, he switched to a nocturnal program of 10 h, 5 times per week, and he slowly returned to school with a cautious rehabilitation program of increasing exercise.

Vascular Access

Among all children receiving HD, a central venous catheter (CVC) is the predominant initial vascular access choice. The International Pediatric HD Network (IPHN) reported the use of an arteriovenous fistula (AVF) in 26% of children initiating HD; this rate was higher in an ESPN/ERA-EDTA study (45%) and much lower (<15%) in a recent USRDS report [18, 60, 61]. An AVF has been associated with better dialysis efficacy, fewer medical complications, less vascular access procedures, and lower costs than a CVC access [60, 61]. It is therefore recommended that when surgical expertise is available, many children starting HD should have an AVF created at least 3 months before anticipated use [62]. However, in some circumstances such as in infants and young children depending on patient size and surgical expertise, those requiring unplanned HD, those with an anticipated short period of dialysis (e.g., <1 year) before (living donor) kidney transplantation, or patient choice, a cuffed CVC is preferentially used [62]. The choice of access thus requires individualization for each patient, and a dedicated vascular access clinic may optimize the timing and quality of the vascular access [62–64]. There is very little data available describing vascular access practices specific to children receiving HHD.

Vascular access training is an essential step when preparing caregivers and patients for HHD and often requires repeated attention, particularly when there is a change in access modality, for example, from CVC to AVF. Vascular access training by highly specialized clinical staff should include correct cannulation methods, proper needle insertion (rope ladder or buttonhole technique for AVF cannulation), care of catheter insertion sites, maintenance of a sterile environment, and identification of signs and symptoms of infection [62, 65]. Low-flow dialysis systems use a double needle/line and a single pump. Therefore, patients require a double lumen CVC or the insertion of two fistula needles.

Dialysis Prescription

One of the main benefits of HHD for families is an increased flexibility to perform HD treatments around their own schedule. As such, a generic "one size fits all" prescription is not appropriate. Each HHD prescription should be tailored to meet the individual patient's needs [27]. It is, in turn, important to assess and define the patient and caregiver's treatment priorities while undertaking HHD. Each dialysis prescription aims to provide "optimal dialysis" rather than just pursuing dialysis adequacy, taking into consideration both the patient's short- and long-term needs (solute balance, symptom control, BP and volume control, growth, nutrition, cardiovascular risk, bone metabolism, education, and quality of life).

HHD prescriptions are modified by changing dialysis duration, frequency, or both (Table 12.4):

- Frequent daily dialysis: 2–3 h of dialysis 6–7 days a week. This regime can be useful for working parents and younger patients who do not tolerate longer sessions and require closer parental monitoring during the session. However, this prescription may not allow freedom from phosphate binders, and due to the high-frequency prescription, this is also the most expensive option.
- Alternate-day prolonged dialysis: 5–6 h of dialysis three to four times a week. The need for phosphate binders and dietary/fluid restrictions is lowered but still remains with this prescription. Dialysis on alternate days can also reduce the burden of HHD by providing a degree of respite.
- Nocturnal dialysis: 8–10 h of dialysis overnight, either daily or on alternate nights. Nocturnal HHD is a gentler, extended HD treatment that takes place at night while the child is asleep and is associated with fewer intradialytic symptoms. Typically, lower dialysis blood flow rates can be utilized, between 100 and

Table 12.4 Pediatric HHD prescriptions compared with conventional HD

Program	Number of sessions per week	Duration (h)	Blood flow rate	Dialysate flow rate	Advantages	Disadvantages
Conventional HD	3–4	3–5	90–200 mL/m^2/min Starting at 90 mL/m^2/min and <100 mL/min for the first sessions	300–800 mL/min	– Most wide-spread and standardized HD modality	– Impact on QoL – Institutionalization – Poor BP and volume control – Inadequate urea clearance – Poor growth
Daily HHD	6–7	2–3	Similar to conventional HD	Similar to conventional HD	– Helpful for working/busy caregivers with a limited window for dialyzing – Best for young children who cannot tolerate long sessions – Children unable to tolerate aggressive UF – Children who are poorly adherent to fluid restrictions – Better phosphate removal than conventional HD	– Rarely allows discontinuation of phosphate binders – Expensive due to higher dialysis consumables cost – Poor social rehabilitaion
Alternate-day prolonged HHD	3–4	5–6	100–200 mL/min starting at 6-8 mL/kg/min	200–300 mL/min	– Reduced fluid and dietary restrictions – Patient and caregiver respite due to days without dialysis	– Seldom allows discontinuation of phosphate binders

(continued)

Table 12.4 (continued)

Program	Number of sessions per week	Duration (h)	Blood flow rate	Dialysate flow rate	Advantages	Disadvantages
Nocturnal HHD	4–7	7–12	100–200 mL/min starting at 6–8 mL/kg/min	200–300 mL/min	– Greatly reduced or elimination of intradialytic symptoms – Often requires no dietary or fluid restrictions – Reduced medications – Excellent removal of phosphate – Excellent volume control – Improved social life	– Anxiety in caregivers and children from fear of disconnection or not hearing machine alarms – Hypophosphatemia – Hypokalemia – Negative calcium balance if 1.5 mmol/L dialysate calcium

HD hemodialysis, *HHD* home hemodialysis, *QoL* quality of life

200 mL/min (starting at 6–8 mL/kg/min) with proportionately lower dialysate flow rates between 200 and 300 mL/min, maintaining a 2:1 dialysate:blood flow ratio. The greater the number of hours dialyzed per week, the gentler the dialysis treatment, with proportionately reduced dialysis symptoms and improved solute and fluid control. Uremic toxins, particularly phosphate and other middle-sized molecules, are more effectively removed compared to conventional HD due to the extended sessions. However, this is a non-selective process, and other essential plasma components are removed as well and can lead to deficiencies that need to be screened for and treated. For nocturnal HHD and to avoid a negative calcium balance, a higher dialysate calcium concentration of 1.75 mmol/L is recommended [5, 27]. Hypophosphatemia is common and can be treated by providing oral supplements or by adding phosphate to the dialysate. This schedule most often allows the patient to stop phosphate binders and dietary restrictions as well as reduce fluid restrictions, thus alleviating to a certain degree the burden of CKD and dialysis.

Use of a low-flow system such as the NxStage System One™ requires specific considerations:

- NxStage™ cartridge selection is largely influenced by the patient's weight.
- Flow fraction is the fixed ratio between the blood flow rate and the dialysis flow rate. The lower the flow fraction, the more saturated the dialysate fluid becomes. Typically, a flow fraction between 30% and 40% is adequate for clearance. This can be reduced to 25% in patients with nocturnal HHD.

Anticoagulation

Unfractionated heparin with a target-activated clotting time of 150–180 s is often used in adults. Recently, dalteparin has also been demonstrated to be a safe and effective alternative anticoagulant when used for pediatric HHD with minimal adverse effects and no evidence of bioaccumulation. The initial dose for dalteparin is 50 UI/kg intravenously as a single bolus at the start of the HHD session. Factor Xa levels should be monitored and not exceed 0.4 at the end of the session [66].

Dialysis Adequacy or Optimal Dialysis

The term "dialysis adequacy" is traditionally based on the measurement of small solute clearance using urea and creatinine and has been associated with survival in several but not all adult studies [67–69]. However, small molecule clearance should be considered as just one metric characterizing dialysis efficacy for children. Outcome parameters to target in an attempt to achieve optimal dialysis in children include the following:

- Urea clearance using urea kinetic modeling. Data specific to the pediatric population are scarce, but it is generally accepted that the recommended delivered dose for adults should be a minimum target for children (Kt/V for a single session ≥0.7 and weekly or standardized Kt/V 2.2) [16, 70]. Metabolic needs in children likely mandate higher clearance requirements [70].
- Fluid and blood pressure control.
- Normal cardiac geometry and function.
- Control of mineral and bone disorders.
- Achievement of target hemoglobin levels.
- Maintenance of residual kidney function.
- Good growth (e.g., normal height velocity) and nutritional status.
- Normal health-related quality of life.
- Psychosocial stability.
- Normal cognitive and developmental assessments.

Complications

Despite the many potential benefits of HHD compared with in-center HD, patient, machine, and/or treatment-related issues remain a concern for healthcare providers, patients, and their caregivers (Table 12.5). Difficulties in troubleshooting the dialysis procedure due to a lack of professional supervision may result in patient- and machine-related complications, highlighting the need for comprehensive training by a specialized multidisciplinary team. The data pertaining to HHD complications in adults is likely to be relevant and applicable to pediatric HHD, but additional issues and complications unique to pediatrics also need to be considered.

Geary et al. described their experience with nocturnal HHD in four children, and very few technical issues were reported. The frequency of these episodes was comparable to the general HD population. Metabolic deficiencies were described, prompting all patients to receive phosphate and calcium supplements in their dialysate, and no fractures or other bone complications were reported. Carnitine deficiency requiring supplementation was also documented in all patients [6]. Hothi et al. described a similar experience in children on nocturnal HD who experienced a rapid lowering of plasma phosphate and PTH levels and concluded that additional dialysate phosphate and possibly calcium may be necessary to prevent bone demineralization due to chronic losses and to prevent over suppression of PTH [47].

The pediatric cross-over study by Laskin et al. showed no statistically significant differences in the number of children that reported adverse effects (access dysfunction, need for a blood transfusion, and clotting of the dialysis circuit) during frequent (five times per week) in-center HD versus thrice-weekly HD treatment periods [71].

Table 12.5 HHD issues and potential solutions

Complications			Solutions
Patient-related	Vascular access	Dysfunction	Vascular checklists
		Thrombosis	Dedicated vascular clinics
		Stenosis	Appropriate access alarm ranges
		Infections	Favor AVF over CVC Correct cannulation methods Strict hygiene at home
		Hemorrhage	Wetness-sensor devices and appropriate alarm ranges
	Nutritional/electrolytes	Hypokalemia	Appropriate dialysate concentration according to potassium monitoring
		Calcium and phosphate deficiency	1.75 mmol/L dialysate calcium for NHD Phosphate supplementation
		Vitamin and carnitine deficiency	Vitamin and carnitine supplementation
	Loss of residual kidney function		
	Psychological	Patient concerns: anxiety, depression Caregiver concerns: anxiety, depression, disturbance to other family members, increased work burden, financial losses Technique failure	Assisted HHD Back-up services Psychological, social, and financial support Respite care Training two or more caregivers Promotion of self-efficacy Assessment and treatment of mood disorders (patients and caregivers)
	Anticoagulation	Undercoagulation: circuit clotting Overcoagulation: bleeding Heparin-induced thrombocytopenia	Development of dialysis platforms that allow for automated saline flushes/boluses which may obviate the need for circuit anticoagulation
Machine-related and procedural	Machine malfunction	Alarm malfunction Pump malfunction Sensor malfunction Power failure	Telehealth technology Regular machine maintenance and auditing After-hours nursing and technologist support Reliable power supply
	UF error	Hypervolemia/hypertension Hypovolemia/hypotension	Appropriate alarm ranges Patient and caregiver training regarding the consequences of UF error Development of machines and strategies adapted for children
	Blood loss	Needle dislodgement CVC disconnection Improper clamp placement	Wetness-sensor devices Patient and caregiver training and promotion of self-efficacy Clear safety messages: "clamp and call"
	Air embolism	Incorrect clamping procedure	Interlink closed connector devices
	Set-up error	Incorrect threading of the tubing to the dialyzer Incorrect priming procedure Incorrect rinse-back procedure	Sufficient staff and patient training Development of a "no blame" culture to encourage adverse event reporting Automated priming and/or rinse-back

AVF arteriovenous fistula, *CVC* central venous catheter, *HHD* home hemodialysis, *NHD* nocturnal hemodialysis, *UF* ultrafiltration

Potential Barriers

In 2017, an online survey was sent to all 221 pediatric dialysis centers which participate in the IPDN to explore the barriers to implementing intensified HD, including HHD. Half of the respondents thought that daily nocturnal dialysis was associated with the best overall patient outcomes. However, only a third stated that their center provided intensified HD, most commonly in the form of short daily HD sessions. The most important barriers to the expansion of intensified HD programs were lack of adequate funding (66%) and shortage of staff (63%), whereas lack of expertise and motivation were reported infrequently as obstacles (21% and 14%, respectively) [9].

As described earlier in the chapter, the availability of HHD is very low in adults and even lower in children. Tong et al. conducted interviews with adult patients receiving in-center HD regarding HHD, many of whom expressed concerns about the potential burden and personal sacrifice HHD would impose on caregivers; in turn, they felt apprehensive about accepting the medical responsibilities of dialysis [72]. Similarly, despite an overall positive experience with children on HHD, the burden of care for the families should not be underestimated. The provision of comprehensive information about HHD to patients and their caregivers and a robust support structure for families, such as access to caregiver respite, the continuous availability of medical and technical advice, and opportunities for peer support, are essential for the implementation of a successful HHD program for children [6, 8, 72, 73].

Transitioning to Adult Care

At some stage, young adults will need to transfer their care from pediatric to adult dialysis units. This can be a particularly stressful time for the young person and their family and if managed poorly can result in adverse clinical outcomes and a failure to establish a strong foundation and trust with key clinical staff within the adult unit. In recognition of the importance of this aspect of patient management, the global pediatric community, and especially those providers who care for children with chronic medical disorders, recommend a transition and transfer process which involves both the pediatric and adult programs and which educates and supports the young person as they increasingly take responsibility for their health [74, 75].

HHD offers many opportunities to proactively engage children and "emerging adults" with their dialysis treatments and kidney care as part of the transition education they require. The education and training program for HHD can become a catalyst to engage the pediatric patient so that they understand their underlying kidney disorder and their dialysis management. Therefore, in this respect, HHD provides an opportunity to encourage the patient to be more competent and confident in advocating for themselves, in a manner that might not occur for the patient who receives in-center HD.

The second essential component of the transition process is securing access to a suitable adult service. This can be a challenge for the pediatric patient who receives

HHD, as it may be difficult to find an adult unit close to home that has an active HHD program and that allows patients to use the same dialysis technology that they have become familiar with. As a result, many young people are compelled to compromise, transitioning to an adult HHD program further away from their home or re-training on a different dialysis system should they wish to remain closer to home. These issues should be addressed during the transition process, well in advance of the actual transfer to adult care.

Case Continued

Eight months after starting HHD, our patient was admitted to the hospital with a chest infection and mild pulmonary edema. His dialysis time was increased to 8 h, 7 times per week, nocturnally; his dialysate potassium was increased to 2 mmol/L and calcium to 1.75 mmol/L; his UF rate was minimized further, the rate determined by his pre-dialysis BP and not his weight, and adjusted to reduce intradialytic BP and heart rate changes. Over the next 12 months, his symptoms resolved, his cardiac function normalized, and he has remained clinically well despite stopping all previous cardiac-related treatments (digoxin, enalapril, and spironolactone).

Conclusion

HHD is a safe and effective dialysis modality for children with ESKD and can be particularly effective and beneficial in patients for whom the provision of PD or conventional HD is associated with less than optimal medical, nutritional, or psychosocial outcomes. Ideally, it should serve as an important treatment option in pediatric dialysis programs. At the same time, recognition of the resources necessary to conduct an HHD program and of the burden of care experienced by families that accompanies the delivery of this therapy at home is exceedingly important, and both issues must be addressed if a pediatric HHD program is to be successful.

Key Points

- Pediatric HHD is provided by very few centers despite promising data regarding the benefits of a home-based intensified HD modality. Further studies addressing the advantages of the therapy and barriers to implementation in children are warranted.
- Optimal management of the pediatric HHD patient requires attention to a variety of issues, including the following:
  - ESKD etiology.
  - Adaptation of technology designed for adults according to patient weight and size.
  - Growth and nutrition.
  - Comorbidities (neurodevelopment, congenital abnormalities, and metabolic disorders).
  - Education.

  - Transition to adult care.
  - Family dynamics and support.
- A successful pediatric HHD program requires a motivated patient and caregiver and a multidisciplinary team with a highly trained HHD medical and nursing team, dietician, social worker, psychologist, and technician.

Conflict of Interest None.

Financial Declaration None.

References

1. Amaral S, Sayed BA, Kutner N, Patzer RE. Preemptive kidney transplantation is associated with survival benefits among pediatric patients with end-stage renal disease. Kidney Int. 2016;90:1100–8.
2. Gillen DL, Stehman-Breen CO, Smith JM, McDonald RA, Warady BA, Brandt JR, et al. Survival advantage of pediatric recipients of a first kidney transplant among children awaiting kidney transplantation. Am J Transplant. 2008;8:2600–6.
3. McDonald SP, Craig JC, Australian and New Zealand Paediatric Nephrology Association. Long-term survival of children with end-stage renal disease. N Engl J Med. 2004;350:2654–62.
4. Neu AM, Sander A, Borzych-Duzalka D, Watson AR, Vallés PG, Ha IS, et al. Comorbidities in chronic pediatric peritoneal dialysis patients: a report of the International Pediatric Peritoneal Dialysis Network. Perit Dial Int. 2012;32:410–8.
5. Hothi DK, Stronach L, Sinnott K. Home hemodialysis in children. Hemodial Int. 2016;20:349–57.
6. Geary DF, Piva E, Tyrrell J, Gajaria MJ, Picone G, Keating LE, et al. Home nocturnal hemodialysis in children. J Pediatr. 2005;147:383–7.
7. Goldstein SL, Silverstein DM, Leung JC, Feig DI, Soletsky B, Knight C, et al. Frequent hemodialysis with NxStage system in pediatric patients receiving maintenance hemodialysis. Pediatr Nephrol. 2008;23:129–35.
8. Silverstein DM. Frequent hemodialysis: history of the modality and assessment of outcomes. Pediatr Nephrol. 2017;32:1293–300.
9. Thumfart J, Müller D, Wagner S, Jayanti A, Borzych-Duzalka D, Schaefer F, et al. Barriers for implementation of intensified hemodialysis: survey results from the International Pediatric Dialysis Network. Pediatr Nephrol. 2018;33:705–12.
10. Culleton BF, Walsh M, Klarenbach SW, Mortis G, Scott-Douglas N, Quinn RR, et al. Effect of frequent nocturnal hemodialysis vs conventional hemodialysis on left ventricular mass and quality of life: a randomized controlled trial. JAMA. 2007;298:1291–9.
11. Rocco MV, Daugirdas JT, Greene T, Lockridge RS, Chan C, Pierratos A, et al. Long-term effects of frequent nocturnal hemodialysis on mortality: the frequent hemodialysis network (FHN) nocturnal trial. Am J Kidney Dis. 2015;66:459–68.
12. Finkelstein FO, Schiller B, Daoui R, Gehr TW, Kraus MA, Lea J, et al. At-home short daily hemodialysis improves the long-term health-related quality of life. Kidney Int. 2012;82:561–9.
13. Jefferies HJ, Virk B, Schiller B, Moran J, McIntyre CW. Frequent hemodialysis schedules are associated with reduced levels of dialysis-induced cardiac injury (myocardial stunning). Clin J Am Soc Nephrol. 2011;6:1326–32.
14. Tennankore KK, Nadeau-Fredette AC, Vinson AJ. Survival comparisons in home hemodialysis: understanding the present and looking to the future. Nephrol Ther. 2021;17S:S64–70.
15. Bell L, Espinosa P. Intensive in-center hemodialysis for children: a case for longer dialysis duration. Hemodial Int. 2003;7:290–5.

16. Ashby D, Borman N, Burton J, Corbett R, Davenport A, Farrington K, et al. Renal association clinical practice guideline on haemodialysis. BMC Nephrol. 2019;20:379.
17. Bonthuis M, Vidal E, Bjerre A, Aydoğ Ö, Baiko S, Garneata L, et al. Ten-year trends in epidemiology and outcomes of pediatric kidney replacement therapy in Europe: data from the ESPN/ERA-EDTA Registry. Pediatr Nephrol. 2021;36:2337–48.
18. USRD Systems. USRDS annual renal data system: 2018 USRDS annual data report. Epidemiology of kidney disease in the United States. Bethesda, MD: National Institutes of Health, National Institute of Diabetes and Digestive and Kidney Diseases; 2018.
19. Chesnaye N, Bonthuis M, Schaefer F, Groothoff JW, Verrina E, Heaf JG, et al. Demographics of paediatric renal replacement therapy in Europe: a report of the ESPN/ERA-EDTA registry. Pediatr Nephrol. 2014;29:2403–10.
20. Harambat J, van Stralen KJ, Kim JJ, Tizard EJ. Epidemiology of chronic kidney disease in children. Pediatr Nephrol. 2012;27:363–73.
21. Kramer A, Boenink R, Stel VS, Santiuste de Pablos C, Tomović F, Golan E, et al. The ERA-EDTA registry annual report 2018: a summary. Clin Kidney J. 2021;14:107–23.
22. USRD Systems. USRDS annual renal data system: 2021 USRDS annual data report. Epidemiology of kidney disease in the United States. Bethesda, MD: National Institutes of Health, National Institute of Diabetes and Digestive and Kidney Diseases; 2021.
23. Chen K, Didsbury M, van Zwieten A, Howell M, Kim S, Tong A, et al. Neurocognitive and educational outcomes in children and adolescents with CKD: a systematic review and meta-analysis. Clin J Am Soc Nephrol. 2018;13:387–97.
24. Mitsnefes MM. Cardiovascular disease risk factors in chronic kidney disease in children. Semin Nephrol. 2021;41:434–8.
25. Müller D, Zimmering M, Chan CT, McFarlane PA, Pierratos A, Uwe Querfeld. Pediatr Nephrol. 2008;23(10):1729–36.
26. de Camargo MFC, Henriques CL, Vieira S et al. Growth of children with end-stage renal disease undergoing daily hemodialysis. Pediatr Nephrol 2014;29:439–44.
27. Hothi DK, Stronach L, Harvey E. Home haemodialysis. Pediatr Nephrol. 2013;28:721–30.
28. Thumfart J, Puttkamer CV, Wagner S, Querfeld U, Müller D. Hemodiafiltration in a pediatric nocturnal dialysis program. Pediatr Nephrol. 2014;29:1411–6.
29. Shroff R, Ledermann S. Long-term outcome of chronic dialysis in children. Pediatr Nephrol. 2009;24:463–74.
30. Rees L, Schaefer F, Schmitt CP, Shroff R, Warady BA. Chronic dialysis in children and adolescents: challenges and outcomes. Lancet Child Adolesc Health. 2017;1:68–77.
31. Foley RN, Parfrey PS, Harnett JD, Kent GM, Murray DC, Barré PE. The prognostic importance of left ventricular geometry in uremic cardiomyopathy. J Am Soc Nephrol. 1995;5:2024–31.
32. Mitsnefes MM, Barletta GM, Dresner IG, Chand DH, Geary D, Lin JJ, et al. Severe cardiac hypertrophy and long-term dialysis: the Midwest Pediatric Nephrology Consortium study. Pediatr Nephrol. 2006;21:1167–70.
33. Hothi DK, Fenton M. The impact of home hemodialysis in children with severe cardiac failure. Hemodial Int. 2020;24:E61–6.
34. Melhem NZ, Yadav P, Stronach L, Hothi DK. Intensified home haemodialysis for managing severe cardiac failure. Pediatr Nephrol. 2015;30:533–6.
35. Movilli E, Gaggia P, Zubani R, Camerini C, Vizzardi V, Parrinello G, et al. Association between high ultrafiltration rates and mortality in uraemic patients on regular haemodialysis. A 5-year prospective observational multicentre study. Nephrol Dial Transplant. 2007;22:3547–52.
36. Navarrete JE, Rajabalan A, Cobb J, Lea JP. Proportion of hemodialysis treatments with high ultrafiltration rate and the association with mortality. Kidney360. 2022;3(8):1359–66. https://kidney360.asnjournals.org/content/early/2022/05/12/KID.0001322022.
37. Hothi DK, Rees L, Marek J, Burton J, McIntyre CW. Pediatric myocardial stunning underscores the cardiac toxicity of conventional hemodialysis treatments. Clin J Am Soc Nephrol. 2009;4:790–7.
38. Hayes W, Hothi DK. Intradialytic hypotension. Pediatr Nephrol. 2011;26:867–79.

39. Lewis KD, Conway J, Cunningham C, Larsen BMK. Optimizing nutrition in pediatric heart failure: the crisis is over and now it's time to feed. Nutr Clin Pract. 2018;33:397–403.
40. McAlister L, Pugh P, Greenbaum L, Haffner D, Rees L, Anderson C, et al. The dietary management of calcium and phosphate in children with CKD stages 2-5 and on dialysis-clinical practice recommendation from the Pediatric Renal Nutrition Taskforce. Pediatr Nephrol. 2020;35:501–18.
41. Spalding EM, Chamney PW, Farrington K. Phosphate kinetics during hemodialysis: evidence for biphasic regulation. Kidney Int. 2002;61:655–67.
42. Fajardo L, Campistrús N, Ríos P, Gómez T. Evolution of serum phosphate in long intermittent hemodialysis. Kidney Int Suppl. 2003;(85):S66–8.
43. Hoppe A, von Puttkamer C, Linke U, Kahler C, Booss M, Braunauer-Kolberg R, et al. A hospital-based intermittent nocturnal hemodialysis program for children and adolescents. J Pediatr. 2011;158:95–9, 99.e1.
44. Franke D, Winkel S, Gellermann J, Querfeld U, Pape L, Ehrich JHH, et al. Growth and maturation improvement in children on renal replacement therapy over the past 20 years. Pediatr Nephrol. 2013;28:2043–51.
45. Bonthuis M, Harambat J, Jager KJ, Vidal E. Growth in children on kidney replacement therapy: a review of data from patient registries. Pediatr Nephrol. 2021;36:2563–74.
46. Fischbach M, Dheu C, Seuge L, Menouer S, Terzic J. In-center daily on-line hemodiafiltration: a 4-year experience in children. Clin Nephrol. 2008;69:279–84.
47. Hothi DK, Harvey E, Piva E, Keating L, Secker D, Geary DF. Calcium and phosphate balance in adolescents on home nocturnal haemodialysis. Pediatr Nephrol. 2006;21:835–41.
48. Fischbach M, Terzic J, Menouer S, Dheu C, Seuge L, Zalosczic A. Daily on line haemodiafiltration promotes catch-up growth in children on chronic dialysis. Nephrol Dial Transplant. 2010;25:867–73.
49. Tjaden L, Tong A, Henning P, Groothoff J, Craig JC. Children's experiences of dialysis: a systematic review of qualitative studies. Arch Dis Child. 2012;97:395–402.
50. Tjaden LA, Maurice-Stam H, Grootenhuis MA, Jager KJ, Groothoff JW. Impact of renal replacement therapy in childhood on long-term socioprofessional outcomes: a 30-year follow-up study. J Pediatr. 2016;171:189–195.e1-2.
51. Hanson CS, Gutman T, Craig JC, Bernays S, Raman G, Zhang Y, et al. Identifying important outcomes for young people with CKD and their caregivers: a nominal group technique study. Am J Kidney Dis. 2019;74:82–94.
52. Jaber BL, Lee Y, Collins AJ, Hull AR, Kraus MA, McCarthy J, et al. Effect of daily hemodialysis on depressive symptoms and postdialysis recovery time: interim report from the FREEDOM (following rehabilitation, economics and everyday-dialysis outcome measurements) study. Am J Kidney Dis. 2010;56:531–9.
53. Kennedy C, Ryan SA, Kane T, Costello RW, Conlon PJ. The impact of change of renal replacement therapy modality on sleep quality in patients with end-stage renal disease: a systematic review and meta-analysis. J Nephrol. 2018;31:61–70.
54. Kraus MA, Fluck RJ, Weinhandl ED, Kansal S, Copland M, Komenda P, et al. Intensive hemodialysis and health-related quality of life. Am J Kidney Dis. 2016;68:S33–42.
55. McFarlane PA, Bayoumi AM, Pierratos A, Redelmeier DA. The quality of life and cost utility of home nocturnal and conventional in-center hemodialysis. Kidney Int. 2003;64:1004–11.
56. Takahashi S. Future home hemodialysis—advantages of the NxStage System One. Contrib Nephrol. 2012;177:117–26.
57. Nadeau-Fredette AC, Tennankore KK, Perl J, Bargman JM, Johnson DW, Chan CT. Home hemodialysis and peritoneal dialysis patient and technique survival in Canada. Kidney Int Rep. 2020;5:1965–73.
58. Rydell H, Ivarsson K, Almquist M, Segelmark M, Clyne N. Improved long-term survival with home hemodialysis compared with institutional hemodialysis and peritoneal dialysis: a matched cohort study. BMC Nephrol. 2019;20:52.
59. Miller BW, Himmele R, Sawin DA, Kim J, Kossmann RJ. Choosing home hemodialysis: a critical review of patient outcomes. Blood Purif. 2018;45:224–9.

60. Borzych-Duzalka D, Shroff R, Ariceta G, Yap YC, Paglialonga F, Xu H, et al. Vascular access choice, complications, and outcomes in children on maintenance hemodialysis: findings from the International Pediatric Hemodialysis Network (IPHN) Registry. Am J Kidney Dis. 2019;74:193–202.
61. Boehm M, Bonthuis M, Noordzij M, Harambat J, Groothoff JW, Melgar ÁA, et al. Hemodialysis vascular access and subsequent transplantation: a report from the ESPN/ERA-EDTA Registry. Pediatr Nephrol. 2019;34:713–21.
62. Shroff R, Calder F, Bakkaloğlu S, Nagler EV, Stuart S, Stronach L, et al. Vascular access in children requiring maintenance haemodialysis: a consensus document by the European Society for Paediatric Nephrology Dialysis Working Group. Nephrol Dial Transplant. 2019;34:1746–65.
63. Chand DH, Swartz S, Tuchman S, Valentini RP, Somers MJG. Dialysis in children and adolescents: the pediatric nephrology perspective. Am J Kidney Dis. 2017;69:278–86.
64. Shroff R, Sterenborg RB, Kuchta A, Arnold A, Thomas N, Stronach L, et al. A dedicated vascular access clinic for children on haemodialysis: two years' experience. Pediatr Nephrol. 2016;31:2337–44.
65. Grewal MK, Mehta A, Chakraborty R, Raina R. Nocturnal home hemodialysis in children: advantages, implementation, and barriers. Semin Dial. 2020;33:109.
66. Lutkin M, Stronach L, Yadav P, Hothi DK. Dalteparin anticoagulation in paediatric home haemodialysis. Pediatr Nephrol. 2018;33:2337–41.
67. Charra B, Calemard E, Ruffet M, Chazot C, Terrat JC, Vanel T, et al. Survival as an index of adequacy of dialysis. Kidney Int. 1992;41:1286–91.
68. Levin NW. Adequacy of dialysis. Am J Kidney Dis. 1994;24:308–15.
69. Steyaert S, Holvoet E, Nagler E, Malfait S, Van Biesen W. Reporting of "dialysis adequacy" as an outcome in randomised trials conducted in adults on haemodialysis. PLoS One. 2019;14:e0207045.
70. Rees L. Assessment of dialysis adequacy: beyond urea kinetic measurements. Pediatr Nephrol. 2019;34:61–9.
71. Laskin BL, Huang G, King E, Geary DF, Licht C, Metlay JP, et al. Short, frequent, 5-days-per-week, in-center hemodialysis versus 3-days-per week treatment: a randomized crossover pilot trial through the Midwest Pediatric Nephrology Consortium. Pediatr Nephrol. 2017;32:1423–32.
72. Tong A, Palmer S, Manns B, Craig JC, Ruospo M, Gargano L, et al. The beliefs and expectations of patients and caregivers about home haemodialysis: an interview study. BMJ Open. 2013;3:e002148.
73. Walker RC, Hanson CS, Palmer SC, Howard K, Morton RL, Marshall MR, et al. Patient and caregiver perspectives on home hemodialysis: a systematic review. Am J Kidney Dis. 2015;65:451–63.
74. Crawford K, Wilson C, Low JK, Manias E, Williams A. Transitioning adolescents to adult nephrology care: a systematic review of the experiences of adolescents, parents, and health professionals. Pediatr Nephrol. 2020;35:555–67.
75. Watson AR, Harden PN, Ferris ME, Kerr PG, Mahan JD, Ramzy MF, et al. Transition from pediatric to adult renal services: a consensus statement by the International Society of Nephrology (ISN) and the International Pediatric Nephrology Association (IPNA). Kidney Int. 2011;80:704–7.

Home Hemodialysis in the Elderly

13

Maroun Azar

Introduction

Elderly patients represent the fastest-growing segment of the end-stage kidney disease (ESKD) population. The COVID-19 pandemic and recent healthcare policies in the United States have incentivized home dialysis therapies, yet a very small proportion of elderly patients with ESKD end up on home hemodialysis (HHD). They often carry higher mortality and morbidity than their younger counterparts and face numerous barriers in making the best treatment choices for ESKD. In this chapter, we review the epidemiology of the elderly ESKD population and discuss special considerations in approaching HHD in the elderly, including geriatric syndromes, vascular access, gaps in the support system, caregiver burden, and the option of conservative (non-dialytic) treatment, with the goal to provide a patient-centered care plan.

Case

An 82-year-old male with type 2 diabetes mellitus, hypertension, atrial fibrillation, coronary artery disease, congestive heart failure new york heart association (NYHA) class II, peripheral artery disease, diverticulitis s/p bowel resection and colostomy, and severe arthritis of the knees had developed chronic kidney disease that progressed over the years to reach stage 5. He had repeatedly avoided discussing ESKD treatment choices and advanced directives, stating that he would never want to go on dialysis. His most recent labs include estimated glomerular filtration rate (eGFR) 12 mL/min/1.73 m², serum potassium 5.4, bicarbonate 18, phosphate 6, albumin 3.2, and Hb 9.2. His medications include aspirin, simvastatin, lisinopril, patiromer, ferric citrate, sodium bicarbonate, torsemide, and an

M. Azar (✉)
Division of Kidney Disease and Hypertension, Brown Medicine, Warren Alpert Medical School of Brown University, Providence, RI, USA
e-mail: maroun.azar@brownphysicians.org

A. Shah et al. (eds.), *Applied Home Hemodialysis*,
https://doi.org/10.1007/978-3-031-77244-3_13

erythropoietin-stimulating agent. During his latest visit, he endorses anorexia, intermittent pruritus, increasing daytime sleepiness, exertional dyspnea, and lower extremity edema. On exam, his blood pressure is 142/64 mmHg; auscultation reveals no cardiac rub and clear lungs. He has +1 pitting bilateral lower extremity edema. He is alert and oriented. He lost 6 lb in the past month and needed assistance to get off the chair and reach his walker. He is now anxious and is having second thoughts about his previous treatment choice. He wants to know more about his options going forward.

While the adjusted incidence of ESKD has decreased since its peak in 2006 and flattened in more recent years, the number of patients initiating dialysis continues to grow, a consequence of an aging population. According to the most recent United States Renal Data System (USRDS) annual report, the incidence of ESKD was highest among patients older than 65 and particularly those older than 75 years of age. Over the past decade, individuals living with a functioning kidney allograft have continued to represent around 30% of the ESKD population, while the incidence and prevalence of home dialysis therapies have somewhat increased. However, as age increases, the percentage of patients utilizing home dialysis decreases. In 2019, 2% of prevalent ESKD patients older than 65 were on home hemodialysis (HHD), compared to 3.4% of ESKD patients 18–44 years old (Fig. 13.1). In addition, epidemiologic studies point to inequities and disparities in care. Whites are more likely to be on HHD compared to other ethnic groups. In New Zealand, 8% of ESKD patients are on HHD [1].

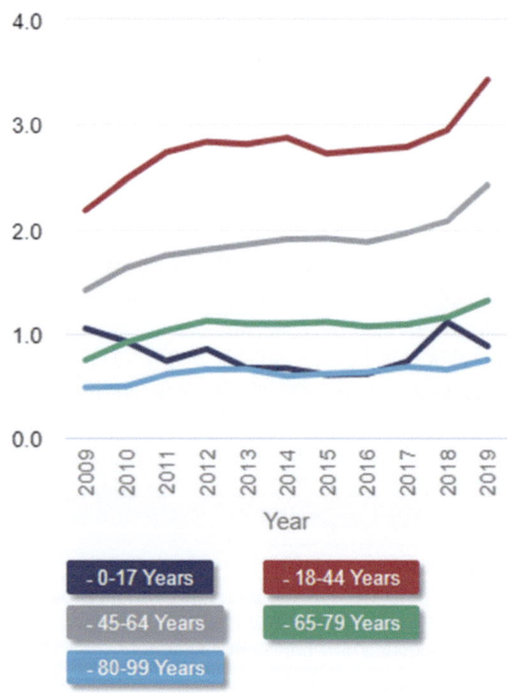

Fig. 13.1 Utilization of home hemodialysis among prevalent patients, stratified by age, 2009–2019 (USRDS 2021 Annual Data Report)

The COVID-19 pandemic has provided incentives to dialyze patients at home. In addition, in the United States, the Executive Order on Advancing American Kidney Health aims at increasing rates of preemptive kidney transplantation and utilization of home dialysis modalities in patients with ESKD. In this current climate, elderly dialysis patients face unique barriers and challenges, many of which have yet to be adequately researched. Nevertheless, HHD can be successful in this age category. An international feasibility study of HHD in patients older than 65 years showed a technique survival of 92%, 83%, and 56% at 1, 2, and 5 years, respectively, with a corresponding event-free survival of 85%, 77%, and 24%, bearing in mind that the median age was 68, with very few octogenarians [2]. An older report showed that mortality in octogenarians and nonagenarians initiating in-center hemodialysis (IHD) or peritoneal dialysis (PD) was very high, about 46% at 1 year [3]. Mortality is certainly expected to be high in older ESKD patients on HHD, but how it compares to IHD or PD remains uncertain. In the frequent hemodialysis network (FHN) trial, the only randomized controlled trial (RCT) comparing adult HHD to standard hemodialysis (HD), there were no patients older than 65 (mean age 48.9 +/− 13.6) [4]. Studies suggesting a survival advantage of HHD over IHD or PD are observational, do not include patients over the age of 70, and suffer from selection bias [5–10]. One study showed similar survival between HHD and automated peritoneal dialysis (APD) (but not continuous ambulatory peritoneal dialysis (CAPD)) but again did not include any older patients [11]. Comparative survival between modalities seems to be the wrong question to ask anyway, especially in the elderly. The decision to initiate HHD versus other modalities must be about other benefits and individualized to suit the patient's goals of care and living situation. Indeed, one survey found that 30% of ESKD patients would not change dialysis modality, even if it increased survival by 100% [12]. The standardized outcomes in nephrology-hemodialysis (SONG-HD) initiative has highlighted important differences in priorities between patients and physicians, such as fatigue, ability to travel, work, sleep, cramps, itching, pain, and caregiver burden [13].

General benefits of HHD are covered in more detail elsewhere in this book and may include better blood pressure control and fluid status, reduced left ventricular hypertrophy, less restrictive diet, better sleep, and physical and mental well-being. Avoiding transportation hassles, spending more time with loved ones, reducing healthcare-acquired infections, and realizing cost savings are particularly relevant to the more vulnerable elderly dialysis patients. Yet, one glance at the "Method to Assess Treatment Choices for Home Dialysis" (MATCH-D), a widely used tool to help clinicians and patients determine candidates for home dialysis (HomeDialysis.org), and it is easy to find many elderly patients facing barriers to HHD. Fortunately, many of these barriers can be overcome, especially if adequate support is available. Here, special considerations in the approach to HHD in the elderly will be discussed.

Geriatric Syndromes

Cognitive, functional impairment, and frailty are common in the chronic kidney disease (CKD) population, increase in prevalence with age, and may worsen after HD, leading to loss of independence. While the literature on these topics specific to HHD is sparse, it is reasonable to extrapolate general concepts from the IHD studies. A systematic review found significant associations between functional or cognitive impairment and frailty with poor outcomes such as mortality and hospitalization [14]. Furthermore, the presence of cognitive and functional impairment may hinder the ability of the elderly ESKD patient to perform HHD independently and safely. A cross-sectional study of HD patients found 13.9%, 36.1%, and 37.3% to have mild, moderate, and severe cognitive impairment, respectively, using a battery of validated neuropsychological tests assessing domains of memory, executive function, and language [15]. In a small study, cognitive function varied acutely during the actual process of dialysis, being worse during the treatment compared to shortly before and the day after [16]. In the FHN trial and an observational extension of its nocturnal arm, frequent HD did not improve cognitive performance at 12 months across a wide range of neuropsychological tests [17, 18]. All of these findings may bear implications for elderly HHD patients. Detecting cognitive impairment and tracking changes over time is important, although the optimal method of doing so remains under research. Many commonly used screening tests have not been validated in CKD patients or show poor sensitivity in this patient population, especially in detecting mild cognitive impairment [19]. The montreal cognitive assessment (MoCA) screening instrument is promising [20, 21].

In a study of functional dependence in prevalent elderly dialysis patients (average age 75), using the Barthel and Lawton Scales for basic and instrumental (activities of daily living (ADL) and instrumental activities of daily living (IADL), respectively), 95% had at least one IADL dependency. 52% were dependent on both IADLs and at least one core ADL [22]. A large US study looked at a national registry of nursing home patients who were starting dialysis and found that dialysis initiation was associated with a sharp decline in functional status. At 1 year, only 13% had maintained their pre-dialysis functional status, while 58% had died [17]. In a much smaller cohort of community elderly 80 years or older living independently, more than 30% had functional loss at 6 months after dialysis initiation regardless of modality, requiring private caregiver support or transfer to a nursing home [23].

In a large cohort of dialysis patients, the prevalence of frailty increased significantly with age, with more than 74% of patients older than 60 meeting frailty criteria. The presence of frailty more than doubled the hazard ratio for 1-year mortality [24]. While it is unclear if exercise training improves mortality and cardiovascular events in the ESKD population, evidence suggests that most forms of exercise programs (resistance +/− aerobic) can probably improve functional capacity, the physical component of health-related quality of life (HRQOL), and depressive symptoms and can possibly improve fatigue and pain [25–27]. In reality, exercise uptake by dialysis patients is low due to many factors, one of which is the lack of encouragement by healthcare providers and patient adoption of the "sick role" [28]. A cultural change that encourages patients to exercise is needed, in addition to the development of exercise equipment that is safe and adapted to use in chairs or recliners.

Vascular Access

Deciding on the optimal vascular access for an elderly patient is a challenging task. Guidelines have pushed the notion of "fistula first, catheter last" [29]. This is based on evidence in the general ESKD population pointing to a survival advantage of arteriovenous fistulas (AVFs). This evidence is based largely on observational studies and is subject to selection bias [30]. Most studies report on the vascular access achieved rather than intended. One possibility is that central venous catheters (CVCs) inherently increase mortality by way of higher infection, hospitalization rate, and access failure, but recent studies found that access-related complications did not explain all the difference in mortality between access types [31, 32]. In observational studies, adjusting for comorbidities that may influence access choice is not perfect and cannot account for differences in illness severity. Supporting this notion, a large USRDS cohort analysis found that the group of patients with a CVC after AVF failure had a significantly lower mortality compared to the group starting with a CVC first. It concluded that patient factors influencing choice of vascular access explained at least two-thirds of the mortality benefit of AVFs [33]. Older ESKD patients carry a higher burden of cardiovascular comorbidities and tend to have lower life expectancy. The survival advantage of AVF may diminish in older patients. An arteriovenous graft (AVG) can be used within days to a couple of weeks and may make more sense in a patient with limited life expectancy. In addition, older patients (and their caregivers) may suffer from decreased vision and manual dexterity and may have tremors, making self-canulation of an AVF or AVG more difficult and even risky. Therefore, a CVC may be acceptable in some cases. Another issue is vascular access primary failure and patency rate. A recent meta-analysis concluded that elderly ESKD patients experience a 79% higher rate of radiocephalic AVF primary failure and a 50% higher rate of failure at 12 months compared to non-elderly. Elbow brachiocephalic AVFs had a 12% higher 12-month patency rate. polytetrafluoroethylene (PTFE) grafts seemed to have an inferior patency rate in the elderly, but this needs to be confirmed by prospective studies [34]. There are currently no formal guidelines related to optimal vascular access in older ESKD patients. Randomized controlled trials are needed. A recent position paper from the Vascular Access Working Group of the Italian Society of Nephrology stresses an individualized multidisciplinary approach [35]. Allon and Lok propose an algorithmic approach to assist in deciding between AVF and AVG, taking into account life expectancy, vascular factors, prior access history, likelihood of access maturation, timing of dialysis, and patient preference [36]. In patients with a very short life expectancy <6 months who still elect to try HHD, a CVC would be more appropriate. But here again, elderly patients may have different perspectives, and survival may not be the only important outcome [37]. Factors affecting the quality of life (QOL) such as needle canulation, ability to bathe, appearance, and burden of access interventions (which may be more frequent in the elderly), should be considered as well. Ongoing research and novel vascular access techniques and materials continue to evolve and may alter our current approach [38].

Gaps in the Support System and Caregiver Burden

Given the frequency of cognitive and functional impairment, many elderly ESKD patients may not be able to perform HHD solo. The assistance they need may vary over a wide spectrum and can range from simply providing reassurance and backup to complete delivery of HHD. Longer training (6–8 weeks) and more professional support may be necessary, especially to overcome barriers to canulation [39]. For most patients, assistance is provided by relatives or friends. A recent report in the general US population estimates some 48 million caregivers provide largely unreimbursed care for a variety of disabled patients and incur substantial out-of-pocket expenses and sacrifice, with even more strain on minority and younger caregivers [40]. Alarmingly, a seminal study by Schulz et al. showed a 63% increase in mortality risk in caregivers experiencing mental or emotional strain compared to non-caregivers [41]. Caregiver burden is much less studied in dialysis patients, let alone elderly HHD patients. Gilbertson et al. have recently reviewed this issue in the dialysis population. They observed that quantitative studies tend to be cross sectional, of poor quality, and very heterogenous in design and outcome measures. Overall, dialysis patient caregiver QOL was worse than in the general population, mostly comparable to that of caregivers of patients with other diseases and better than the QOL of the patients that they care for. The majority of caregivers were female spouses. 12.6% were illiterate. About a third were employed outside of their caregiving role. Caregiving ranged from 26 to 69 h a week. In HHD, caregivers tended to be relatively younger compared to those caring for patients on PD or IHD. It was not possible, however, to draw definitive conclusions related to their QOL in comparison to other modalities [42]. In the FHN trial, the higher caregiver burden in nocturnal HHD compared to IHD did not reach statistical significance. Furthermore, the study looked at perceived caregiver burden by the patients themselves rather than actual burden of their unpaid caregivers [43]. In another study in nocturnal HHD, global burden scores were relatively low in caregivers, and 25% had depression. However, there was no control group [44]. Selection bias can be a problem in HHD studies as the average patient age tends to be younger with less comorbidities. Studies do not account for disease severity and change over time. Sicker patients may not respond to surveys or participate in studies. Scales used in studies are variable and may not capture subtle emotions and relationships. More quantitative and qualitative studies, along with interventional studies aimed at reducing caregiver burden in the HHD population are needed. Very few have examined interventions in IHD and PD, with positive results, including an educational program, a continuous care model, and supportive and cognitive behavioral therapy

[45–47]. It is also worth noting that even though elderly HHD patients may need more support, training them to do as much as possible rather than fully relying on their partner may alleviate caregiver burden [48]. Some have advocated to replace the term caregiver with "care partner" in support of this philosophy [49]. Respite care should be frequently offered to these care partners as needed. This may be in the form of a paid and trained home assistant or temporary in-center dialysis. The latter is less ideal as it changes dialysis modality but is more common since private dialysis care is not typically subsidized and patients may not be able to afford a private dialysis assistant.

Assisted HHD—(HHD provided by paid trained professionals via a structured program) is limited to very few geographical areas at this time and not reimbursed in the United States. It is an area of growing interest and research and can take many forms, including home assisted HHD, transitional care units [50], mobile units [51], and nursing home HHD [52]. This topic is discussed in more detail elsewhere in this book.

The COVID-19 pandemic has made it possible to provide HHD patients care via telehealth and bill for it. It is not clear how this will change post-pandemic, but the latter has reignited interest in telehealth and highlighted some benefits and challenges. Benefits may include closer patient monitoring, decreased travel time and costs, especially in rural areas, more participation by family members, and less exposure to healthcare infections. These benefits are particularly relevant to the vulnerable elderly population. Challenges and barriers include Internet connectivity and compatible devices, patient technology literacy (especially in the elderly), health insurance portability and accountability act (HIPAA) compliant platforms, and physical exam limitations. Refinement in technology platforms, outcomes research, and changes in healthcare regulations will guide the future of telehealth in home dialysis [53].

Decision-Making Process and the Option of Non-dialytic or Conservative Management

Given the high mortality and morbidity of older patients with advanced CKD, it is not always clear if any form of dialysis would significantly improve their survival or QOL. For the elderly patient and their loved ones to make the best choice regarding ESKD treatment, an honest discussion about prognosis and expectations with the different treatment options is crucial. Notwithstanding variation in patient and family attitudes among different cultures, research suggests that patients want this. One survey found that the vast majority of advanced CKD patients wanted to hear about prognosis and treatment options, including the possibility of withdrawal from dialysis. Less than 18% wanted to live as long as possible, even if the price was prolonged pain and suffering [54]. Another survey found that 97% of patients wanted to be given life expectancy information—even if their prognosis was poor—and patients specifically wanted their physician to disclose this information without prompting [55]. One survey found that patients were more likely to choose dialytic therapy (DT) versus conservative management (CM) if it increased life expectancy, could be done day or evening rather than just day, and if subsidized transport was available. More would choose CM versus DT if DT meant more hospital days and more restrictions on travel. Patients would trade off 7 months of life expectancy to reduce hospital visits and 15 months of life expectancy to increase ability to travel [56]. In practice though, ESKD patients often risk being marginalized in these important decisions [57] and can then be left with misconceptions and regrets.

The Renal Physicians Association has published its revised guidelines "Shared Decision-Making in the Appropriate Initiation of and Withdrawal from Dialysis" [58].

A review by Tamura et al. provides a useful framework for individualizing decisions in elderly ESKD patients by considering life expectancy, risks and benefits of competing treatments (including "number needed to treat" comparisons), and patient preferences, which can then be applied to assist in choosing a dialysis modality, a dialysis vascular access (and whether to refer for transplantation) [59].

While no RCT has compared dialytic therapies (DT) to CM, a number of retrospective studies shed some light on this issue. In a UK cohort of elderly ESKD patients, the survival advantage of DT was lost in patients with high comorbidity burden or ischemic heart disease [60]. When adjusting for age >75, diabetes mellitus, and comorbidities, a larger UK observational study only showed a marginal, non-statistically significant 4 months survival advantage of DT versus CM [61]. Looking at survival from a different perspective, another UK observational study showed longer survival on DT versus CM, but when removing hospital days and time spent on dialysis and transportation from the equation, this survival advantage shrank to just a few months [62].

The ability to estimate the life expectancy of ESKD patients is useful to assist in this complex decision-making. A number of prognostic tools have emerged for this purpose. While they should not be used to deny or impose treatments, they can be useful in risk stratification and in guiding the conversation. Cohen et al., who had previously developed and validated a popular 6-month HD mortality tool based on the "surprise question" (would I, the clinician, be surprised if this patient died in the next 6 months?) [63], subsequently developed and validated a predictive model for 6 and 12-month mortality in adults with advanced CKD not on dialysis. The model uses age and functional status measured by Karnofsky performance score (KPS) and the surprise question [64]. Couchoud et al. developed and validated a 3-month and a 3-year predictive model in incident ESKD patients (PD and HD) [65, 66].

Expectations regarding other outcomes of importance need to be set. Symptoms associated with ESKD are often vague, difficult to quantify objectively, and difficult to distinguish from symptoms that can be attributed to conditions coexisting with ESKD or side effects of medications used to manage these conditions. Uremic symptoms, sleep, and depression may not necessarily improve with DT and may even worsen in many. Nutrition may improve, only to decline again with dialysis vintage [67].

In patients who chose CM, one study showed that functional status tended to be stable in the last year of life but declined sharply in the last month, although the KPS used may have lacked the sensitivity to track small changes over time [68]. Patients undergoing CM can experience a sharp increase in symptom burden in the last 2 months of life [69, 70]. QOL was assessed in a UK cohort of mostly elderly patients with ESKD treated with DT versus CM: CM patients were older, more dependent, had higher comorbidities, poorer physical health, and more anxiety at baseline. Mental health, depression symptoms, and global satisfaction with life were similar in all modality groups at baseline. Physical health and anxiety scores changed little during follow-up in both groups. Satisfaction with life scores decreased significantly after dialysis initiation and did not subsequently recover, but did not change over time in the CM group [71]. A recent systematic review looking at long-term outcomes in patients with advanced CKD who chose CM was published. Acknowledging significant heterogeneity and limitations, select findings include a median survival range of 1–41 months, 1–2 hospital admissions, 7–8 clinic visits, and 2 emergency department visits per year. Mental health improved over 8–24 months, and QOL was maintained until late in the course. Of those who died, 20–76% had received hospice care, 27–68% died in a hospital, and 12–71% died at home. A significant number were hospitalized and/or received an invasive procedure during the final month of life [72]. Therefore, while patients who elect CM can remain stable for a long time, it is important to prepare and anticipate escalating palliative support along the disease trajectory as symptoms can escalate toward the end.

A comprehensive geriatric exam would be ideal to evaluate the functional age of elderly ESKD patients, risk stratify them, and assist in individualizing diagnostic and therapeutic interventions. It can be done at baseline and repeated serially. A recent paper describing two different models of incorporating geriatric assessment into a nephrology clinic supports this notion [73]. A geriatric assessment typically evaluates cognition, functional status, mental health, comorbidity burden, nutrition, hearing, vision, incontinence, social support, and medication review. The busy nephrologist may opt to use simple tools that do not consume much time, such as the "Mini-COG" and the "Timed Get Up and Go Test," to screen for cognitive impairment and frailty, respectively, acknowledging that other tools are more sensitive and specific. Similarly, ADLs and IADLs can be assessed by the validated Barthel and Lawton scales. The Beck Depression Inventory is the most studied depression screening tool in ESKD but is long. The shorter version (BDI-FS) may be a good initial screening option [74]. The patient health questionnaire (PHQ-2) and PHQ-9 are widely used but are less well studied in this population. A small selection of useful and easy-to-administer tools is suggested in Table 13.1.

A patient-centered approach requires a candid discussion of all the above considerations and aligning the treatment plan with the patient's goals of care. This may require tailoring the HHD prescription to account for individual factors and preferences beyond traditional measures such as dialyzer clearance of urea, time on dialysis, volume of distribution of urea (KT/V) and phosphate control. Particularly for KT/V, guidelines aiming for a specific target do not account for elderly patients and their specific metabolic characteristics. A frail older ESKD patient may have lower food intake and muscle mass and therefore not need as much clearance as a younger, healthier patient. For some, starting with less frequent and shorter HD may be

Table 13.1 Useful and easy administer tools

Screening tool	Domains assessed	Where to find
6 and 12 months mortality in CKD patients calculator (from [64])	Mortality in patients with CKD stage IV or V	QxMD (app or online)
3-month mortality of incident elderly ESRD patients calculator (from [65])	Risk of early death in elderly patients starting dialysis	QxMD (app or online)
Montreal Cognitive Assessment (MoCA)	Short term memory Visuospatial abilities Executive function Attention, concentration, and working memory Language Orientation to time and place	Mocatest.org
Patient Health Questionaire (PHQ-9)	Depression	phqscreeners.com
Barthel or Katz index	Activities of daily living	Mdcalc.com/www.alz.org
Lawton scale	Instrumental activities of daily living	Neurotoolkit.com

appropriate and may preserve residual kidney function [75] with less risk of hypotension, myocardial, and cerebral ischemia. This incremental HD approach is discussed separately in this book. Conversely, an elderly patient who struggles with significant fluid overload may benefit from frequent HHD, which allows for smaller ultrafiltration rates and less related ischemic complications.

A recent paper proposes framing this patient-centered approach within three attainable goals of care: dialysis as bridging (to kidney transplant) or long-term maintenance treatment, dialysis as final treatment destination, and active medical management without dialysis, whereas elderly ESKD patients with poor prognosis may be better suited by avoiding dialysis and relying on appropriate palliative support [76].

Current standard outcome targets for elderly patients on HD, including HHD, are often at odds with their preferences and goals of care. Our current healthcare structure needs to adapt to allow for optimal patient-centered care. A recent opinion paper proposes improving our assessment of ESKD care quality by recommending a balanced score card that includes three elements: population-based best clinical practice, patient perceptions of his or her care, and individually crafted patient goals of care [77]. In the United States, the new kidney care models launched recently under the framework of the Advancing American Kidney Health initiative hold some promise in seeking to align incentives with patient-centered goals [78].

Back to Our Case

The patient agreed to a visit to discuss goals of care in the presence of his 80-year-old wife and 50-year-old son. He was interested in knowing his prognosis, even if poor. Based on his age, high number of comorbidities, and impaired functional status, it was clear his risk of death in the next 3–12 months is quite high with or without dialysis, ranging approximately between 25% and 45% using the predictive models discussed above. What mattered most to the patient was to be able to attend the wedding of his beloved granddaughter in 8 months. He was willing to make some sacrifices to achieve that goal, after which QOL would take priority over survival. He also hoped he could breathe more comfortably. Cognitive screening and discussion with his family did not reveal any cognitive impairment. He did require assistance in bathing but was able to perform other ADLs independently. His hearing and vision were adequate. He lived at least 90 min from the closest dialysis center. It was important for him to minimize transportation and maximize time with loved ones. His wife had many health issues but was able to live independently with minor assistance in IADLs. He had no pets, and his house had adequate storage space. His son lived across the street and worked from home. He was available and willing to assist with HHD. The patient understood that dialysis may or may not achieve his goals or improve all his symptoms. He decided he would give HHD a try and was encouraged to perform it as independently as possible. Given limited life expectancy and the lack of pre-existing vascular access, a CVC was placed as his permanent access. He also had residual kidney function, and an initial prescription of HHD 3–4 times a week was deemed appropriate. Both patient and son underwent training for 5 weeks, after which the patient started performing HHD independently. His son was present for backup during machine setup and treatment initiation in the evening. His wife continued to cook and did her best to follow the kidney diet. His weekly KT/V was 2.2, serum phosphate was 5.9, and serum potassium and bicarbonate were normal. His appetite improved, and he gained 5 lb back. His dyspnea and edema resolved. He still had occasional mild pruritus that was relieved with topical treatment. With home physical therapy (PT), he was able to stand up and use his walker independently. 24/7 professional support was readily available. He made it to his granddaughter's wedding. Over the following weeks, as his residual function continued to decline, some of his symptoms and edema returned, along with worsening metabolic complications. It became clear he needed more frequent HHD or, alternatively, a higher dose of IHD, but he felt it would be too much and decided to withdraw from dialysis. Hospice care was arranged to address his end-of-life symptoms. He died at home a week later, his wife and son by his bedside as he had wished.

Key Points

- QOL, not survival, is the most important outcome for most elderly patients with ESKD.
- HHD is an underutilized treatment option for elderly patients with ESKD but poses unique challenges that require consideration:
  - Geriatric syndromes: cognitive impairment and frailty are very common, leading to increased dependency.
  - Optimal vascular access: may not necessarily be AVF and needs to be individualized.
  - Availability of a care partner, attention to care partner burnout.
- Conservative non-dialytic management may be more appropriate for some elderly patients with ESKD.
- Validated screening and prognostic tools can assist in risk stratification and help in shared decision-making.

References

1. U.S.R.D. System. USRDS annual data report: epidemiology of kidney disease in the United States. Bethesda, MD: National Institutes of Health, National Institute of Diabetes and Digestive and Kidney Diseases; 2021.
2. Cornelis T, et al. An international feasibility study of home haemodialysis in older patients. Nephrol Dial Transplant. 2014;29(12):2327–33.
3. Kurella M, et al. Octogenarians and nonagenarians starting dialysis in the United States. Ann Intern Med. 2007;146(3):177–83.
4. F.H.N.T. Group, et al. In-center hemodialysis six times per week versus three times per week. N Engl J Med. 2010;363(24):2287–300.
5. Nitsch D, et al. Outcomes in patients on home haemodialysis in England and Wales, 1997-2005: a comparative cohort analysis. Nephrol Dial Transplant. 2011;26(5):1670–7.
6. Marshall MR, et al. Home hemodialysis and mortality risk in Australian and New Zealand populations. Am J Kidney Dis. 2011;58(5):782–93.
7. Marshall MR, et al. Survival on home dialysis in New Zealand. PLoS One. 2014;9(5):e96847.
8. Nadeau-Fredette AC, et al. An incident cohort study comparing survival on home hemodialysis and peritoneal dialysis (Australia and New Zealand Dialysis and Transplantation Registry). Clin J Am Soc Nephrol. 2015;10(8):1397–407.
9. Weinhandl ED, Gilbertson DT, Collins AJ. Mortality, hospitalization, and technique failure in daily home hemodialysis and matched peritoneal dialysis patients: a matched cohort study. Am J Kidney Dis. 2016;67(1):98–110.
10. Rydell H, et al. Improved long-term survival with home hemodialysis compared with institutional hemodialysis and peritoneal dialysis: a matched cohort study. BMC Nephrol. 2019;20(1):52.
11. Bitar W, et al. Similar survival on home hemodialysis and automated peritoneal dialysis: an inception cohort study. Nephrol Dial Transplant. 2021;37:1545.
12. Bass EB, et al. How strong are patients' preferences in choices between dialysis modalities and doses? Am J Kidney Dis. 2004;44(4):695–705.
13. Tong A, et al. Establishing core outcome domains in hemodialysis: report of the standardized outcomes in nephrology-hemodialysis (SONG-HD) consensus workshop. Am J Kidney Dis. 2017;69(1):97–107.
14. Kallenberg MH, et al. Functional and cognitive impairment, frailty, and adverse health outcomes in older patients reaching ESKD-A systematic review. Clin J Am Soc Nephrol. 2016;11(9):1624–39.
15. Murray AM, et al. Cognitive impairment in hemodialysis patients is common. Neurology. 2006;67(2):216–23.
16. Murray AM, et al. Acute variation in cognitive function in hemodialysis patients: a cohort study with repeated measures. Am J Kidney Dis. 2007;50(2):270–8.
17. Kurella Tamura M, et al. Functional status of elderly adults before and after initiation of dialysis. N Engl J Med. 2009;361(16):1539–47.
18. Dixon BS, et al. Cognitive changes associated with switching to frequent nocturnal hemodialysis or renal transplantation. BMC Nephrol. 2016;17:12.
19. Vanderlinden JA, et al. Quantifying cognitive dysfunction across the spectrum of end-stage kidney disease: a systematic review and meta-analysis. Nephrology (Carlton). 2019;24(1):5–16.
20. Drew DA, et al. Evaluation of screening tests for cognitive impairment in patients receiving maintenance hemodialysis. J Am Soc Nephrol. 2020;31(4):855–64.
21. Tiffin-Richards FE, et al. The Montreal Cognitive Assessment (MoCA)—a sensitive screening instrument for detecting cognitive impairment in chronic hemodialysis patients. PLoS One. 2014;9(10):e106700.
22. Cook WL, Jassal SV. Functional dependencies among the elderly on hemodialysis. Kidney Int. 2008;73(11):1289–95.

23. Jassal SV, Chiu E, Hladunewich M. Loss of independence in patients starting dialysis at 80 years of age or older. N Engl J Med. 2009;361(16):1612–3.
24. Johansen KL, et al. Significance of frailty among dialysis patients. J Am Soc Nephrol. 2007;18(11):2960–7.
25. Bernier-Jean A, et al. Exercise training for adults undergoing maintenance dialysis. Cochrane Database Syst Rev. 2022;1:CD014653.
26. Gomes Neto M, et al. Intradialytic exercise training modalities on physical functioning and health-related quality of life in patients undergoing maintenance hemodialysis: systematic review and meta-analysis. Clin Rehabil. 2018;32(9):1189–202.
27. Chung YC, Yeh ML, Liu YM. Effects of intradialytic exercise on the physical function, depression and quality of life for haemodialysis patients: a systematic review and meta-analysis of randomised controlled trials. J Clin Nurs. 2017;26(13–14):1801–13.
28. Kontos PC, et al. Factors influencing exercise participation by older adults requiring chronic hemodialysis: a qualitative study. Int Urol Nephrol. 2007;39(4):1303–11.
29. Vascular Access 2006 Work Group. Clinical practice guidelines for vascular access. Am J Kidney Dis. 2006;48(Suppl 1):S248–73.
30. Ravani P, et al. Associations between hemodialysis access type and clinical outcomes: a systematic review. J Am Soc Nephrol. 2013;24(3):465–73.
31. Ravani P, et al. Examining the association between hemodialysis access type and mortality: the role of access complications. Clin J Am Soc Nephrol. 2017;12(6):955–64.
32. Quinn RR, et al. The effect of predialysis fistula attempt on risk of all-cause and access-related death. J Am Soc Nephrol. 2017;28(2):613–20.
33. Brown RS, Patibandla BK, Goldfarb-Rumyantzev AS. The survival benefit of "fistula first, catheter last" in hemodialysis is primarily due to patient factors. J Am Soc Nephrol. 2017;28(2):645–52.
34. Lazarides MK, et al. A meta-analysis of dialysis access outcome in elderly patients. J Vasc Surg. 2007;45(2):420–6.
35. Lomonte C, et al. The vascular access in the elderly: a position statement of the Vascular Access Working Group of the Italian Society of Nephrology. J Nephrol. 2016;29(2):175–84.
36. Allon M, Lok CE. Dialysis fistula or graft: the role for randomized clinical trials. Clin J Am Soc Nephrol. 2010;5(12):2348–54.
37. Xi W, et al. Patient attitudes towards the arteriovenous fistula: a qualitative study on vascular access decision making. Nephrol Dial Transplant. 2011;26(10):3302–8.
38. Viecelli AK, Lok CE. Hemodialysis vascular access in the elderly-getting it right. Kidney Int. 2019;95(1):38–49.
39. Ward FL, Faratro R, McQuillan RF. Self-cannulation of the vascular access in home hemodialysis: overcoming patient-level barriers. Semin Dial. 2018;31(5):449–54.
40. Skufca L, Rainville C. Caregiving out-of-pocket costs study 2021. Washington, DC: AARP Research; 2021.
41. Schulz R, Beach SR. Caregiving as a risk factor for mortality: the caregiver health effects study. JAMA. 1999;282(23):2215–9.
42. Gilbertson EL, et al. Burden of care and quality of life among caregivers for adults receiving maintenance dialysis: a systematic review. Am J Kidney Dis. 2019;73(3):332–43.
43. Suri RS, et al. Effects of frequent hemodialysis on perceived caregiver burden in the Frequent Hemodialysis Network trials. Clin J Am Soc Nephrol. 2014;9(5):936–42.
44. Rioux JP, Narayanan R, Chan CT. Caregiver burden among nocturnal home hemodialysis patients. Hemodial Int. 2012;16(2):214–9.
45. Mollaoglu M, Kayatas M, Yurugen B. Effects on caregiver burden of education related to home care in patients undergoing hemodialysis. Hemodial Int. 2013;17(3):413–20.
46. Rahim A, et al. Effects of a continuous care model on perceived quality of life of spouses of haemodialysis patients. East Mediterr Health J. 2009;15(4):944–50.
47. Hener T, Weisenberg M, Har-Even D. Supportive versus cognitive-behavioral intervention programs in achieving adjustment to home peritoneal kidney dialysis. J Consult Clin Psychol. 1996;64(4):731–41.

48. Lowry MR, Atcherson E. Spouse-assistants' adjustment to home hemodialysis. J Chronic Dis. 1984;37(4):293–300.
49. Bennett PN, Schatell D, Shah KD. Psychosocial aspects in home hemodialysis: a review. Hemodial Int. 2015;19(Suppl 1):S128–34.
50. Bowman B, et al. Improving incident ESKD care via a transitional care unit. Am J Kidney Dis. 2018;72(2):278–83.
51. Sims J, et al. The effect of holiday haemodialysis treatments on patient mood, adverse symptoms and subjective wellbeing using the Big Red Kidney Bus. Nephrology (Carlton). 2017;22(2):107–13.
52. Bellin EY, et al. Epidemiology of nursing home dialysis patients—a hidden population. Hemodial Int. 2021;25(4):548–59.
53. Lew SQ, et al. Telehealth for home dialysis in COVID-19 and beyond: a perspective from the American Society of Nephrology COVID-19 Home Dialysis Subcommittee. Am J Kidney Dis. 2021;77(1):142–8.
54. Davison SN. End-of-life care preferences and needs: perceptions of patients with chronic kidney disease. Clin J Am Soc Nephrol. 2010;5(2):195–204.
55. Fine A, et al. Nephrologists should voluntarily divulge survival data to potential dialysis patients: a questionnaire study. Perit Dial Int. 2005;25(3):269–73.
56. Morton RL, et al. Factors influencing patient choice of dialysis versus conservative care to treat end-stage kidney disease. CMAJ. 2012;184(5):E277–83.
57. Dahlerus C, et al. Patient perspectives on the choice of dialysis modality: results from the empowering patients on choices for renal replacement therapy (EPOCH-RRT) study. Am J Kidney Dis. 2016;68(6):901–10.
58. https://www.renalmd.org/store/ViewProduct.aspx?ID=7014408.
59. Tamura MK, Tan JC, O'Hare AM. Optimizing renal replacement therapy in older adults: a framework for making individualized decisions. Kidney Int. 2012;82(3):261–9.
60. Murtagh FE, et al. Dialysis or not? A comparative survival study of patients over 75 years with chronic kidney disease stage 5. Nephrol Dial Transplant. 2007;22(7):1955–62.
61. Chandna SM, et al. Survival of elderly patients with stage 5 CKD: comparison of conservative management and renal replacement therapy. Nephrol Dial Transplant. 2011;26(5):1608–14.
62. Carson RC, et al. Is maximum conservative management an equivalent treatment option to dialysis for elderly patients with significant comorbid disease? Clin J Am Soc Nephrol. 2009;4(10):1611–9.
63. Cohen LM, et al. Predicting six-month mortality for patients who are on maintenance hemodialysis. Clin J Am Soc Nephrol. 2010;5(1):72–9.
64. Schmidt RJ, et al. Derivation and validation of a prognostic model to predict mortality in patients with advanced chronic kidney disease. Nephrol Dial Transplant. 2019;34(9):1517–25.
65. Couchoud CG, et al. Development of a risk stratification algorithm to improve patient-centered care and decision making for incident elderly patients with end-stage renal disease. Kidney Int. 2015;88(5):1178–86.
66. Dusseux E, et al. A simple clinical tool to inform the decision-making process to refer elderly incident dialysis patients for kidney transplant evaluation. Kidney Int. 2015;88(1):121–9.
67. Cabrera VJ, et al. Symptom management of the patient with CKD: the role of dialysis. Clin J Am Soc Nephrol. 2017;12(4):687–93.
68. Murtagh FE, Addington-Hall JM, Higginson IJ. End-stage renal disease: a new trajectory of functional decline in the last year of life. J Am Geriatr Soc. 2011;59(2):304–8.
69. Murtagh FE, et al. Trajectories of illness in stage 5 chronic kidney disease: a longitudinal study of patient symptoms and concerns in the last year of life. Clin J Am Soc Nephrol. 2011;6(7):1580–90.
70. O'Connor NR, Kumar P. Conservative management of end-stage renal disease without dialysis: a systematic review. J Palliat Med. 2012;15(2):228–35.
71. Da Silva-Gane M, et al. Quality of life and survival in patients with advanced kidney failure managed conservatively or by dialysis. Clin J Am Soc Nephrol. 2012;7(12):2002–9.

72. Wong SPY, et al. Long-term outcomes among patients with advanced kidney disease who forgo maintenance dialysis: a systematic review. JAMA Netw Open. 2022;5(3):e222255.
73. Hall RK, et al. Incorporating geriatric assessment into a nephrology clinic: preliminary data from two models of care. J Am Geriatr Soc. 2016;64(10):2154–8.
74. Kondo K, et al. Depression screening tools for patients with kidney failure: a systematic review. Clin J Am Soc Nephrol. 2020;15(12):1785–95.
75. Obi Y, et al. Incremental hemodialysis, residual kidney function, and mortality risk in incident dialysis patients: a cohort study. Am J Kidney Dis. 2016;68(2):256–65.
76. Vandecasteele SJ, Kurella Tamura M. A patient-centered vision of care for ESKD: dialysis as a bridging treatment or as a final destination? J Am Soc Nephrol. 2014;25(8):1647–51.
77. Kliger AS. Quality measures for dialysis: time for a balanced scorecard. Clin J Am Soc Nephrol. 2016;11(2):363–8.
78. Kshirsagar AV, et al. Keys to driving implementation of the new kidney care models. Clin J Am Soc Nephrol. 2022;17:1082.

Fertility and Pregnancy Considerations for Patients on Home Hemodialysis

14

Stephanie Braunthal, Kenneth K. Chen, and Ankur Shah

Background, Epidemiology, and Outcomes

Fertility and pregnancy must be considered in patients with End-Stage Kidney Disease (ESKD). Point prevalence per million United States residents with ESKD ages 22–44 years in 2018 was 1024.3, the total likely being greater when accounting for the full age range of fertility [1]. Renal dysfunction has a significant impact on reproductive physiology [2], though gynecologic disorders are often underrecognized in patients with chronic kidney disease (CKD) [3]. Both uremia and reduced clearance of gonadotropin-releasing hormone (GnRH), luteinizing hormone (LH), and prolactin disrupt the pulsatile nature of the hypothalamic-pituitary-axis (HPA) that regulates the menstrual cycle [2, 4]. Menstrual irregularities in patients with CKD occur when the glomerular filtration rate (GFR) is less than 15 mL/min, and patients are likely anovulatory at the point of ESKD [4]. Subsequent imbalances of estrogen and progesterone noted in hemodialysis patients lead to endometrial abnormalities [5]. This, in combination with anovulation, depression, and anemia, contributes to the estimated 84% of women on hemodialysis who report sexual dysfunction [6, 7]. Renal transplant restores fertility within a few months post-operatively [8].

The first pregnancy with a successful outcome in a patient with ESKD on hemodialysis was reported by Confortini et al. in 1971 [9]. Renal failure has historically been thought to cause infertility, though over the past several decades, there has been an increase in both conception and live birth rates [10–12]. Most recent data

S. Braunthal · K. K. Chen
Division of Obstetric Medicine, Department of Medicine, Warren Alpert Medical School of Brown University, Providence, RI, USA
e-mail: stephanie_braunthal@brown.edu; kenneth_k_chen@brown.edu

A. Shah (✉)
Warren Alpert Medical School, Brown University, Providence, RI, USA
e-mail: Ankur.shah@brownphysicians.org

A. Shah et al. (eds.), *Applied Home Hemodialysis*,
https://doi.org/10.1007/978-3-031-77244-3_14

from the Australia and New Zealand Dialysis and Transplant (ANZATA) Registry report an increase in the rate of pregnancies per 1000 person-years from 0.54 to 3.3 between 1976 and 2008 [10]. A meta-analysis of pregnant patients on dialysis suggests that there were more than 600 cases from 2000 to 2014, a more than sixfold increase from what was reported in a similar study earlier in the decade that included a literature review from 2000 to 2008 [11]. A survey of almost 200 nephrologists practicing in the United States suggests that the live birth rate from 2010 to 2015 is just under 80%, compared to under 40% in the 1980s and 1990s [12, 13]. The improvements are attributed to a combination of intensified and nocturnal hemodialysis prescriptions, increased clearance, and the use of erythropoietin stimulating agents in the management of chronic anemia [7].

Although there has been incremental success in the ability to conceive and birth live infants, ESKD remains a significant risk factor for obstetric complications. A retrospective cohort of dialyzed and transplanted ESKD patients followed in the ANZATA Registry from 1991 to 2013 suggests that patients with ESKD are at higher risk for pregnancy induced hypertension, cesarian section, neonatal and perinatal death, pre-term delivery, low birth weight, small for gestational age, low Apgar scores, neonatal ICU stay, and congenital abnormalities compared to those without renal replacement therapy. Of the renal replacement patients, there was a statistically significant increased odds of low birthweight (<2500 g) in those receiving dialysis [14]. Additional risks include early pregnancy loss/miscarriage, anemia, infections, polyhydramnios, hemorrhage, and death [15]. A comparison of a more intensively dialyzed Canadian cohort from 2000 to 2013 to a standardly dialyzed American cohort from 1990 to 2011 demonstrated dose response improvement in live births and reduction in both pre-term delivery and small for gestational age in those who were dialyzed at least 36 h per week, compared to those dialyzed 20 h or less [16]. The aforementioned meta-analysis reviewing 681 pregnancies in 641 patients from 2000 to 2014 found similar correlations with the number of hours spent dialyzing to improving the likelihood of term delivery and weight of the baby [11].

Renal Physiology in Pregnancy

Nephrologists caring for reproductive-aged patients with advanced renal disease requiring hemodialysis are key to providing counseling and management preconception, during pregnancy, and postpartum. Optimizing patients during these periods requires an understanding of renal physiology in pregnancy and the way that that renal disease and pregnancy interface.

In normal pregnancy, there are profound changes in the balance of estrogen, progesterone, relaxin, beta-Human chorionic gonadotropin (HCG), and myriad other hormones that affect the Renin-angiotensin-aldosterone (RAAS) system, as well as Antidiuretic Hormone (ADH) secretion and metabolism, which engender increases in blood volume, reductions in oncotic pressure, systemic relaxation of smooth muscle, and vasodilation. Clinically, patients present with higher heart rates and a parabolic trend in their blood pressures, with nadirs in the second trimester at approximately 20 weeks gestation and vasogenic edema [17–21].

In patients without renal dysfunction, the kidney will expand by 1–1.5 cm, and there is dilation of the collection system causing a physiologic hydronephrosis, the latter of which is also thought to be due to mechanical compression as seen on imaging studies [22–24]. GFR increases by approximately 50% [25], and there is reduced reabsorption at the proximal tubule of glucose, total protein, albumin, uric acid, and amino acids [21, 26]. Notably, protein excretion in pregnancy is higher than in the non-pregnant state, with less than 300 mg/24 h considered normal. Plasma osmolality decreases to approximately 270 mOsm/kg, serum sodium decreases by 4–5 mEq/L, and total body potassium increases, though its excretion remains constant [21]. Increases in minute ventilation and subsequent excretion of bicarbonate lead to chronic respiratory alkalosis with metabolic compensation [27].

Additional physiologic changes that nephrologists should be aware of are pregnancy's effects on anemia and bone metabolism. There is a physiologic anemia secondary to a mismatch in the rate of blood volume expansion to red blood cell mass turnover, which is often exacerbated by increased iron demands from the fetus and poor oral intake causing deficiency [28]. Maternal Parathyroid Hormone (PTH) secretion increases, as does calcium absorption, and nutritional demand for vitamin D [29].

For patients with CKD not yet on renal replacement therapy, there is some concern that pregnancy can cause progression of the disease; however, studies are conflicting [30, 31].

Management Considerations

Optimization of ESKD patients for pregnancy includes a focus on blood pressure, nutrition, volume status, solutes, proteinuria, and anemia. Nephrologists should also be aware of measures taken to prevent and recognize preeclampsia, as well as anticipated schedules for fetal monitoring.

Assessment of Dry Weight and Volume Status

Weight gain in pregnancy accounts for growth of the fetus, placenta, amniotic fluid, blood volume, and growth of the uterus and other maternal tissues [32]. Weight gain recommendations have been dictated in a 2009 Institute of Medicine report: approximately 1 lb per week beginning in the second trimester for a singleton fetus; half a pound per week for those with a BMI ≥30 [33].

Dry weight is expectedly difficult to assess given the dynamic weight and cardiovascular changes throughout the gestational period. A combination of maternal blood pressure, amniotic fluid index, and plasma atrial natriuretic peptide (ANP) may be used to help titrate dialysis prescriptions. One successful approach has been to target post-hemodialysis plasma ANP to <100 pg/mL in earlier trimesters and to

150–200 pg/mL in the third trimester [34, 35]. Brain natriuretic peptide (BNP), while also higher than normal in pregnancy, has demonstrated a lower association with poor adverse outcomes when ≤100 pg/mL [36–38].

Solute Clearance

Intensifying dialysis can help mitigate the maternal and fetal risks in pregnancy. More frequent dialysis or increased hours per session enhances solute clearance and offers better control of fluid, electrolytes, and nitrogenous waste products compared to conventional thrice-weekly dialysis. Long, frequent dialysis in excess of 36 h per week is recommended in pregnancy in the absence of residual kidney function with a target BUN <35 to 50 mg/dL. Nocturnal home hemodialysis is an ideal method of dialysis to achieve this goal. This creates a more stable internal environment better suited to support pregnancy. Additionally, European guidelines recommend hemodialysis be initiated when maternal urea concentration is 47.6–56 mg/dL. A number of published studies demonstrate the correlation between both weekly duration of dialysis and gestational age at delivery, birth weight, and live birth rate, as well as the inverse correlation between maternal urea concentration and birth outcomes [11, 39–42]. In a meta-regression of these studies, including 681 pregnancies, a linear relationship was demonstrated between dialysis time, pre-term delivery, and SGA. SGA was also associated with the number of treatments per week. The authors concluded, "The main determinant of outcomes on Hemodialysis (HD) is the dialysis schedule." The use of Kt/v urea is not validated in pregnancy.

Blood Pressure

Blood pressure should be controlled to <140/90 mmHg. Historically, there has been little consensus as to which threshold to control blood pressure in pregnancy [43], though recent results of the chronic hypertension and pregnancy (CHAP) trial, a large, multicenter randomized trial published in April 2022, present compelling evidence to control preexisting hypertension to tighter control, and the Society of Maternal-Fetal Medicine recently drafted recommendations to reflect this [44, 45].

Data remains controversial regarding the safety profiles of many antihypertensive agents during pregnancy [43], though the American College of Obstetricians and Gynecologists (ACOG) provides guidance on dosing, indications, and side effects of commonly used oral and intravenous medications in pregnancy. In non-emergent situations, oral labetalol, extended release nifedipine, or methyldopa may be used as the first line, with hydrochlorothiazide as the second line. For emergent lowering, intravenous labetalol, hydralazine, or immediate release oral nifedipine may be used. Angiotensin-converting enzyme (ACE) inhibitors and angiotensin-receptor blockers (ARB) are contraindicated due to teratogenicity noted with exposure during the second and third trimesters [46].

Should patients require antihypertensive agents postpartum, many are continued on oral labetalol and extended release nifedipine, as both have been demonstrated to pass through breast milk at low enough levels that there would be an unlikely effect on the infant. If there is an indication for an ACE inhibitor, enalapril is the best studied and is also present at low enough levels to provide reassurance regarding neonatal safety [46]. ARBs are less well studied, but if necessary, losartan may be considered [47].

Preeclampsia Detection and Prevention

The ACOG defines preeclampsia as:

- Systolic blood pressure of ≥140 mmHg or a diastolic blood pressure of ≥90 mmHg on at least two occasions, 4 h apart BEFORE 20 weeks gestation.

OR

- Systolic blood pressure ≥160 mmHg or a diastolic blood pressure ≥110 mmHg (may be taken minutes apart) BEFORE 20 weeks gestation.

AND

- Proteinuria, as defined by ≥300 mg of protein in a 24 h urine collection, protein/creatinine ratio of ≥0.3, or dipstick of 2+ (if other modalities are unavailable).

OR, in the absence of proteinuria, hypertension (defined above) must be accompanied by any of the following:

- Platelets ≤100 × 10^9/L.
- Renal insufficiency—serum creatinine ≥1.1 mg/dL or doubling of the serum creatinine in the absence of other renal dysfunction.
- Impaired liver function—aminotransferases elevated to twice the upper limit of normal.
- Pulmonary edema.
- New headache that does not respond to medication or can be explained by alternate etiology.
- Visual symptoms.

Severe range blood pressure or any of the non-proteinuria features will classify preeclampsia as that with severe features. If the patient has hypertension prior to 20 weeks gestation, the patient is considered to be a chronic hypertensive, and the development of any proteinuria or any of the severe features earns the title of superimposed preeclampsia [48].

Superimposed preeclampsia is difficult to define in patients with underlying kidney disease, as renal markers of proteinuria and serum creatinine are unreliable, and there is no consensus on the diagnostic criteria [49]. In hemodialysis patients, missed or inadequate sessions may lead to sudden increases in blood pressure or pulmonary edema that may have to be differentiated. Special attention must thus be paid to platelets, liver function, and neurologic symptoms [46]. Research is underway to analyze the sFlt-1/PlGF ratio, markers of angiogenic and antiangiogenic imbalance associated with the development of preeclampsia, and has shown some evidence of helping differentiate preeclampsia in patients with underlying CKD; however, it is not part of the diagnostic criteria at this time [49, 50].

Preeclampsia with severe features often requires a magnesium sulfate infusion for neuroprotection from eclamptic seizures [48]. Patients with underlying renal disease are at increased risk for magnesium toxicities, and there should be careful monitoring of both magnesium levels and clinical symptoms (e.g., loss of patellar reflexes, respiratory depression, cardiac arrest) for any ESKD patient who requires treatment, with prompt dialysis should any occur. The ACOG outlines suggested protocols for renal dosing in non-dialysis-dependent patients [48].

Strategies to prevent preeclampsia in high-risk individuals include daily low-dose aspirin, ideally started before 16 weeks gestation, as well as high-dose calcium (1 g/day) [50].

Anemia

Iron deficiency anemia may be treated by oral or intravenous supplementation. Intravenous is typically reserved for the second trimester after 13 weeks of gestation [51]. Erythropoietin has a good safety profile [52], though attention should be made to its hypercoagulable side effects. Red blood cell transfusions may be used for severe anemia [50].

Nutrition

To account for the increased protein demands in pregnancy, as well as amino acids, phosphorus, and water soluble vitamins lost in diasylate in intensified hemodialysis regimens, dietary protein should be 1.5–1.8 g/kg/day, diet may be liberalized, including phosphorus, and folic acid supplementation should be at least 5 mg/day [4, 50].

Fetal Surveillance

Given the increased risk of stillbirth, the ACOG recommends consideration of once to twice weekly antenatal fetal surveillance for those with moderate to severe renal disease, with potential increases for those with ESKD on hemodialysis [53].

Postpartum Considerations

In the postpartum period, 6–8 L of total body water will shift from the extravascular to intravascular space, as well as increased sodium excretion due to RAAS-related excess of sodium. Normal daily diuresis in the first 2 weeks postpartum is up to 3000 cc/day. Mechanical and psychological stress place those who make urine at elevated retention. This, in combination with slow correction of the physiologic caliceal dilation, engenders an increased risk of urinary tract infection during the 6–8 weeks after delivery [54].

Target volume status postpartum depends on the patient's desire to breastfeed. Diuresis is one method to suppress lactation [55]; thus, careful consideration should be made to not remove too much fluid. Not a lot of data exists regarding the implications of hemodialysis on the quality of the breastmilk. One case-control study of a lactating woman whose breastmilk was analyzed pre- and post-hemodialysis beginning 10 days postpartum and compared to six healthy age-matched controls demonstrated similar nutrient levels (protein, triglycerides, cholesterol) and immunoglobulins compared to breastmilk of healthy women. There was some suggestion that the electrolyte, creatinine, and urea changes pre- and post-dialysis made lactating post-treatment more favorable [56].

Key Points

- Fertility and pregnancy outcomes have improved for patients on dialysis in recent decades, but risks remain higher than in the general population.
- Intensive hemodialysis regimens of >36 h per week are associated with better pregnancy outcomes.
- Blood pressure should be controlled to <140/90 mmHg using pregnancy-safe medications.
- Diagnosing preeclampsia is challenging in ESKD patients and requires close monitoring.
- Dry weight assessments and dialysis prescriptions need frequent adjustment during pregnancy.

References

1. https://nccd.cdc.gov/ckd/detail.aspx?Qnum=Q68&Strat=Year%2c+Age#refreshPosition.
2. Ahmed SB, Ramesh S. Sex hormones in women with kidney disease. Nephrol Dial Transplant. 2016;31(11):1787–95. https://doi.org/10.1093/ndt/gfw084.
3. Cochrane R, Regan L. Undetected gynaecological disorders in women with renal disease. Hum Reprod. 1997;12(4):667–70. https://doi.org/10.1093/humrep/12.4.667.
4. Tangren J, Nadel M, Hladunewich MA. Pregnancy and end-stage renal disease. Blood Purif. 2018;45(1–3):194–200. https://doi.org/10.1159/000485157. Epub 2018 Jan 26. PMID: 29478065.

5. Matuszkiewicz-Rowińska J, Skórzewska K, Radowicki S, Niemczyk S, Sokalski A, Przedlacki J, Puka J, Świtalski M, Wardyn K, Grochowski J, Ostrowski K. Endometrial morphology and pituitary-gonadal axis dysfunction in women of reproductive age undergoing chronic haemodialysis—a multicentre study. Nephrol Dial Transplant. 2004;19(8):2074–7. https://doi.org/10.1093/ndt/gfh279.
6. Strippoli GF, Collaborative Depression and Sexual Dysfunction (CDS) in Hemodialysis Working Group, Vecchio M, Palmer S, De Berardis G, Craig J, Lucisano G, Johnson D, Pellegrini F, Nicolucci A, Sciancalepore M, Saglimbene V, Gargano L, Bonifati C, Ruospo M, Navaneethan SD, Montinaro V, Stroumza P, Zsom M, Torok M, et al. Sexual dysfunction in women with ESRD requiring hemodialysis. Clin J Am Soc Nephrol. 2012;7(6):974–81. https://doi.org/10.2215/CJN.12601211.
7. Chou J, Kiebalo T, Jagiello P, Pawlaczyk K. Multifaceted sexual dysfunction in dialyzing men and women: pathophysiology, diagnostics, and therapeutics. Life (Basel). 2021;11(4):311. https://doi.org/10.3390/life11040311.
8. Wang GC, Zheng JH, Xu LG, Min ZL, Zhu YH, Qi J, Duan QL. Measurements of serum pituitary-gonadal hormones and investigation of sexual and reproductive functions in kidney transplant recipients. Int J Nephrol. 2010;2010:612126. https://doi.org/10.4061/2010/612126.
9. Confortini P, Galanti G, Ancona G, et al. Full term pregnancy and successful delivery in a patient on chronic haemodialysis. Proc Eur Dial Transplant Assoc. 1971;8:74–80.
10. Shahir AK, Briggs N, Katsoulis J, Levidiotis V. An observational outcomes study from 1966–2008, examining pregnancy and neonatal outcomes from dialysed women using data from the ANZDATA Registry. Nephrology. 2013;18:276–84.
11. Piccoli GB, Minelli F, Versino E, Cabiddu G, Attini R, Vigotti FN, Rolfo A, Giuffrida D, Colombi N, Pani A, Todros T. Pregnancy in dialysis patients in the new millennium: a systematic review and meta-regression analysis correlating dialysis schedules and pregnancy outcomes. Nephrol Dial Transplant. 2016;31(11):1915–34. https://doi.org/10.1093/ndt/gfv395.
12. Sachdeva M, Barta V, Thakkar J, Sakhiya V, Miller I. Pregnancy outcomes in women on hemodialysis: a national survey. Clin Kidney J. 2017;10(2):276–81. https://doi.org/10.1093/ckj/sfw130.
13. Hou SH. Frequency and outcome of pregnancy in women on dialysis. Am J Kidney Dis. 1994;23(1):60–3. https://doi.org/10.1016/s0272-6386(12)80813-4. PMID: 8285199.
14. Hewawasam E, Davies CE, Gulyani A, Li Z, Clayton PA, Sullivan E, McDonald SP, Jesudason S. Factors influencing fertility rates in Australian women receiving kidney replacement therapy: analysis of linked ANZDATA registry and perinatal data over 22 years. Nephrol Dial Transplant. 2022;37(6):1152–61. https://doi.org/10.1093/ndt/gfab157. PMID: 33848341.
15. Bruno Vecchio RC, Del Negro V, Savastano G, Porpora MG, Piccioni MG. Dialysis on pregnancy: an overview. Women. 2021;1(1):60–9. https://doi.org/10.3390/women1010005.
16. Hladunewich MA, Hou S, Odutayo A, Cornelis T, Pierratos A, Goldstein M, Tennankore K, Keunen J, Hui D, Chan CT. Intensive hemodialysis associates with improved pregnancy outcomes: a Canadian and United States cohort comparison. J Am Soc Nephrol. 2014;25(5):1103–9. https://doi.org/10.1681/ASN.2013080825. Epub 2014 Feb 13. PMID: 24525032; PMCID: PMC4005313.
17. Berkane N, Liere P, Oudinet JP, et al. From pregnancy to preeclampsia: a key role for estrogens. Endocr Rev. 2017;38(2):123–44.
18. Conrad KP. Maternal vasodilation in pregnancy: the emerging role of relaxin. Am J Physiol Regul Integr Comp Physiol. 2011;301(2):R267–75.
19. Kodogo V, Azibani F, Sliwa K. Role of pregnancy hormones and hormonal interaction on the maternal cardiovascular system: a literature review. Clin Res Cardiol. 2019;108:831. https://doi.org/10.1007/s00392-019-01441-x.
20. Lumbers ER, Pringle KG. Roles of the circulating renin-angiotensin-aldosterone system in human pregnancy. Am J Physiol Regul Integr Comp Physiol. 2014;306(2):R91–R101.
21. Cheung KL, Lafayette RA. Renal physiology of pregnancy. Adv Chronic Kidney Dis. 2013;20(3):209–14.

22. Bailey RR, Rolleston GL. Kidney length and ureteric dilatation in the puerperium. J Obstet Gynaecol Br Commonw. 1971;78(1):55–61. https://doi.org/10.1111/j.1471-0528.1971.tb00191.x. PMID: 5557675.
23. Ugochinyere IF, Chiamaka NS, Obinna AE, Chukwunyelu AA-M, Amechi AJ. Sonographic assessment of renal volume in normotensive pregnant women and women with pregnancy-induced hypertension in Enugu Metropolis. J Diagn Med Sonogr. 2021;37(5):442–9. https://doi.org/10.1177/87564793211021094.
24. Lin YJ, Ou YC, Tsang LC, Lin H. Diagnostic value of magnetic resonance imaging for successful management of a giant hydronephrosis. J Obstet Gynaecol. 2012;33(1):89–91.
25. Krutzén E, Olofsson P, Bäck SE, Nilsson-Ehle P. Glomerular filtration rate in pregnancy: a study in normal subjects and in patients with hypertension, preeclampsia and diabetes. Scand J Clin Lab Invest. 1992;52(5):387–92. https://doi.org/10.3109/00365519209088374. PMID: 1514017.
26. Davison JM, Hytten FE. The effect of pregnancy on the renal handling of glucose. Br J Obstet Gynaecol. 1975;82(5):374–81. https://doi.org/10.1111/j.1471-0528.1975.tb00652.x. PMID: 1137700.
27. Carlin A, Alfirevic Z. Physiological changes of pregnancy and monitoring. Best Pract Res Clin Obstet Gynaecol. 2008;22(5):801–23. https://doi.org/10.1016/j.bpobgyn.2008.06.005. Epub 2008 Aug 28. PMID: 18760680.
28. American College of Obstetricians and Gynecologists' Committee on Practice Bulletins—Obstetrics. Anemia in pregnancy: ACOG practice bulletin, number 233. Obstet Gynecol. 2021;138(2):e55–64. https://doi.org/10.1097/AOG.0000000000004477. PMID: 34293770.
29. Pitkin RM. Calcium metabolism in pregnancy: a review. Am J Obstet Gynecol. 1975;121(5):724–37. https://doi.org/10.1016/0002-9378(75)90481-0. PMID: 1090175.
30. Piccoli GB, Cabiddu G, Attini R, Vigotti FN, Maxia S, Lepori N, Tuveri M, Massidda M, Marchi C, Mura S, Coscia A, Biolcati M, Gaglioti P, Nichelatti M, Pibiri L, Chessa G, Pani A, Todros T. Risk of adverse pregnancy outcomes in women with CKD. J Am Soc Nephrol. 2015;26(8):2011–22. https://doi.org/10.1681/ASN.2014050459. Epub 2015 Mar 12. PMID: 25766536; PMCID: PMC4520166.
31. Zhang JJ, Ma XX, Hao L, Liu LJ, Lv JC, Zhang H. A systematic review and meta-analysis of outcomes of pregnancy in CKD and CKD outcomes in pregnancy. Clin J Am Soc Nephrol. 2015;10(11):1964–78. https://doi.org/10.2215/CJN.09250914. Epub 2015 Oct 20. PMID: 26487769; PMCID: PMC4633792.
32. Kominiarek MA, Rajan P. Nutrition recommendations in pregnancy and lactation. Med Clin North Am. 2016;100(6):1199–215. https://doi.org/10.1016/j.mcna.2016.06.004. PMID: 27745590; PMCID: PMC5104202.
33. Moore Simas TA, Waring ME, Sullivan GM, Liao X, Rosal MC, Hardy JR, Berry RE Jr. Institute of Medicine 2009 gestational weight gain guideline knowledge: survey of obstetrics/gynecology and family medicine residents of the United States. Birth. 2013;40(4):237–46. https://doi.org/10.1111/birt.12061. PMID: 24344704; PMCID: PMC3974574.
34. Arai H, Mori KP, Yokoi H, et al. Intensified hemodialysis for complicated pregnancy in a primigravida with advanced maternal age: a case report with literature review focusing on appropriate hemodialysis management during pregnancy. Ren Replace Ther. 2020;6:47. https://doi.org/10.1186/s41100-020-00296-7.
35. Shahnazi M, Sayyah Meli M, Hamoony F, Sadrimehr F, Ghatre Samani F, Koshavar H. The effects of intravenous hydration on amniotic fluid volume and pregnancy outcomes in women with term pregnancy and oligohydramnios: a randomized clinical trial. J Caring Sci. 2012;1(3):123–8. https://doi.org/10.5681/jcs.2012.018. PMID: 25276686; PMCID: PMC4161079.
36. Singh K, Sikka P, Suri V, Prasad R, Khullar M, Vijayvergiya R. Brain natriuretic peptide in pregnant women with heart disease. Obstet Med. 2020;13(1):25–9. https://doi.org/10.1177/1753495X18819351. Epub 2019 Feb 2. PMID: 32284729; PMCID: PMC7133100.

37. Tanous D, Siu SC, Mason J, Greutmann M, Wald RM, Parker JD, Sermer M, Colman JM, Silversides CK. B-type natriuretic peptide in pregnant women with heart disease. J Am Coll Cardiol. 2010;56(15):1247–53. https://doi.org/10.1016/j.jacc.2010.02.076. PMID: 20883932.
38. Elkayam U. Clinical characteristics of peripartum cardiomyopathy in the United States: diagnosis, prognosis, and management. J Am Coll Cardiol. 2011;58(7):659–70. https://doi.org/10.1016/j.jacc.2011.03.047. PMID: 21816300.
39. Barua M, Hladunewich M, Keunen J, Pierratos A, McFarlane P, Sood M, Chan CT. Successful pregnancies on nocturnal home hemodialysis. Clin J Am Soc Nephrol. 2008;3:392–6.
40. Asamiya Y, Otsubo S, Matsuda Y, Kimata N, Kikuchi K, Miwa N, Uchida K, Mineshima M, Mitani M, Ohta H, Nitta K, Akiba T. The importance of low blood urea nitrogen levels in pregnant patients undergoing hemodialysis to optimize birth weight and gestational age. Kidney Int. 2009;75:1217–22.
41. Haase M, Morgera S, Bamberg C, Halle H, Martini S, Hocher B, Diekmann F, Dragun D, Peters H, Neumayer HH, Budde K. A systematic approach to managing pregnant dialysis patients—the importance of an intensified haemodiafiltration protocol. Nephrol Dial Transplant. 2005;20:2537–42.
42. Hladunewich MA, Hou S, Odutayo A, Cornelis T, Pierratos A, Goldstein M, Tennankore K, Keunen J, Hui D, Chan CT. Intensive hemodialysis associates with improved pregnancy outcomes: a Canadian and United States cohort comparison. J Am Soc Nephrol. 2014;25:1103–9.
43. Braunthal S, Brateanu A. Hypertension in pregnancy: pathophysiology and treatment. SAGE Open Med. 2019;7:2050312119843700. https://doi.org/10.1177/2050312119843700. PMID: 31007914; PMCID: PMC6458675.
44. Tita AT, Szychowski JM, Boggess K, Dugoff L, Sibai B, Lawrence K, Hughes BL, Bell J, Aagaard K, Edwards RK, Gibson K, Haas DM, Plante L, Metz T, Casey B, Esplin S, Longo S, Hoffman M, Saade GR, Hoppe KK, Foroutan J, Tuuli M, Owens MY, Simhan HN, Frey H, Rosen T, Palatnik A, Baker S, August P, Reddy UM, Kinzler W, Su E, Krishna I, Nguyen N, Norton ME, Skupski D, El-Sayed YY, Ogunyemi D, Galis ZS, Harper L, Ambalavanan N, Geller NL, Oparil S, Cutter GR, Andrews WW, Chronic Hypertension and Pregnancy (CHAP) Trial Consortium. Treatment for mild chronic hypertension during pregnancy. N Engl J Med. 2022;386(19):1781–92. https://doi.org/10.1056/NEJMoa2201295. PMID: 35363951.
45. SMFM_Statement_CHAP_draft_April_2022.pdf (elsevierhealth.com).
46. American College of Obstetricians and Gynecologists' Committee on Practice Bulletins—Obstetrics. ACOG practice bulletin no. 203: chronic hypertension in pregnancy. Obstet Gynecol. 2019;133(1):e26–50. https://doi.org/10.1097/AOG.0000000000003020. PMID: 30575676.
47. Kearney L, Wright P, Fhadil S, Thomas M. Postpartum cardiomyopathy and considerations for breastfeeding. Card Fail Rev. 2018;4(2):112–8. https://doi.org/10.15420/cfr.2018.21.2. PMID: 30206487; PMCID: PMC6125711.
48. Gestational hypertension and preeclampsia: ACOG practice bulletin summary, number 222. Obstet Gynecol. 2020;135(6):1492–95. https://doi.org/10.1097/AOG.0000000000003892. PMID: 32443077.
49. Wiles K, Chappell LC, Lightstone L, Bramham K. Updates in diagnosis and management of preeclampsia in women with CKD. Clin J Am Soc Nephrol. 2020;15(9):1371–80. https://doi.org/10.2215/CJN.15121219. Epub 2020 Apr 2. PMID: 32241779; PMCID: PMC7480554.
50. Hui D, Hladunewich MA. Chronic kidney disease and pregnancy. Obstet Gynecol. 2019;133(6):1182–94. https://doi.org/10.1097/AOG.0000000000003256. PMID: 31135733.
51. Achebe MM, Gafter-Gvili A. How I treat anemia in pregnancy: iron, cobalamin, and folate. Blood. 2017;129(8):940–9. https://doi.org/10.1182/blood-2016-08-672246. Epub 2016 Dec 29. PMID: 28034892.
52. Sienas L, Wong T, Collins R, Smith J. Contemporary uses of erythropoietin in pregnancy: a literature review. Obstet Gynecol Surv. 2013;68(8):594–602. https://doi.org/10.1097/OGX.0b013e3182a2d51c. PMID: 23921673.
53. Indications for outpatient antenatal fetal surveillance. Obstet Gynecol. 2021;137(6):e177–97. https://doi.org/10.1097/AOG.0000000000004407.

54. Chauhan G, Tadi P. Physiology, postpartum changes. In: StatPearls. Treasure Island, FL: StatPearls Publishing; 2022. https://www.ncbi.nlm.nih.gov/books/NBK555904/.
55. Cominos DC, van der Walt A, van Rooyen AJ. Suppression of postpartum lactation with furosemide. S Afr Med J. 1976;50(8):251–2. PMID: 3858.
56. Balzer MS, Gross MM, Lichtinghagen R, Haller H, Schmitt R. Got milk? Breastfeeding and milk analysis of a mother on chronic hemodialysis. PLoS One. 2015;10(11):e0143340. https://doi.org/10.1371/journal.pone.0143340. PMID: 26571490; PMCID: PMC4646653.

International Applications of Home Hemodialysis: Barriers and How They Can Be Overcome

15

Jordan Thorne, David Clark, and Karthik Tennankore

Introduction

With its advent in the 1960s, home hemodialysis (HHD) has long been an option for patients with kidney failure. HHD is defined as hemodialysis performed in the home environment by patients or paid/unpaid caregivers. HHD allows for treatment flexibility both in the frequency (days/week) and duration of therapy [1]. Both conventional HHD prescriptions (typically 3 times/week for 4 h each session) and intensive prescriptions (short daily, long, long-frequent, and nocturnal) exist [2]. Irrespective of the schedule, patients receiving HHD have been shown to have either similar or superior patient-important outcomes compared with peritoneal dialysis (PD) or facility-based hemodialysis. These benefits include facilitation of employment or a reduction in weekly commute times [3]. Whether it is fostering patient independence or tailoring prescriptions to a patient's lifestyle, home dialysis modalities have been demonstrated to improve overall patient quality of life compared to facility-based hemodialysis [4].

While advantageous, HHD does present many challenges, especially as patients adapt to being independent for their care at home. Perhaps most crucially, thus far HHD has not been demonstrated as a sustainable long-term dialysis option in many lower income countries. This is explained by many factors, including policy and governmental roadblocks and a lack of adequate reimbursement and incentives to providers. There is also an inevitable up-front increased cost that is borne by the patient as they initiate HHD, that without reimbursement and community support,

J. Thorne
Department of Medicine, Dalhousie University and Nova Scotia Health, Halifax, NS, Canada
e-mail: jordan.thorne@nshealth.ca

D. Clark · K. Tennankore (✉)
Department of Medicine, Dalhousie University and Nova Scotia Health, Halifax, NS, Canada

Division of Nephrology, Nova Scotia Health, Halifax, NS, Canada
e-mail: david.clark@nshealth.ca; karthikk.tennankore@nshealth.ca

A. Shah et al. (eds.), *Applied Home Hemodialysis*,
https://doi.org/10.1007/978-3-031-77244-3_15

deters many patients. In addition, there are a paucity of formal legislation and government incentive programs designed to encourage HHD implementation, particularly in lower income countries. Policy aside, HHD continues to be a relatively unfamiliar option for many patients with kidney failure. In addition, patients themselves may be hesitant to adopt HHD due to a number of factors including concerns about how to manage technical challenges, a fear of catastrophic events, a desire to avoid overmedicalization of the home, and a perception that adoption of HHD will lead to isolation from nearby medical support. Patient-perceived barriers to HHD are made even more significant when considering the gaps in education for providers. Many nephrology fellowship programs provide little exposure to HHD either through didactic training or hands-on care of patients receiving HHD. In addition to patient and provider barriers, infrastructure requirements for HHD also deter HHD growth across countries and contribute to the disparity of access globally. These include limited space in the home to store equipment safely, limited access to a quality water source, and difficulties providing enough energy to sustain HHD.

While these challenges may impair the adoption of HHD across the world, there are potential solutions that can be gleaned from HHD programs that have been successful. Education gaps can be addressed by formal pre-dialysis education programs, training supports for patients and their caregivers, as well as increased supports for patients during their initial transition home. Concerns around the risk of adverse events may be alleviated through patient and provider education around the safety of HHD, the use of novel HHD technological support, and respite programs designed to provide support to HHD patients and their caregivers in times of need. Finally, there is a need to focus on changes to policy and the provision of incentives to maximize the use of HHD, and these changes need to consider novel ways to maintain environmental sustainability.

This chapter will discuss international applications of HHD, reviewing the current barriers that make HHD implementation more challenging and the unique and emerging approaches different regions have taken to address these barriers. Furthermore, we will highlight current or evolving efforts to address the lack of international growth of HHD as a viable treatment option for patients with kidney failure. Finally, we will summarize this chapter with a framework for nephrologists and policymakers who wish to expand HHD access, particularly in regions without established programs, drawing on expert opinion and existing literature. The recent COVID-19 pandemic has demonstrated the risks of exposing vulnerable kidney failure patients to facility-based dialysis, where highly communicable infections can severely impact the health of dialysis patients [5]. As the global population continues to live longer and kidney failure continues to become more prevalent, the international demand for dialysis will continue to grow, and supporting HHD expansion will be of critical importance.

Global Prevalence of HHD

The prevalence of kidney failure continues to rise, and it is estimated that 14.5 million individuals will require kidney replacement therapy by 2030 [6]. Hemodialysis (especially facility-based hemodialysis) continues to dominate, and although the incidence of dialysis use has remained stable or slightly decreased in high-income countries, it has been increasing in low-middle-income countries [7]. However, while the prevalence of kidney failure has increased globally [8], the use of HHD has lagged behind. Historically, HHD was a prevailing treatment option, in the face of a smaller total dialysis population. In the United States, HHD use was as high as 40% (in the 1970s), but this has since fallen to 1% over the last several years [9]. Worldwide, the distribution of dialysis modalities varies significantly, with countries such as New Zealand, Australia, and France leading the way at approximately 8–13% HHD use as a proportion of prevalent dialysis therapy [10, 11]. In addition to the fact that HHD is more commonly used in higher income countries, there is a trend to higher HHD uptake in countries with nationalized health services, or single-payer systems [12]. However, outside of Australia and New Zealand, the global prevalence of HHD is considerably lower. In an international survey study, 45% (69/154) of countries reported that HHD was available in most (≥50% of centers) or some (<50% of centers) and unavailable in 55%, but the proportions were even lower in low-income countries [13]. In the most recent United States Renal Data System (USRDS) report comparing the international prevalence of dialysis modalities, no participating country had a prevalent use of 10% or more [10] and many reported that no patients were receiving HHD. Overall, despite the benefits, HHD remains largely underutilized across most countries.

Educational Barriers to Home Hemodialysis and Potential Solutions

Patient-Focused

To prepare patients for HHD, physicians and nurses need to foster patient and caregiver independence, as there are many insecurities patients can understandably experience when transitioning home. Patients may be intimidated by the technical complexity of HHD machinery, have a fear of cannulation or vascular access, or be concerned about making mistakes in technique leading to severe adverse events [14]. Given the variability in comfort patients may experience when transitioning home, a program individually tailored to one's concerns is ideal. There have been many efforts to better characterize the HHD patient experience. One example includes Kidney Care UK's Annual Patient Reported Measures (PREM) reports, which help interdisciplinary nephrology teams better understand patient experiences, and identify improvements that can be made from a patient's perspective. The 2020 PREM Report [15] identified patient communication, the need for shared decision-making, and increased support as the areas most in need of improvement for HHD. While these are relevant to all kidney failure patients, patients on HHD face unique challenges compared to those undergoing facility-based hemodialysis [16]. As a result, there must be an emphasis on effective pre-dialysis HHD education followed by a robust support system for patients once they are independent at home.

It is well established that predialysis patient education around modality options is lacking. Even in a more contemporary survey of patients (from 2017 to 2019) conducted in Europe, 25% received no information on dialysis modalities prior to dialysis initiation. Even more concerning was the discrepancy in patient-perceived education prior to the initiation of kidney replacement therapy. Overall, a total of 42% felt they received no information on HHD, but this ranged from a high of 52% in lower GDP countries to a low of 27% in higher GDP countries. This, coupled with the observation that those from low-GDP countries had less satisfaction with their dialysis treatment [17], suggests that there may be an unmet need. Respondents to this survey also emphasized the impact both family members and allied health professionals have on their eventual treatment of choice, further supporting the use of a shared decision model (SDM) in pre-dialysis education. Pre-dialysis SDM's often involve patient decision aids that, while variable in the scope and description [18], promote patient autonomy in making healthcare decisions [19]. SDM use in pre-dialysis education is being studied in multiple clinical trials taking place across the United States, including the feasibility of enhanced dialysis education intervention for chronic kidney disease patients (CKD-EDU) trial [20], and the shared decision-making in dialysis (DIAL-SDM) trial [21].

Acknowledging that the provision of education is a major determinant of dialysis choice, comprehensive pre-dialysis education must include options for home dialysis. Principles such as "home first," (as stated by the National Kidney Foundation–Kidney Disease Outcomes Quality Initiative), may be helpful to frame pre-dialysis modality discussions [22]. In addition, pre-dialysis education programs continue to be used with success across nephrology programs internationally (Fig. 15.1). One example is the GUIDE program in the Netherlands, a structured pre-dialysis program that has been shown to increase rates of home dialysis [23]. This program begins with Category 4 CKD patients and includes a home visit from a social worker, followed by assessments of the patient's values, functional status, and social supports to identify a form of renal replacement therapy best suited for them. Programs such as these are crucial to increase awareness toward HHD, as this modality often aligns with the desire of patients to maintain freedom and flexibility and to minimize travel for dialysis.

One of the major contributors to the lack of education about dialysis modality options relates to the timing of dialysis and the presence or absence of predialysis care. Patients experiencing unplanned dialysis initiation have been shown to be less likely to transition to HHD [24]. This is where transitional care units (TCU) may help to facilitate the transition to HHD. TCUs are specialized facility-based hemodialysis units staffed with an allied health team trained in providing home dialysis modality training. Focusing on incident dialysis patients, TCUs typically consist of a structured program ranging on the order of weeks to a few months, where patients

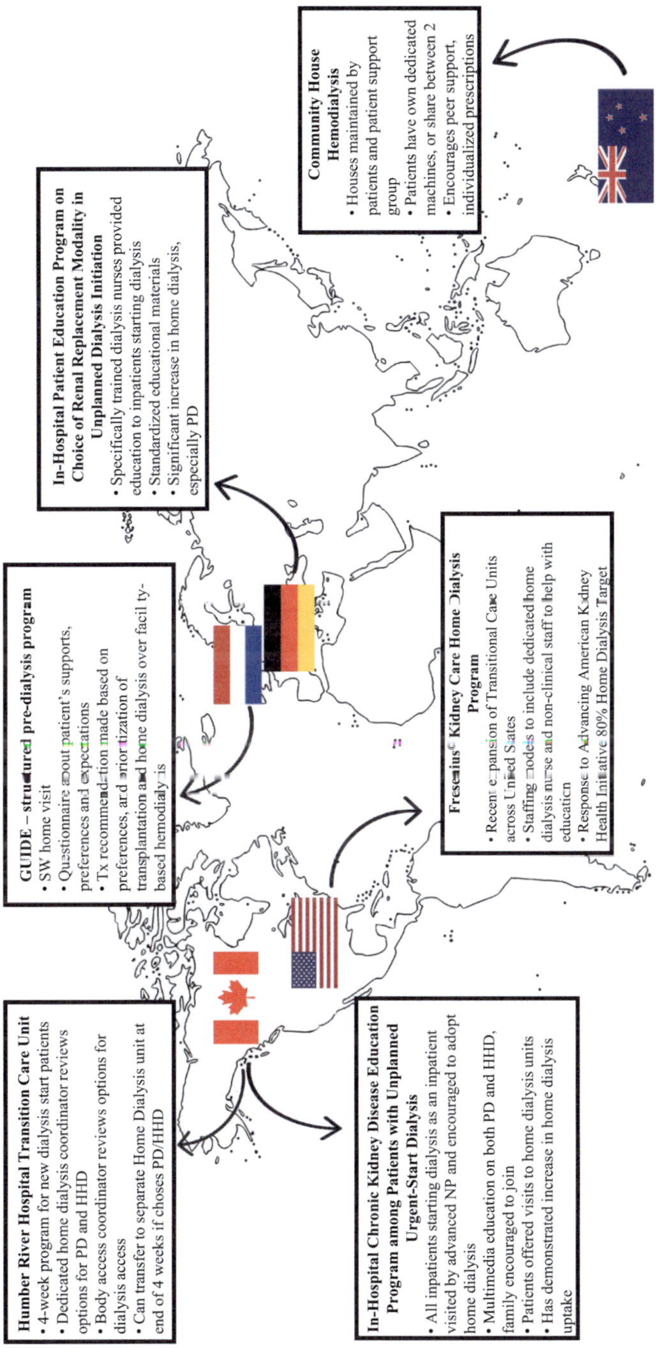

Fig. 15.1 International approaches to HHD promotion and patient support. *PD* peritoneal dialysis, *HHD* home hemodialysis

learn the skills required to begin HHD and develop the confidence to do so along the way [25]. TCU programs have been demonstrated as a tool that, in combination with peer support programs, can increase home dialysis uptake, especially in a population of unplanned dialysis starts [26]. In addition to TCUs, inpatient education programs directed to those who are still in hospital after initiating chronic hemodialysis in an unplanned fashion are also valuable at enhancing the uptake of HHD. In Canada, one example of an acute inpatient education program resulted in significantly less patients remaining on in-center hemodialysis and an increase in home dialysis uptake [27]. This program used nurse practitioners to encourage home dialysis options to inpatients undergoing new dialysis starts and incorporated personal support persons in the discussion as well.

In addition to direct education, the importance of preserving a patient's personal support network is crucial. One such example is Community House Hemodialysis in New Zealand [28]. Specifically designed for communities that have more socioeconomic barriers to HHD, this community house model encourages autonomy while maintaining patient support through the use of peers. Community houses offer a private space where patients have access to their own machines, while simultaneously allowing interaction between individuals. These models may be more supportive to HHD utilization for some cultures. One further example of efforts to engage patients in their own communities includes the Waswanipi Home Hemodialysis Pilot Program in Quebec, Canada. This program focuses on a Cree community with a population of 1400, where kidney failure patients must travel 7 h round trip by car to the nearest dialysis center. Participants receive a 2-week intensive HHD education program before being provided with equipment and virtual support. In more rural communities, this offers the potential to save many hours of patient time, as well as valuable transportation resources [29].

Provider-Focused

While standardized patient and peer support programs can increase patient comfort with HHD, there is also a need for provider education. Recent surveys of American Nephrology fellows revealed trainees lack confidence with home dialysis, especially HHD [30]. Less than half of the trainees felt comfortable with HHD competencies, including writing and adjusting prescription, vascular access, water quality, and machine knowledge. Only 59% of trainees regularly attended a home dialysis continuity clinic, where HHD also appears to be underrepresented. Three-quarters of trainees indicated their clinics contained patients only on PD or mostly on PD, but only a paucity included HHD. In a qualitative study, nephrologists recognized their lack of knowledge, fears, and concerns about home dialysis and how these concerns influenced patient modality selection [31]. Similarly, knowledge about HHD as a viable treatment option for patients with social or medical barriers is limited for other nephrology care practitioners. In a survey of facility-based dialysis nurses, facility-based nurses felt that facility-based hemodialysis was preferred for patients of lower socioeconomic status, limited education, advanced age, those without English as their primary language, and those without social supports. This was in stark contrast to the views of home dialysis nurses, who overwhelmingly supported PD or HHD options [32].

How might these misperceptions of patient eligibility and concerns be alleviated? The development of novel training programs that combine expert knowledge from a variety of Nephrology programs to engage providers on innovations in HHD may be a viable solution. One example of this is Project Extension for Community Healthcare Outcome (ECHO) [33], which is an educational model that uses videoconferencing to connect care providers from across the United States. This platform uses a virtual curriculum that focuses on home dialysis management through a variety of case-based examples. Virtual curricula focusing on home dialysis are not only more easily accessible to learners, it can also be used in the education and development of allied health staff. Incorporating physicians, dialysis nurses, technicians, and social workers in case-based learning focusing on clinical scenarios ranging from vascular access to the management of site infections can improve both the knowledge and staff (at a programmatic level) in regions far removed from these expert hubs.

While expanding upon the knowledge base of providers at established home dialysis programs is important for ongoing patient recruitment, there also exists a need to educate practitioners without formal programs about how to start their own programs. One example of this is the explore home dialysis (EHD) program, created by the University Health Network in Toronto, Ontario, Canada. This immersive experiential learning program is focused on exposing physicians, educators, and nurses from various international backgrounds to a curriculum focused on home dialysis clinical encounters, core curriculum teaching, simulation, and concept testing [34]. Programs such as EHD are critical to provide nephrologists, administrators, and policymakers with the skills to develop a program from the ground up.

Finally, it is also imperative to educate other nephrology care providers who may be exposed to patients wishing to transition to HHD but are not otherwise deemed eligible. In a small continuing nurses education initiative that focused on barriers to home dialysis and how to overcome them (including assisted home dialysis, modified HHD prescriptions, and novel aids to help patients with physical disabilities), perceptions shifted such that more nurses were in favor of home dialysis when given a list of perceived barriers [35]. Therefore, with the appropriate staff education, it would be expected that more patients would be identified as potentially eligible, further increasing the probability of patients transitioning to HHD.

Understanding the Cost of HHD

Acknowledging the disproportionate amount of health care funding allocated toward kidney failure across nations, the cost and cost-effectiveness of dialysis therapy continue to be a key issue for countries worldwide [36]. In reviewing the economic assessment of dialysis modalities, an important consideration is the perspective taken for analyses, (either that of the patient, healthcare provider, or payer) [37], and the country in which the analysis was conducted. In the developed world, HHD is more cost-effective compared with facility-based HD, corroborated by robust economic reviews [38–41]. However, substantial global variation in the reimbursement of dialysis expenses has limited the generalizability of conclusions drawn from economic reviews conducted in higher income countries. This is compounded by the fact that there are a paucity of robust economic evaluations of dialysis care (including HHD) in lower income countries [36, 37, 40].

Thus far, most economic analyses of HHD performed in developed countries have examined the costs of providing this therapy from the payer perspective. Despite variability in analytic approaches and results, it is collectively agreed that HHD is less costly than facility-based HD given the need for fewer human resources and lower facility management expenses [39, 40, 42–46]. Other trended differences in both direct and indirect dialysis costs (comparing HHD to facility-based HD) have been reported [47–53]; Table 15.1 summarises some economic analyses of HHD programs within Canada [38–43, 46–48, 52, 53] serving as but one example of a developed nation with a single-payer universal healthcare system that funds all dialysis care. Cost benefits of HHD over facility-based HD as reported in developed nations are often contingent on elapsed therapy time [38–40, 49–52]. Facility-based hemodialysis costs are stable over time, as the cost to provide hemodialysis in a center is relatively constant. Kidney-specific medications, human resources, hospitalizations, consumables, and facility costs are the primary cost drivers for facility-based hemodialysis. Conventional HHD and intensive/frequent HHD costs in year

Table 15.1 Trended differences in both direct and indirect dialysis costs in Canada: comparing conventional facility-based hemodialysis and HHD [38–43, 46–48, 52, 53]

Dialysis cost	Conventional facility-based hemodialysis (thrice weekly)	Home hemodialysis[a]	
		Conventional (thrice weekly)	Intensive/ frequent
Direct			
Machine, scales, chairs	+	+	+
Consumables/supplies	+	+	++
Patient training	N/A	+++	+++
Human resources (nursing, technician, social work, dietician, etc.)	+++	+	+
Renal medications	++	++	+
Dialysis monitoring and laboratory costs	+	+	+
Facility costs	+++	+	+
Home renovations	N/A	++	++
Utility costs	+	+	++
Hospitalization	++	++	+
Indirect[b]			
Transportation to/from dialysis	++	N/A	N/A
Lost productivity (patient and/ or caregiver)	+++	++	+

[a] Conventional machine/equipment platforms
[b] Assumed trends; identified area of need for further study

1 are greater than those in subsequent years, as the costs of HHD reduce in subsequent years after capital investments and training have been paid for, highlighting the importance of patient selection and avoidance of early technique failure. Conventional and frequent HHD costs are driven by kidney-specific medications, capital investment (machines, home renovations), patient training, and consumables (more for frequent HHD) [38–40].

To date, there remains a paucity of data on the economic effect of dialysis modalities as analyzed from the patients' perspective [37]. Varied types of healthcare coverage provided within/across nations are again a source of considerable heterogeneity for the personal financial impact of dialysis on patients. For patients undergoing HHD, relevant reported costs include expenses incurred during training and ongoing utility costs (i.e., water and electricity) [53, 54], which can represent a substantial cost burden if transferred to the patient and not otherwise funded by the provider program [53]. A lack of reimbursement for assumed out-of-pocket HHD costs has been identified as both unjust and a deterrent for patient selection of HHD [55, 56]. Other gaps in the literature include the impact on employment in the household and attendant economics when a patient performs HHD, as well as averted costs of recurring transportation [54]. In general, HHD is assumed to increase home and workforce productivity and reduce transportation costs borne by patients or their families as compared with facility-based HD [38].

Appreciating that costs are an issue when considering HHD as a treatment option, the use of economic incentives to increase the use of HHD, including those directed toward patients and nephrologists is a continued area of study. Several countries have implemented reimbursement programs to offset patient disincentives of HHD where they may exist within their respective funding models for dialysis care. Notable examples include subsidies for water or electricity costs in select Canadian Provinces [53, 56], Australian States [57], and opportunities for patients to apply for subsidy programs to offset patient-borne costs of HHD in France [42]. Although it is unknown if the practice of providing subsidies to patients to cover such costs increases the use of HHD, it is of collective global opinion by HHD experts and health economists that such subsidies should exist to avoid unjust inequities related to patient costs of dialysis care [53, 56]. Similarly, in lieu of the uncertainty regarding the impact of physician remuneration on the use of HHD (owing to a lack of controlled trial evidence and significant heterogeneity in how nephrologists are remunerated) international consensus suggests that physician reimbursement for HHD be equitable to facility-based hemodialysis [42].

Understanding the impact of funding model structure on the use of HHD is made difficult by both significant global variation and sheer number of existing models for reimbursement of dialysis care [36, 42, 58]. Example funding models for dialysis care in high-income nations include the provision of global budgets (fixed amount of funding per dialysis facility), fee-for-service (payment for each service), activity-based funding (payments based on the number and type of dialysis patients and expected resource consumption), pay-for-performance (payments based on meeting care targets, quality, or safety) or a mixture of methods [58]. Of these options, limited evidence exists for the activity-based funding model to facilitate the implementation of best kidney care practices, including the expansion of HHD [59]. However, local socioeconomic, environmental, and funding lever factors are all presumed to impact the success of funding models to permit increased use of HHD, and therefore may vary considerably across jurisdictions [42].

Acknowledging the varied payment systems for dialysis worldwide, and that payers may have difficulty synthesizing the published literature to ascertain local relevancy; Komenda and colleagues [40] detailed costing models which highlight the component cost drivers of HHD versus other dialysis modalities. These models may serve to address variability in costs that exist across countries; decision-makers can adjust component costs accordingly if attempting to use the model to estimate costs in their own setting. Such information could then be used to inform coverage policy development, especially if developing payment systems that encourage HHD [40].

Policy and HHD: Roadblocks Beyond Cost

The discontinuation rate of HHD among patients has been reported at almost 25% after 1 year [60], and there are barriers that legislation can address beyond cost to improve both the uptake and maintenance of HHD. In the United States, for example, there is ongoing advocacy to improve HHD patient quality of life. These include efforts to provide family leave for patients, to support family members to undergo HHD training, and to facilitate mobile phlebotomy units to prevent time-consuming visits to facility-based clinics [61]. In addition, there is a need to further support telehealth modalities for home dialysis patients. In 2018, the United States Senate's Creating High-Quality Results and Outcomes Necessary to Improve Chronic (CHRONIC) Care Act attempted to address financial and infrastructural barriers to telehealth through changes to Medicare reimbursement policy [62]. Outside of the United States, efforts to change policy to support HHD uptake vary from country to country. In Hong Kong for example, while a PD-first policy has been in place since 1985 and has been successful in reducing the expensive costs of facility-based hemodialysis, incentives to choose HHD have been driven by local health authorities rather than regional legislation [63]. In Singapore, tiered subsidy programs have been designed to increase home dialysis uptake, along with specific promotional community programs and the funding of community patient outreach support programs to encourage HHD [63]. While government support varies globally, a focus on incentivizing patients and providers to choose HHD must go beyond cost. Supporting patients to take the necessary time for training and follow-up care and facilitating the involvement of support persons in the care of HHD patients is needed to further ease the transition from training to treatment.

Infrastructure and Natural Resources

While HHD has been shown to be more cost-effective compared to facility-based hemodialysis [38], there are still significant resource considerations that must be discussed prior to initiation. These pertain to the need for reliable infrastructure patients require to successfully undergo HHD including water and access to a reliable source of energy. This includes access to a power grid capable of providing 2–5 kWh of energy consumption and large volumes of clean water per treatment [53]. In addition, these supplies must be reliable. Even with modern plumbing and a stable municipal electrical and water supply, supplementation with backup generators, booster pumps for feed waterlines and thermostatic mixing valves may be required to meet HHD technical requirements [64]. As a result, novel technologies to address these barriers and the evolving carbon footprint [65] have emerged to facilitate more sustainable HHD. In particular, the amount of water required for hemodialysis is significant, especially if drawing from a smaller municipal source. Approximately 60–90% of "source water" (drinking-quality water) is rejected through the generation of high-purity dialysis water. With hemodialysis machines requiring an average of 150 L of dialysis water, this leads to clean water requirements exceeding the range of 500 L per treatment [66].

Decreasing water consumption with HHD would not only reduce the need for patients to access municipal water supply but would also reduce costs associated with retrofitting homes with the necessary purification and storage facilities. The need to purify a municipal water source has led to the development of reverse osmosis systems for HHD that remove metals and microbes through pumping water at high pressures across a semipermeable membrane [66]. This water treatment process is unfortunately quite inefficient, resulting in over three-quarters of the consumed water being discarded as waste [53]. As a result, more recent HHD systems such as the NxStage System One™ and PureFlow™ have aimed for slower dialysate rates, requiring less purified water, or, alternatively, pre-mixed dialysate fluid bags that avoid the need for a water source. The NxStage System One™ and PureFlow™ perform "water-efficient" dialysis, running slower flow rates of 100–300 mL over longer runs of 6–8 h. This creates a more compact and potentially affordable platform for HHD [67]. However, while the potential benefits of lower flow dialysate systems are evident in terms of water consumption, ensuring adequate clearance may require higher dialysate flow and/or more frequent or longer treatments. Furthermore, although pre-mixed dialysate bags may avoid issues of water contamination or lack of water to support HHD, they come with an additional cost that may not be easily supported on a large scale, especially for lower income countries.

While lower flow HHD systems are more efficient, there remains significant dialysis-derived water that is treated as "waste." This includes predialysis effluent known as "reject water" from the reverse osmosis treatment process, and spent dialysate effluent that has passed through the dialysis system [68]. In recognition of this loss of water, there has been a recent initiative to recycle dialysis effluent. In particular, spent dialysis water may have agricultural benefits [69]. One example of the application of effluent recycling in a rural setting exists in the Australian Outback in Kiwirrkurra. In this particular indigenous community, rejected water from community dialysis hubs is collected in large plastic tanks and delivered to residential gardens [70]. This process has even contributed to the local economy, creating employment opportunities for locals.

Ideally, a process that is "waste-free" would be available, and this is where novel solutions such as sorbent dialysis may play a role. Sorbent dialysis technology consists of a water-free cartridge containing activated charcoal, urease, and zirconium compounds that is completely self-contained and requires no water source [71]. While the described mechanism at its core is over 50 years old [72], its application toward a potential portable, compact and sustainable home dialysis modality has led to a resurgence in the form of "wearable" or "portable" artificial kidneys (WAK and PAK). Groups in the United States, Switzerland, and Netherlands have been working on clinical trials using sorbent dialysis technology in cartridges on belts or in rolling suitcases prioritizing flexible treatment regimens and portability [73] (Fig. 15.2).

Prioritizing more sustainable water practices should also align with an overall goal of delivering environmentally sustainable HHD, especially given its significant associated carbon footprint. Connor and colleagues identified that traditional HHD systems produced more greenhouse gas emissions than facility-based hemodialysis [77], and only with NxStage™ systems with low flow rates and longer run times were emissions comparable to conventional HD. This study took into account a variety of factors in estimating total emissions, including staff and patient travel, material consumption, construction, waste management and even follow-up appointments. The notion that HHD carries potentially a larger carbon footprint than facility-based HD has led to a variety of strategies to reduce emissions including expanded use of solar-powered hemodialysis. Besides the environmental impact, groups in Australia have demonstrated that solar-assisted group HHD hubs can decrease energy consumption and lower costs by over 75% [78] (Fig. 15.2). In addition, professional societies in Australia and New Zealand have developed The Green Nephrology Action Team [79], which provides information to patients and providers highlighting waste reduction, sustainable water consumption, and alternative power sources. To summarize, emerging technologies that aim to reduce the required water resources or utilize other forms of power (i.e., solar energy) may support further growth of HHD, especially in countries where these resources issues prevail. However, if the costs of these newer technologies are prohibitive, expansion will not occur.

Conclusion and Future Directions

Drawing on the barriers that prevent the growth of HHD across the globe, it is imperative to develop and design a systematic approach, focused on expanding the utilization of home dialysis. In an International roundtable meeting, several key

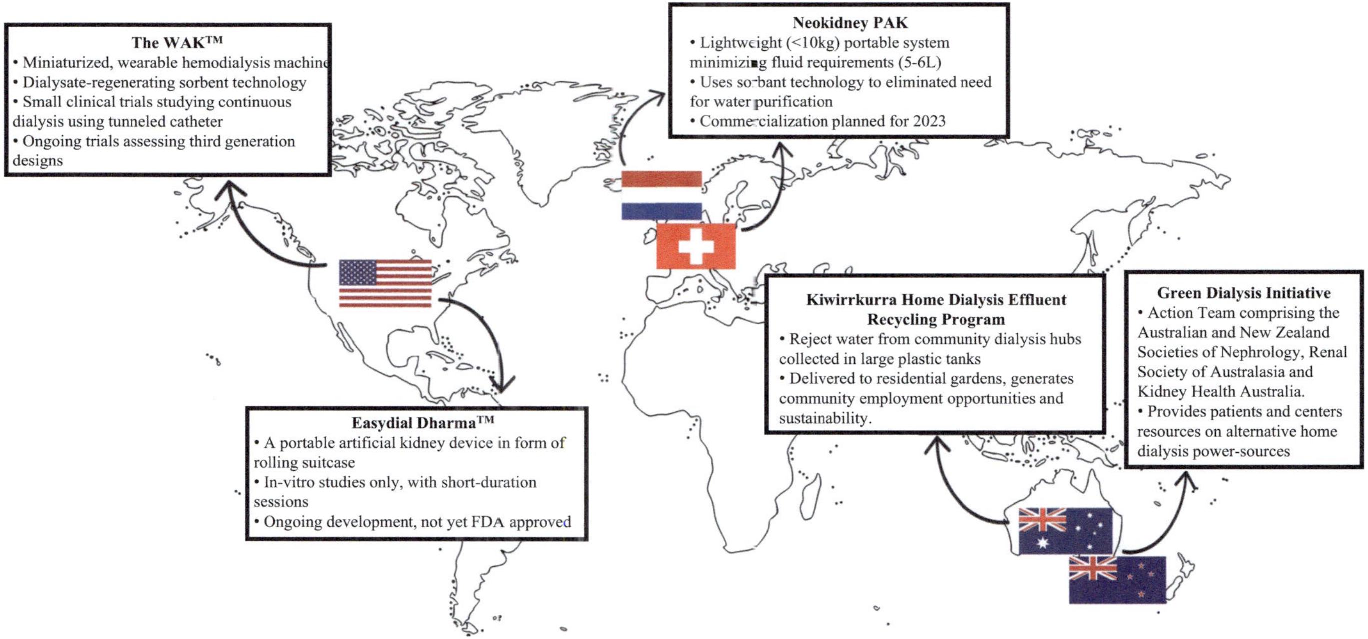

Fig. 15.2 International approaches to natural resource conservation and HHD technological innovation. *WAK* wearable artificial kidney, *PAK* portable artificial kidney

action items were identified as critical to improve the expansion of HHD to eligible patients with kidney failure. These included (1) the development of international standards (focussing on education and training), (2) empowering patients, (3) a culture of support, and (4) mitigation of institutional or governmental roadblocks. If there is an emphasis on addressing resource limitations, costs (borne by both provider and patient), and novel technologies that may allow regions without clean water or stable electrical grids to support HHD, these steps may be helpful in engaging countries to place a greater emphasis on HHD [80].

The current landscape of HHD globally varies significantly by region. While we have highlighted some novel solutions groups have used to facilitate HHD in their communities, a shared vision moving forward on addressing barriers to HHD is needed to guide practitioners wishing to implement HHD programming for their patients with kidney failure. To increase the number of patients starting with or transitioning to HHD, we will require a holistic approach that empowers patients to be active participants in the management of their kidney failure. Facilitating this will require systematic approaches to overcome major barriers they face along the way (Fig. 15.3).

One possible approach would be to grow a HHD program based on lessons learned from peritoneal dialysis programs. Providing education for both patients and providers, ensuring multidisciplinary team involvement and potentially working toward outcome-based incentives, are all strategies that have been used in PD programs and that may be applied to HHD [81]. Inevitably the development and further growth of a more comprehensive HHD program will require significant investment and should be partnered with legislation to ensure its success. One example of this is the Advancing American Kidney Health Initiative that received federal support in an effort to improve kidney health in the United States. Specifically, this involves novel payment models to prioritize transplant and home dialysis modalities for patients with kidney failure. Along with government support, professional guidelines to guide practice will also help to grow HHD. Many of these guidelines are publicly available (for example the British Columbia Renal Agency in Canada [82]) providing a starting point to direct global HHD program implementation. Broad collaboration with experts around the world, (for example, the International Home Dialysis Roundtable) is another avenue to help stakeholders without robust HHD exposure learn how to develop and sustain a program.

In conclusion, international applications of HHD (as outlined in this chapter) provide multiple micro- and macro-level strategies to inform stakeholders and overcome barriers to HHD. We must embrace these strategies to ensure that HHD is both available and sustainable for all eligible patients with kidney failure.

Key Points

- Despite the benefits, HHD remains largely underutilized across most countries.
- Educational barriers to HHD can be both patient and provider-focused, and include a lack of awareness, inconsistency of effective pre-dialysis programming, and HHD technical complexity.

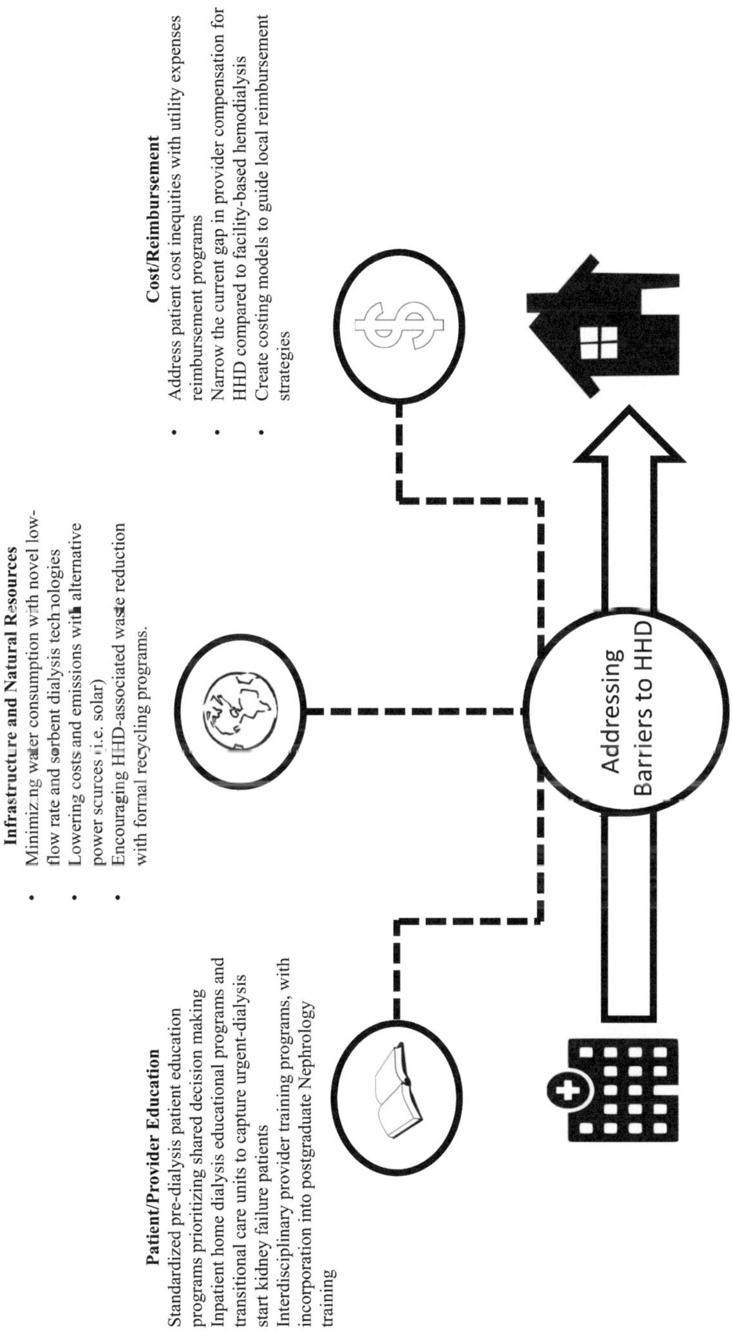

Fig. 15.3 Addressing barriers to HHD

- Local socioeconomic, environmental, and funding level factors vary significantly and remain a key barrier to HHD for countries worldwide.
- Novel technologies and creative water-conservation strategies will be key to improve the environmental sustainability of HHD and minimize infrastructure costs.
- There are many examples of unique micro- and macro-level strategies to address barriers to HHD that can be embraced and adapted locally to ensure HHD is available for all eligible patients with kidney failure.

References

1. Tennankore K, Na Y, Wald R, Chan C, Perl J. Short daily-, nocturnal- and conventional-home hemodialysis have similar patient and treatment survival. Kidney Int. 2017;93(1):188–94. https://doi.org/10.1016/j.kint.2017.06.014.
2. Tennankore K, Nadeau-Fredette AC, Chan CT. Intensified home hemodialysis: clinical benefits, risks and target populations. Nephrol Dial Transplant. 2014;29(7):1342–9. https://doi.org/10.1093/ndt/gft383.
3. Walker RC, Howard K, Morton RL, Palmer SC, Marshall MR, Tong A. Patient and caregiver values, beliefs and experiences when considering home dialysis as a treatment option: a semi-structured interview study. Nephrol Dial Transplant. 2016;31(1):133–41. https://doi.org/10.1093/ndt/gfv330.
4. Chuasuwan A, Pooripussarakul S, Thakkinstian A, Ingsathit A, Pattanaprateep O. Comparisons of quality of life between patients underwent peritoneal dialysis and hemodialysis: a systematic review and meta-analysis. Health Qual Life Outcomes. 2020;18(1):191. Published 2020 Jun 18. https://doi.org/10.1186/s12955-020-01449-2.
5. Nogueira GM, Oliveira MS, Moura AF, Cruz CMS, Moura-Neto JA. COVID-19 in dialysis units: a comprehensive review. World J Virol. 2021;10(5):264–74. https://doi.org/10.5501/wjv.v10.i5.264.
6. McCullough KP, Morgenstern H, Saran R, Herman WH, Robinson BM. Projecting ESRD incidence and prevalence in the United States through 2030. J Am Soc Nephrol. 2019;30(1):127–35. https://doi.org/10.1681/ASN.201805053.
7. Himmelfarb J, Vanholder R, Mehrotra R, Tonelli M. The current and future landscape of dialysis. Nat Rev Nephrol. 2020;16(10):573–85. https://doi.org/10.1038/s41581-020-0315-4.
8. Jain AK, Blake P, Cordy P, Garg AX. Global trends in rates of peritoneal dialysis. J Am Soc Nephrol. 2012;23(3):533–44. https://doi.org/10.1681/ASN.2011060607.
9. Rivara MB, Mehrotra R. The changing landscape of home dialysis in the United States. Curr Opin Nephrol Hypertens. 2014;23(6):586–91. https://doi.org/10.1097/MNH.0000000000000066.
10. United States Renal Data System. 2020 USRDS annual data report: epidemiology of kidney disease in the United States. Bethesda, MD: National Institutes of Health, National Institute of Diabetes and Digestive and Kidney Diseases; 2020.
11. Australian Bureau of Statistics. Australian demographic statistics, Jun 2020, time series spreadsheets, cat. no. 3101.0, viewed 4 Jan 2021; 2020.
12. MacGregor M, Agar J, Blagg C. Home haemodialysis—international trends and variation. Nephrol Dial Transplant. 2006;7:1934–45. https://doi.org/10.1093/ndt/gfl093.
13. Htay H, Bello AK, Levin A, et al. Hemodialysis use and practice patterns: an international survey study. Am J Kidney Dis. 2021;77(3):326–335.e1. https://doi.org/10.1053/j.ajkd.2020.05.030.
14. Hanson CS, Chapman JR, Craig JC, et al. Patient experiences of training and transition to home haemodialysis: a mixed-methods study. Nephrology. 2017;22(8):631–41.

15. The Renal Association, Kidney Care UK. Patient reported experience of kidney care in the UK; 2020.
16. Walker RC, Hanson CS, Palmer SC, et al. Patient and caregiver perspectives on home hemodialysis: a systematic review. Am J Kidney Dis. 2015;65(3):451–63. https://doi.org/10.1053/j.ajkd.2014.10.020.
17. de Jong RW, Stel V, Rahmel A, Murphy M, Vanholder R, Massy Z, Jager K. Patient-reported factors influencing the choice of their kidney replacement treatment modality. Nephrol Dial Transplant. 2021;37:477. https://doi.org/10.1093/ndt/gfab059.
18. Winterbottom A, Mooney A, Russon L, Hipkiss V, Ziegler L, Williams R, Finderup J, Bekker H. Kidney disease pathways, options and decisions: an environmental scan of international patient decision aids. Nephrol Dial Transplant. 2020;35:2072–82. https://doi.org/10.1093/ndt/gfaa102.
19. Yu X, Nakayama M, Wu MS, Kim YL, Mushahar L, Szeto CC, Schatell D. Shared decision-making for a dialysis modality. Kidney Int Rep. 2022;7(1):15–27. https://doi.org/10.1016/j.ekir.2021.10.019.
20. Feasibility of enhanced dialysis education (EDU) intervention for chronic kidney disease (CKD) patients (CKD-EDU). ClinicalTrials.gov. NCT03465449. https://clinicaltrials.gov/ct2/show/NCT03465449.
21. Shared decision making in dialysis (DIAL-SDM). ClinicalTrials.gov. NCT04392440. https://clinicaltrials.gov/ct2/show/NCT04392440.
22. Chan CT, Collins K, Ditschman EP, et al. Overcoming barriers for uptake and continued use of home dialysis: an NKF-KDOQI conference report. Am J Kidney Dis. 2020;75(6):926–34. https://doi.org/10.1053/j.ajkd.2019.11.007.
23. de Maar JS, de Groot MA, Luik PT, Mui KW, Hagen EC. GUIDE, a structured pre-dialysis programme that increases the use of home dialysis. Clin Kidney J. 2016;9(6):826–32. https://doi.org/10.1093/ckj/sfw037.
24. Hanko J, Jastrzebski J, Nieva C, White L, Li G, Zalunardo N. Dedication of a nurse to educating suboptimal haemodialysis starts improved transition to independent modalities of renal replacement therapy. Nephrol Dial Transplant. 2011;26(7):2302–8. https://doi.org/10.1093/ndt/gfq669. Epub 2010 Nov 11. PMID: 21071546.
25. Hussein WF, Bennet PN, Schiller B. Innovations to increase home hemodialysis utilization: the transitional care unit. Am J Kidney Dis. 2021;28(2):178–83. https://doi.org/10.1053/j.ackd.2021.02.009.
26. Morfín JA, Yang A, Wang E, Schiller B. Transitional dialysis care units: a new approach to increase home dialysis modality uptake and patient outcomes. Semin Dial. 2018;31(1):82–7. https://doi.org/10.1111/sdi.12651.
27. Rioux JP, Cheema H, Bargman JM, Watson D, Chan CT. Effect of an in-hospital chronic kidney disease education program among patients with unplanned urgent-start dialysis. Clin J Am Soc Nephrol. 2011;6(4):799–804. https://doi.org/10.2215/CJN.07090810.
28. Marshall MR, van der Schrieck N, Lilley D, et al. Independent community house hemodialysis as a novel dialysis setting: an observational cohort study. Am J Kidney Dis. 2013;61(4):598–607. https://doi.org/10.1053/j.ajkd.2012.10.020.
29. https://www.creehealth.org/services/home-hemodialysis-pilot.
30. Gupta N, Taber-Hight EB, Miller BW. Perceptions of home dialysis training and experience among US nephrology fellows. Am J Kidney Dis. 2021;77(5):713–718.e1. https://doi.org/10.1053/j.ajkd.2020.09.014.
31. de Jong RW, Stel VS, Heaf JG, Murphy M, Massy ZA, Jager KJ. Non-medical barriers reported by nephrologists when providing renal replacement therapy or comprehensive conservative management to end-stage kidney disease patients: a systematic review. Nephrol Dial Transplant. 2021;36(5):848–62. https://doi.org/10.1093/ndt/gfz271.
32. Tennankore KK, Hingwala J, Watson D, et al. Attitudes and perceptions of nephrology nurses towards dialysis modality selection: a survey study. BMC Nephrol. 2013;14:192. https://doi.org/10.1186/1471-2369-14-192.

33. Becevic M, Mutrux R, Edison K. Show-Me ECHO: complex disease care capacity-building telehealth program. Stud Health Technol Inform. 2016;226:233–6.
34. Morita PP, Huynh K, Zakir A, et al. Supporting the establishment of new home dialysis programs through the explore home dialysis program. Kidney Int Rep. 2018;4(2):293–300. Published 2018 Oct 29. https://doi.org/10.1016/j.ekir.2018.10.019.
35. Phillips M, Wile C, Bartol C, et al. An education initiative modifies opinions of hemodialysis nurses towards home dialysis. Can J Kidney Health Dis. 2015;2:16. Published 2015 Apr 28. https://doi.org/10.1186/s40697-015-0051-z.
36. Just PM, de Charro FT, Tschosik EA, Noe LL, Bhattacharyya SK, Riella MC. Reimbursement and economic factors influencing dialysis modality choice around the world. Nephrol Dial Transplant. 2008;23(7):2365–73.
37. Blake PG, Just PM. Economics of dialysis. In: Hörl WH, Koch KM, Lindsay RM, et al., editors. Replacement of renal function by dialysis. Dordrecht: Springer Netherlands; 2004. p. 1455–86.
38. Klarenbach SW, Tonelli M, Chui B, Manns BJ. Economic evaluation of dialysis therapies. Nat Rev Nephrol. 2014;10(11):644–52.
39. Klarenbach S, Tonelli M, Pauly R, Walsh M, Culleton B, So H, et al. Economic evaluation of frequent home nocturnal hemodialysis based on a randomized controlled trial. J Am Soc Nephrol. 2014;25(3):587–94.
40. Komenda P, Gavaghan MB, Garfield SS, Poret AW, Sood MM. An economic assessment model for in-center, conventional home, and more frequent home hemodialysis. Kidney Int. 2012;81(3):307–13.
41. McFarlane PA, Pierratos A, Redelmeier DA. Cost savings of home nocturnal versus conventional in-center hemodialysis. Kidney Int. 2002;62(6):2216–22.
42. Manns BJ, Mendelssohn DC, Taub KJ. The economics of end-stage renal disease care in Canada: incentives and impact on delivery of care. Int J Health Care Finance Econ. 2007;7(2–3):149–69.
43. Kroeker A, Clark WF, Heidenheim AP, Kuenzig L, Leitch R, Meyette M, et al. An operating cost comparison between conventional and home quotidian hemodialysis. Am J Kidney Dis. 2003;42(1 Suppl):49–55.
44. Agar JW, Knight RJ, Simmonds RE, Boddington JM, Waldron CM, Somerville CA. Nocturnal haemodialysis: an Australian cost comparison with conventional satellite haemodialysis. Nephrology. 2005;10(6):557–70.
45. Baboolal K, McEwan P, Sondhi S, Spiewanowski P, Wechowski J, Wilson K. The cost of renal dialysis in a UK setting—a multicentre study. Nephrol Dial Transplant. 2008;23(6):1982–9.
46. Komenda P, Copland M, Makwana J, Djurdjev O, Sood MM, Levin A. The cost of starting and maintaining a large home hemodialysis program. Kidney Int. 2010;77(11):1039–45.
47. McFarlane P, Komenda P. Economic considerations in frequent home hemodialysis. Semin Dial. 2011;24(6):678–83.
48. Beaudry A, Ferguson TW, Rigatto C, Tangri N, Dumanski S, Komenda P. Cost of dialysis therapy by modality in Manitoba. Clin J Am Soc Nephrol. 2018;13(8):1197–203.
49. Wong CKH, Chen J, Fung SKS, Mok MMY, Cheng YL, Kong I, et al. Direct and indirect costs of end-stage renal disease patients in the first and second years after initiation of nocturnal home haemodialysis, hospital haemodialysis and peritoneal dialysis. Nephrol Dial Transplant. 2019;34(9):1565–76.
50. Lockridge RS, Albert J, Anderson H, Barger T, Coffey L, Craft V, et al. Nightly home hemodialysis: fifteen months of experience in Lynchburg, Virginia. Home Hemodial Int. 1999;3(1):23–8.
51. Mohr PE. The economics of daily dialysis. Adv Ren Replace Ther. 2001;8(4):273–9.
52. Krahn MD, Bremner KE, de Oliveira C, Dixon SN, McFarlane P, Garg AX, et al. Home dialysis is associated with lower costs and better survival than other modalities: a population-based study in Ontario, Canada. Perit Dial Int. 2019;39(6):553–61.

53. Nickel M, Rideout W, Shah N, et al. Estimating patient-borne water and electricity costs in home hemodialysis: a simulation. CMAJ Open. 2017;5(1):E61–5. Published 2017 Feb 10. https://doi.org/10.9778/cmajo.20160108.
54. Weinhandl ED. Economic impact of home hemodialysis. Adv Chronic Kidney Dis. 2021;28(2):136–42.
55. Walker RC, Howard K, Tong A, Palmer SC, Marshall MR, Morton RL. The economic considerations of patients and caregivers in choice of dialysis modality. Hemodial Int. 2016;20(4):634–42.
56. The Kidney Foundation of Canada. The burden of out-of-pocket costs for Canadians with kidney failure. 2018. https://www.kidney.ca/burden.
57. The Home Network. Financial support for home dialysis. 2021. https://thehomenetwork.weebly.com/uploads/4/9/5/5/4955455/financial_fact_sheets_australia__reviewed_2021_.pdf.
58. Vanholder R, Davenport A, Hannedouche T, Kooman J, Kribben A, Lameire N, et al. Reimbursement of dialysis: a comparison of seven countries. Am J Kidney Dis. 2012;23(8):1291–8.
59. Levin A, Lo C, Noel K, Djurdjev O, Amano EC. Activity-based funding model provides foundation for province-wide best practices in renal care. Healthc Q. 2013;16(4):49–54.
60. Seshasai RK, Mitra N, Chaknos CM, et al. Factors associated with discontinuation of home hemodialysis. Am J Kidney Dis. 2016;67(4):629–37. https://doi.org/10.1053/j.ajkd.2015.11.003.
61. Liu F, Srivatana V, Salenger P. Policies to support home dialysis patients: patients need help too. Am J Kidney Dis. 2022;79(5):746–9. https://doi.org/10.1053/j.ajkd.2021.06.029.
62. Gajarawala SN, Pelkowski JN. Telehealth benefits and barriers. J Nurse Pract. 2021;17(2):218–21. https://doi.org/10.1016/j.nurpra.2020.09.013.
63. Tang SCW, Yu X, Chen HC, et al. Dialysis care and dialysis funding in Asia. Am J Kidney Dis. 2020;75(5):772–81. https://doi.org/10.1053/j.ajkd.2019.08.005.
64. Agar JW, Perkins A, Heaf JG. Home HD—setup in the home. Hemodial Int. 2015;19:S93–S111. https://doi.org/10.1111/hdi.12290.
65. Nagai K, Suzuki H, Ueda A, Agar JWM, Itsubo N. Assessment of environmental sustainability in renal healthcare. J Rural Med. 2021;16(3):132–8. https://doi.org/10.2185/jrm.2020-049.
66. Dheda S, Eps CV, Hawley C, Johnson DW. Water treatment for centre and home-based haemodialysis. In: Updates in hemodialysis. London: IntechOpen; 2015. https://doi.org/10.5772/59380.
67. Bieber SD, Young BA. Home hemodialysis: core curriculum 2021. Am J Kidney Dis. 2021;78(6):876–85. https://doi.org/10.1053/j.ajkd.2021.01.025.
68. Agar JW. Reusing dialysis wastewater: the elephant in the room. Am J Kidney Dis. 2008;52(1):10–2. https://doi.org/10.1053/j.ajkd.2008.04.005.
69. Tarrass F, Benjelloun M, Benjelloun O. Recycling wastewater after hemodialysis: an environmental analysis for alternative water sources in arid regions. Am J Kidney Dis. 2008;52(1):154–8. https://doi.org/10.1053/j.ajkd.2008.03.022.
70. https://homedialysis.org/news-and-research/blog/80-a-holiday-gift-to-the-planet-from-the-outback.
71. Agar JW. Review: understanding sorbent dialysis systems. Nephrology (Carlton). 2010;15(4):406–11. https://doi.org/10.1111/j.1440-1797.2010.01321.x.
72. Gordon A, Greenbaum MA, Marantz LB, McArthur MJ, Maxwell MH. A sorbent based low volume recirculating dialysate system. Trans Am Soc Artif Intern Organs. 1969;15:347–52.
73. van Gelder MK, Mihaila SM, Jansen J, et al. From portable dialysis to a bioengineered kidney. Expert Rev Med Devices. 2018;15(5):323–36. https://doi.org/10.1080/17434440.2018.1462697.
74. Gura V, Rivara MB, Bieber S, et al. A wearable artificial kidney for patients with end-stage renal disease. JCI Insight. 2016;1(8):e86397. https://doi.org/10.1172/jci.insight.86397.
75. https://www.nextkidney.com/.
76. https://www.diality.com/.

77. Connor A, Lillywhite R, Cooke MW. The carbon footprints of home and in-center maintenance hemodialysis in the United Kingdom. Hemodial Int. 2011;15(1):39–51. https://doi.org/10.1111/j.1542-4758.2010.00523.x.
78. Agar JW, Perkins A, Tjipto A. Solar-assisted hemodialysis. Clin J Am Soc Nephrol. 2012;7(2):310–4. https://doi.org/10.2215/CJN.09810911.
79. https://www.greendialysis.org/.
80. Mendu ML, Divino-Filho JC, Vanholder R, et al. Expanding utilization of home dialysis: an action agenda from the first international home dialysis roundtable. Kidney Med. 2021;3(4):635–43. Published 2021 May 25. https://doi.org/10.1016/j.xkme.2021.04.004.
81. Ahmad M, Wallace EL, Jain G. Setting up and expanding a home dialysis program: is there a recipe for success? Kidney360. 2020;1(6):569–79. Published 2020 May 1. https://doi.org/10.34067/KID.0000662019.
82. http://www.bcrenal.ca/health-professionals/clinical-resources/home-hemodialysis.

Home Hemodialysis During a Pandemic and Disaster Management

16

Gopa Green, Tanuja Yalamarti, Shahrzad Zonoozi, and Graham Edwin Abra

In this chapter, experiences from various home hemodialysis (HHD) programs around the globe in the face of natural disasters will be highlighted. Additionally, HHD during the Coronavirus-19 (COVID-19) pandemic along with outcomes will be discussed. The chapter closes with specific disaster management guidance relevant to HHD. The collective experiences and lessons learned from the above may better inform dialysis program strategies to successfully maintain HHD during periods of crisis [1, 2].

Case

A 54-year-old man with a history of end-stage kidney disease secondary to IgA nephropathy complicated by hypertension has been treated with HHD for the past 4 years. He is listed for a kidney transplant and has been dialyzing successfully five times per week for 3 h each session. He lives in a suburban area in a single-family home with his wife and two daughters. Local media and emergency response systems alert his community late in the evening after a lightning storm to a large fast-moving wildfire that is threatening residences approximately three miles from the patient's home.

G. Green
US Renal Care, Plano, TX, USA
e-mail: GreenG@usrenalcare.com

T. Yalamarti
Division of Critical Care, Department of Medicine, Stanford University School of Medicine, Stanford, CA, USA
e-mail: yalamart@stanford.edu

S. Zonoozi
Virginia Nephrology Group, Arlington, VA, USA

G. E. Abra (✉)
Division of Nephrology, Department of Medicine, Stanford University School of Medicine, Stanford, CA, USA
e-mail: gabra@stanford.edu

A. Shah et al. (eds.), *Applied Home Hemodialysis*,
https://doi.org/10.1007/978-3-031-77244-3_16

General Disaster Management Guidance

Detailed anticipatory planning is necessary to ensure dialysis patient safety during a disaster. Dialysis centers may be nonoperational and dialysis patients may need to be treated elsewhere. Patients on HHD may have disruptions in their home environments that make dialyzing there more challenging or impossible. After disasters, transportation networks can be disrupted, and patients and dialysis facilities may need to rely on help from emergency responders or military personnel. Fortunately, many disasters, such as hurricanes, wildfires, blizzards, and floods, can be predicted days ahead of time. The approach for different disaster scenarios also varies. For disasters such as tornadoes, hurricanes, or wildfires, citizens must evacuate their homes and seek shelter in other locations. Other events such as severe ice or snowstorms require citizens to shelter in place [3].

In response to the need to improve communication during natural disasters the Kidney Community Emergency Response (KCER) Coalition was set up in 2006. This partnership helps facilitate effective responses to disasters that affect patients with end-stage kidney disease (ESKD). KCER has developed a strategic plan for disaster responses to address the specific needs of dialysis patients, including implementation and dissemination of best practices at the state, local, and individual levels [4]. This organization, along with the National Kidney Foundation (NKF), publishes and disseminates information to dialysis clinics and patients regarding the necessary steps for disaster preparedness.

The KCER Coalition recommends pre-disaster identification of alternative dialysis facilities and renal emergency diet education. It further provides guidance on the preparation of early evacuation plans including the preservation of medical documentation and ensuring adequate medication supplies [5]. Patients should be counseled on steps necessary to shelter in place to prolong survival time without dialysis treatment. Specific KCER recommendations for patients include (Table 16.1): renal emergency diet education and adherence, a strict fluid intake regimen, stockpiling of non-perishable and appropriate foods, storage of 2 weeks of extra medical supplies, acquisition and storage of a potassium-binding resin, and availability of contact information for local police, fire, electric, water, and emergency services [3]. NKF also provides a list of dialysis-specific and general disaster preparedness items for patients to have ready in advance of a potential crisis.

Two groups of researchers [6, 7] conducted surveys of adults requiring care at dialysis centers after hurricanes Katrina and Sandy to assess general disaster and dialysis-specific preparedness utilizing the Department of Homeland Security general checklist and NKF's dialysis-specific checklist. Irrespective of their sociodemographic characteristics, most subjects were found to be unprepared for a disaster. Analysis of the data further showed that having access to alternate dialysis in an integrated system, access to transportation, and a stable social situation may be the most important factors in avoiding missed dialysis treatments. Such investigations should prompt quality improvement initiatives that focus on education at the level of the dialysis center to review these checklists with patients and assist with pre-disaster planning.

Table 16.1 Key recommendations of the KCER coalition

For patients with kidney failure	For nephrology providers	For federal, state, and local emergency providers
Keep updated lists at all times Medications and allergies, major health problems, physician, and dialysis facility Names and contact information, emergency contact information, including kidney care team Out-of-state contact if available and the KCER emergency number (888-33-KIDNEY) Emergency diet; emergency supply kit	**Make an emergency plan** Appoint a leader and deputy to oversee preparation and operations List emergency telephone numbers for patients and staff Procure and maintain emergency equipment and supplies Plan evacuation of patients and staff Secure equipment, supplies, and records if evacuation is needed. In the event of a disaster, report facility open/closed status to the ESRD network and daily nephrology disaster conference call (number to be publicized at the time of the disaster) Help each patient develop an emergency plan as shown in the first column	**Planning** Include a kidney community representative in disaster planning Include provisions for kidney failure patients in all plans and involve ESRD networks in planning Encourage early evacuation of kidney failure patients
Planning Create a personal evacuation plan Evacuate early if authorities advise evacuation Make alternate plans for transportation to your regular dialysis facility		**Addressing the needs of dialysis facilities** List facilities as high-priority locations for restoration of services such as power, water, and telephone Facilitate delivery of supplies Assist with security, generators, and fuel Give priority to dialysis personnel for limited supplies such as housing and gasoline Make arrangements for patients and staff to pass roadblocks and travel during curfews Assist in identifying alternate dialysis sites when dialysis units close
		Addressing needs of kidney patients in evacuee shelters Ask all evacuees about kidney failure, and make the resumption of regular dialysis the highest priority Provide renal failure diet as indicated Concentrate dialysis patients in particular shelters near dialysis units with appropriate capacity Group dialysis patients in a particular area of the shelter to assist with monitoring and transportation

In September 2016, the Centers for Medicare & Medicaid Services (CMS) released the *Emergency Preparedness Requirements for Medicare and Medicaid Participating Providers and Suppliers Final Rule* (https://www.cms.gov/Medicare/Provider-Enrollment-and-Certification/SurveyCertEmergPrep/Emergency-Prep-Rule). Per this CMS rule, providers must demonstrate completion of risk assessments, written disaster plans, policies, and procedures and ongoing training and testing of these plans with staff and partners in the community. These requirements fall under new conditions of participation/conditions for coverage and if they are not met, providers and suppliers risk citation and consequent loss of Medicare or Medicaid reimbursement.

Natural Disasters Experience

Natural events such as floods, hurricanes, wildfires, earthquakes, and pandemics have the potential to pose a significant threat to human health and safety alongside damage to property and infrastructure. When natural events occur in communities without the ability to cope with them, they have the potential to become disasters and can lead to significant morbidity and mortality. With increasing global surface temperatures, the possibility of more droughts and powerful storms is also increased. Rising sea levels expose locations at higher altitudes to the power of erosive forces of waves and currents. With a growing population and changing climates, the increasing threat of natural disasters places all communities at risk.

Dialysis is a life-sustaining treatment for dialysis-dependent patients. These patients are unable to tolerate prolonged lapses in treatment and are more vulnerable to the effects of natural disasters. Climate change and rising global temperatures may lead to increases in natural disasters in the upcoming years. Patients receiving in-center dialysis rely on a highly trained workforce to deliver treatments whereas those on HHD are more self-reliant in performing treatments. Herein we will look at experiences with natural disasters and dialysis-dependent patients, focusing on those on HHD where specific information about this subset of ESKD patients is available.

Earthquakes

The 1995 earthquake striking the city of Kobe, Japan led to extensive damage to electricity and water facilities. While awaiting restoration of services, water was supplied to dialysis units by tank trucks or the use of equipment converting seawater into fresh water. While awaiting resumption of dialysis, patients were managed with oral potassium exchange resins and dietary advice [8, 9].

In the aftermath of the 2009 earthquake in L'Aquila, Italy, tents were used to allow the resumption of dialysis for patients opting to return to the area [10].

The Christchurch earthquake in 2011 in New Zealand led to 42 hemodialysis patients and support personnel being flown to another city for resumption of care due to power outages and lack of clean water. Of note, patients who could manage HHD independently were prioritized to be repatriated at home [11]. Following the Christchurch earthquake, a document entitled "Planning guide for a dialysis emergency" was created to provide an approach to managing dialysis patients in a natural disaster. Based on this experience, almost all HHD machines were fitted with an ultra-filter, and all urban water was chlorinated and a carbon filter was added [11].

In addition to immediate health risks, there is also a significant emotional and psychological burden associated with natural disasters for vulnerable populations. In Turkey, following the 1999 Marmara earthquake, one study reported that in patients on chronic dialysis, the most severe problem encountered was psychiatric complications. During one of the aftershocks, all patients receiving dialysis disconnected bloodlines on their own and ran out of the building despite bleeding [12]. It is important to consider the need for additional support services when managing patients during and in the aftermath of natural disasters.

Floods

During the 2011 floods in Queensland, Australia, patients on chronic dialysis were contacted and asked to ensure they had dialysis supplies and medications for at least 1 week and assessed for the need for evacuation [13]. Prior to Cyclone Yasi, patients were evacuated to safe areas where they could receive dialysis. Following Cyclone Yasi, key areas for improvement were found to be the sharing of patient information and the lack of up-to-date prescriptions [14].

Wildfires

During recent years, the frequency of wildfires has increased worldwide. Wildfire smoke exposure has been associated with increased mortality among patients with ESKD receiving in-center hemodialysis [15]. The provision of high-efficiency air purifiers in dialysis centers and N-95 masks to vulnerable patients to combat the potential adverse respiratory effects of prolonged smoke exposure may be beneficial in mitigating these effects. Public safety power shut-offs during wildfire seasons, at times prolonged over multiple days, have also affected dialysis centers, staff, and patients in the North San Francisco Bay Area of California. Having alternate plans for dialysis centers, partnerships with non-affiliated providers, and evacuation and communication plans are key components for preparedness. HHD systems that use pre-packaged therapy fluid do not require any special plumbing or reverse osmosis system and can be used in emergency situations when the water supply may be interrupted. Generators for home backup use may allow uninterrupted HHD even during power shut-offs for limited periods of time.

Hurricanes

Hurricane Katrina caused unprecedented urban destruction to the greater New Orleans healthcare system when it made landfall in 2005. More than 1800 deaths were attributable to loss of access to healthcare facilities, disproportionately affecting economically disadvantaged patients with chronic illnesses. Nearly 2500 ESKD patients on hemodialysis and peritoneal dialysis who received their usual care in 43 local facilities in Southern Louisiana were relocated to facilities in Baton Rouge, Houston, and Atlanta, often after having missed multiple dialysis treatments, in some cases for more than a week. Widespread closures of dialysis facilities and more permanent relocations of patients after the storm led to an 18% reduction in the ESKD population in this area 2 months after the storm with 148 dialysis patient deaths recorded within the first month. Nearly 6000 physicians were also displaced after Hurricane Katrina in both Louisiana and neighboring Mississippi, highlighting the need for both public and private support to rebuild healthcare infrastructure after a large-scale disaster [4].

In 2012, Hurricane Sandy hit greater New York with the resultant loss of public services. Despite the availability of predictions allowing for early planning and preparation, there were disruptions to routine dialysis services. This led to a surge as patients sought treatment in alternative locations including local hospitals [16]. Disruptions to dialysis treatments have deleterious effects. In one study analyzing claims data from CMS, it was found that in comparison with patients with ESKD living in states unaffected by Hurricane Sandy, those living in affected areas had a higher 30-day mortality rate [17]. A group led by investigators at the US Department of Health and Human Services suggested a role for early dialysis (defined as additional pre-emptive treatments before the storm necessitates evacuations) in improving outcomes for patients affected by Hurricane Sandy [18].

During Hurricane Sandy, KCER held daily teleconferences and helped facilitate the identification and transportation of patients needing dialysis. In 2013, the US Department of Health and Human Services released emPOWER Map—a software which allows emergency services to rapidly locate those who have submitted Medicare claims for equipment using electricity including HHD machines [19].

Pandemics

COVID-19, caused by the severe acute respiratory syndrome coronavirus 2 (SARS-CoV-2), has led to a pandemic with far-reaching consequences since early 2020. Patients receiving in-center hemodialysis are more susceptible to the spread of infectious diseases; furthermore, patients with ESKD have weakened immune systems and are at risk for more severe illness [20]. For patients with ESKD on dialysis, strategies used to allow ongoing dialysis care included cohorting patients under investigation and establishment of specific shifts or centers for patients with confirmed COVID-19 infection.

The use of home dialysis modalities can help maintain social distancing, reduce costs and issues with transportation, and minimize exposures by reducing the need for in-person clinic visits during a pandemic. Telemedicine has been successfully utilized for follow-up visits in the home dialysis population. While patients on home dialysis have higher mortality rates from COVID-19 infection in comparison to the general population, they have a lower mortality risk when compared to in-center dialysis patients [21].

In a study from France, using data from the French Biomedicine Agency, between March 1 and June 15, 2020, 7 of the 423 patients with HHD in France were diagnosed with COVID-19 [22]. The incidence was noted to be less than that observed in patients on in-center hemodialysis (reported to be 3.8%) but similar to patients treated with peritoneal dialysis. In view of this, the report calls for increased investment in HHD and a return to the concept of "home dialysis first." In another study from Italy, the investigators reported that during the pandemic, increased needs required tailoring of in-center hemodialysis and the use of home dialysis modalities can allow for increased flexibility and personalization of treatments (Table 16.2) [23].

The Kidney Community Emergency Response (KCER) coalition, National Kidney Foundation (NKF), American Association of Kidney Patients (AAKP), Department of Health (DoH), Red Cross and the National Forum of End-Stage Renal Disease (ESRD) Networks have resources available for patients and clinicians to aid with disaster management.

Table 16.2 Lessons from the pandemic and considerations regarding home dialysis treatments [23]

	Best practices	Barriers	Suggestions
Home dialysis treatment	Limit exposure to the hospital setting	Isolation Acute intradialytic problems Dialysis prescriptions	Reinforcement of telemedicine
Home biochemical controls	Practical, reducing the need for going to a laboratory or hospital	Standard pre- and post-dialysis controls may be difficult to organize	Frequency of controls would not be reduced
Family involvement	Important psychosocial support	The burden may be heavy and create tension	Psychosocial aid could be needed
Residual kidney function	Better preserved in tailored dialysis	Slow loss of kidney function could go unnoticed	Consider not only remote monitoring
Assisted home dialysis	Limited exposure to the hospital setting and no travel time	May fail to guarantee privacy	Attention on potential carriers
Reduction of travel time and carbon footprint	"Green" advantages	Waste management needs to be organized in advance	Limited need to travel is an advantage in a "lockdown"

Specific Disaster Management Guidance for Patients on HHD

HHD provides many benefits during natural disasters including self-sufficient patients, lack of need for additional workforce, and less risk of spread of infectious disease. It is important to ensure backup plans are in place for dialysis at local in-center facilities for these patients in case of an evacuation, though some patients may be able to maintain themselves on HHD if they utilize a portable dialysis device and continue to have access to power and necessary supplies. However, it is important to keep in mind that natural disasters often disrupt in-center operations and a surge in demand for treatment slots at centers that remain open can make it challenging for patients on HHD to find dialysis care. In addition to in-center facilities, hemodialysis can be done in-home dialysis center training rooms with HHD machines. Ideally, each dialysis facility should develop affiliation agreements with both local and regional partners that should be accessible to HHD patients. Dialysis centers should maintain additional supplies which could be used if there are issues leading to delivery or supply chain interruption for patients. Along with plans to evacuate patients, each dialysis center should also have plans for the evacuation of refrigerated medications (erythrocyte stimulating agents, vaccines, etc.) in a cooler or other insulated container in order to avoid having to discard medications in the event of a power outage or prolonged evacuation.

Patients should also be prepared to continue dialysis at home in situations where the medical supply chains could be affected. Systems requiring bagged or pre-mixed dialysate may mandate the need for additional stockpiling of supplies in advance. Having at least an extra week's worth of supplies and dialysate mitigates risk and can avoid the transition to in-center dialysis. Manufacturers of some HHD devices have recommendations for supplies for non-medical emergencies which are helpful to review periodically. Registration with utility companies may aid with the prioritization of restoration of services to patients on HHD. It is helpful to assess if patients on HHD have generators or other backup power systems during home visits. There may be local or state programs for rebates or reimbursements for patients for these systems. The use of virtual care for remote monitoring and integrating telehealth into an existing practice will also allow medication review, education, and support for patients and caregivers as well as coordination between healthcare team members [24] during disasters or pandemics while Internet connectivity remains available.

In some disasters, a boil-water advisory may be issued by local authorities when the water supply is thought to be contaminated by pathogens or toxic chemicals. Depending on the HHD device being used, pre-mixed dialysate or transition to in-center dialysis may be appropriate for devices that rely on the local water supply for dialysate production.

All chronic dialysis patients will benefit from receiving education and developing an action plan for what to do in the event of a disaster with a specific focus on what to do if there are disruptions to the water or electricity supply. Regular conduction of disaster drills to test emergency and communications plans and assess HHD patients and staff's ability to coordinate care should be incorporated in dialysis centers. If there are delays in receiving maintenance dialysis, it may be helpful for dialysis-dependent patients to have a potassium-binding agent, along with diuretics in those with residual kidney function, to be taken at the instruction of their nephrologist as well as information regarding an emergency dialysis diet.

Case Revisited

The patient and his family evacuate from his home due to the advancing wildfire. They are able to bring his portable HHD system along with 1 week of pre-packaged dialysate and ancillary supplies with them. They evacuate to a pre-designated friend's home approximately 50 miles away that the patient had identified during routine dialysis center disaster planning 4 months prior. In addition to dialysis supplies, the patient also carries a printed list of essential medications, at least a week's supply of the medications, personal medical and insurance information, important contact numbers, and appropriate non-perishable low potassium and phosphorus foods. The center staff contact the patient by phone to ensure he has been able to safely evacuate and make plans for him to dialyze at an in-center dialysis facility at a safe distance from the wildfire should he be unable to treat with HHD at his friend's home for any reason.

Conclusion

With increasing population, climate change, and globalization, the threat of natural disasters is ever present and rising. Dialysis-dependent patients are particularly vulnerable to the effects of natural disasters, as the dialysis procedure requires both functional infrastructure and a skilled workforce. In general, disasters fall into two categories: those where evacuation is needed and those where there is a stay-at-home order. With appropriate preparation and planning, HHD can be continued in certain circumstances, especially when there is a stay-at-home order, with minimal disruption in a safe manner allowing continued treatments for dialysis dependent patients. HHD can be particularly advantageous at times when isolation is necessary, such as during the COVID-19 pandemic. Preparation remains key: early assessment and evaluation of potential impacts, implementation of appropriate management strategies, and efficient use of resources can help mitigate the effects of disasters.

References

1. Jones KE, Patel NG, Levy MA, Storeygard A, Balk D, Gittleman JL, et al. Global trends in emerging infectious diseases. Nature. 2008;451(7181):990–3.
2. Madhav N, Oppenheim B, Gallivan M, Mulembakani P, Rubin E, Wolfe N. Pandemics: risks, impacts, and mitigation. In: Jamison DT, Gelband H, Horton S, Jha P, Laxminarayan R, et al., editors. Disease control priorities: improving health and reducing poverty. Washington, DC: International Bank for Reconstruction and Development/The World Bank; 2017.
3. Howard E, Wiseman K. Emergency and disaster planning: patient education and preparation. Nephrol Nurs J. 2001;28:527–8.
4. Kopp JB, Ball LK, Cohen AC, Kenney RJ, Lempert KD, Miller PE, Muntner P, Qureshi N, Yelton SA. Kidney patient care in disasters: emergency planning for patients and dialysis facilities. Clin J Am Soc Nephrol. 2007;2:825–38.
5. Kleinpeter MA, Norman LD, Krane NK. Dialysis services in the hurricane-affected areas in 2005: lessons learned. Am J Med Sci. 2006;332:259–63.
6. Foster M, Brice JH, Shofer F, Principe S, Dewalt D, Falk R, Ferris M. Personal disaster preparedness of dialysis patients in North Carolina. Clin J Am Soc Nephrol. 2011;6:2478–84. PMID: 21852660.

7. Murakami N, Siktel HB, Lucido D, Winchester JF, Harbord NB. Disaster preparedness and awareness of patients on hemodialysis after Hurricane Sandy. Clin J Am Soc Nephrol. 2015;10:1389–96.
8. Fukagawa M. Nephrology in earthquakes: sharing experiences and information. Clin J Am Soc Nephrol. 2007;2:803–8.
9. Naito H. The basic hospital and renal replacement therapy in the Great Hanshin Earthquake. Ren Fail. 1997;19(5):701–10. https://doi.org/10.3109/08860229709109036.
10. Bonomini M, Stuard S, Dal Canton A. Dialysis practice and patient outcome in the aftermath of the earthquake at L'Aquila, Italy, April 2009. Nephrol Dial Transplant. 2011;26(8):2595–603. https://doi.org/10.1093/ndt/gfq783. Epub 2011 Jan 19. PMID: 21248293.
11. Irvine J, Buttimore A, Eastwood D, Kendrick-Jones J. Earthquakes and dialysis: our experience. Nephrology. 2014;19:296–303. https://doi.org/10.1111/nep.12222.
12. Sever MS, Erek E, Vanholder R, Koc M, Yavuz M, Aysuna N, Ergin H, Ataman R, Yenicesu M, Canbakan B, Demircan C, Lameire N. Lessons learned from the catastrophic Marmara earthquake: factors influencing the final outcome of renal victims. Clin Nephrol. 2004;61(6):413–21. https://doi.org/10.5414/cnp61413. PMID: 15224805.
13. Johnson DW, Hayes B, Gray NA, Hawley C, Hole J, Mantha M. Renal services disaster planning: lessons learnt from the 2011 Queensland floods and North Queensland cyclone experiences. Nephrology (Carlton). 2013;18(1):41–6. https://doi.org/10.1111/nep.12008.
14. McArdle J. Cyclone Yasi: dialysis mission impossible. Ren Soc Australasia J. 2011;7(2):76–8. Gale Academic OneFile, link.gale.com/apps/doc/A265192668/AONE?u=anon~21ada3a2&sid=googleScholar&xid=114b8ebe. Accessed 11 Mar 2022.
15. Xi Y, Kshirsagar AV, Wade TJ, Richardson DB, Brookhart MA, Wyatt L, Rappold AG. Mortality in US hemodialysis patients following exposure to wildfire smoke. J Am Soc Nephrol. 2020;31(8):1824–35. https://doi.org/10.1681/ASN.2019101066.
16. Lin CJ, Pierce LC, Roblin PM, Arquilla B. Impact of Hurricane Sandy on hospital emergency and dialysis services: a retrospective survey. Prehosp Disaster Med. 2014;29(4):374–9. https://doi.org/10.1017/S1049023X14000715.
17. Kelman J, Finne K, Bogdanov A, Worrall C, Margolis G, Rising K, MaCurdy TE, Lurie N. Dialysis care and death following Hurricane Sandy. Am J Kidney Dis. 2015;65(1):109–15. https://doi.org/10.1053/j.ajkd.2014.07.005.
18. Lurie N, Finne K, Worrall C, Jauregui M, Thaweethai T, Margolis G, Kelman J. Early dialysis and adverse outcomes after Hurricane Sandy. Am J Kidney Dis. 2015;66:507–12, ISSN 0272-6386.
19. Davis M, Kopp JB. Preparing for disasters for patients on dialysis. Clin J Am Soc Nephrol. 2015;10(8):1316–7. https://doi.org/10.2215/CJN.07340715.
20. Stern LD, Waikar S. Time to expand access and utilization of home dialysis: lessons from the COVID-19 pandemic. Mayo Clin Proc. 2020;95(7):1323–4. https://doi.org/10.1016/j.mayocp.2020.04.038.
21. Hsu CM, Weiner DE, Aweh G, Salenger P, Johnson DS, Lacson E Jr. Epidemiology and outcomes of COVID-19 in home dialysis patients compared with in-center dialysis patients. J Am Soc Nephrol. 2021;32(7):1569–73. Advance online publication. https://doi.org/10.1681/ASN.2020111653.
22. Michel PA, Piccoli GB, Couchoud C, Fessi H. Home hemodialysis during the COVID-19 epidemic: comment on the French experience from the viewpoint of a French home hemodialysis care network. J Nephrol. 2020;33(6):1125–7. https://doi.org/10.1007/s40620-020-00893-z.
23. Cozzolino M, Piccoli GB, Ikizler TA, Ronco C. The COVID-19 infection in dialysis: are home-based renal replacement therapies a way to improve patient management? J Nephrol. 2020;33(4):629–31. https://doi.org/10.1007/s40620-020-00784-3.
24. Scarpioni R, Manini A, Chiappini P. Remote patient monitoring in peritoneal dialysis helps reduce risk of hospitalization during covid-19 pandemic. J Nephrol. 2020;11:1–2.

Green Nephrology in Home Haemodialysis

17

Elaine Phua, Carol Pollock, and Yvonne Shen

Introduction

Haemodialysis (HD) is a resource-intensive form of treatment. It requires large amounts of water and energy and generates a considerable amount of waste. Whilst decades have been spent developing and improving haemodialysis provision and outcomes in patients, the study of and emphasis placed on the impact these actions have on the environment has been largely overlooked. Green nephrology has become a topic of growing interest in the last two decades. This chapter highlights the impact haemodialysis has on the environment, suggests methods for conservation in the home haemodialysis setting, illustrated by real-world examples and discusses developments still required in this area. As global demand for dialysis increases, healthcare providers have a growing role to play in environmental sustainability: conserving natural resources and protecting global ecosystems to meet today's needs without compromising the needs of future generations. A forward-looking approach to this issue seeks to improve air and water quality, provide

E. Phua (✉)
Department of Renal Medicine, Royal North Shore Hospital, St Leonards, NSW, Australia

C. Pollock
Department of Renal Medicine, Royal North Shore Hospital, St Leonards, NSW, Australia

University of Sydney, Camperdown, NSW, Australia

Kolling Institute of Medical Research, St Leonards, NSW, Australia
e-mail: carol.pollock@sydney.edu.au

Y. Shen
Department of Renal Medicine, Royal North Shore Hospital, St Leonards, NSW, Australia

University of Sydney, Camperdown, NSW, Australia

Sydney Dialysis Centre, St Leonards, NSW, Australia
e-mail: Yvonne.Shen@health.nsw.gov.au

A. Shah et al. (eds.), *Applied Home Hemodialysis*,
https://doi.org/10.1007/978-3-031-77244-3_17

renewable energy sources and reduce landfills, which preserves access to food and water, education and job opportunities and finally, sanitation and healthcare.

Background

Over the last century, the world has undergone significant population growth with an increase in per-capita consumption, industrialisation and technological innovation. Issues with governance have impacted land and water availability, ecosystems including plant and animal biodiversity and climate change [1]. A media release on a review of over 15,000 scientific and government sources by the Intergovernmental Science-Policy Platform on Biodiversity and Ecosystem Services (IPBES) in 2019 highlights the significant changes the planet has undergone in the last few decades. Three-quarters of land-based and 66% of marine-based environments have been altered by human actions, more than a third of the earth's land surface and three-quarters of freshwater resources are now devoted to livestock production and agriculture, urban areas have more than doubled since 1992 and plastic pollution has increased tenfold since 1980 with 300–400 million tonnes of heavy metals and toxins released from industrial facilitates into the earth's waters annually. Greenhouse gas (GHG) emissions have doubled since 1980, raising average global temperatures by at least 1.26 °F (0.7 °C) and is expected to rise further by 8.64 °F (4.8 °C) by 2100 [1–3].

The costs of global warming and its negative impact on health outcomes are widely recognised [4]. Almost a quarter of total global deaths, 13.6 million of deaths per year in 2016 (24%), are due to modifiable environmental risks [5, 6]. Increasingly warm climates lead to an increased risk of acute kidney injury and burden of stone disease and environmental toxins have been associated with kidney disease [2, 7, 8]. The environmental impact on the incidence of kidney disease is seen in chronic kidney disease of unknown cause (CKDu), a disease pattern strongly linked to environmental factors and is unrelated to classical causes of kidney disease likely diabetes, hypertension or glomerular disease. It is seen disproportionately in young males living in hot, agricultural communities, who are impacted by heat and dehydration, exposure to pesticides, heavy metals and infections, and are disadvantaged by other social determinants of health. It has been recognised in Central America, Sri Lanka and Central India, with expected increase in prevalence with changing climate conditions [9–11]. The estimated number of patients worldwide receiving dialysis in 2018 was 3.362 million with 2.99 million (89%) receiving HD, a much smaller proportion (11%) receiving peritoneal dialysis. Only 1% of patients receiving HD perform this at home [12]. The number of patients receiving dialysis rose by about 6% worldwide in 2018 with higher growths in lower income countries compared with higher income countries and this number is expected to increase further [12, 13]. This increases the already insatiable demand for potable water and energy and leads to increases in waste generation and carbon emissions. We are being drawn into a vicious cycle of watching the burden of chronic kidney disease place an increasing demand for natural resources for treatment, leading to an increased environmental burden which in turn, further impacts the health outcomes of current and future generations [8]. The impact of climate change on health can be direct (heatwaves, floods, bushfires and altered air quality), indirect (altered distributions of infectious diseases and aeroallergens, food insecurity, increase in vector-borne diseases, and changes in water quality and flows) and deferred (displacement and social unrest) [2]. The risks that climate change pose to social and environmental determinants of health and vice versa are impossible to ignore [4, 14].

Home HD has the benefit of reduced environmental impact and cost on the healthcare system [15–17], with the added benefit that any steps made towards environmental sustainability can begin on a smaller scale involving just one patient, their household and their machine. The provision of home HD involves a few stages—shared decision-making between patient and clinician, education and training, evaluation of the patient's home environment and the individualised approach to the set-up of water and energy supply for dialysis to take place at home depending on location and resource-availability [18–20]. A multi-disciplinary approach and an understanding of the essentials of home HD provision are required to reach the goal of green dialysis in the home setting.

Water

Water scarcity refers to the long-term phenomenon where the level of demand exceeds supply which can lead to displacement and adverse health outcomes. Less than 3% of the world's water resources are freshwater [21]. As its supply wanes from mishandling and contamination of freshwater supplies, demand for it grows to meet the needs of urbanisation and a growing population. In fact, global demand for water is expected to increase by 20–30% per year by 2050 and water scarcity is expected to impact two-thirds of the world's population by that time [22]. Water is an essential part of HD and is sourced mostly from municipal water, and to a lesser extent, non-municipal sources like lakes, reservoirs, bore and tank water [23]. It has to undergo treatment (sedimentation, flocculation, softening, oxidation and disinfection and carbon filtration) to become potable water, or water suitable for drinking [24–26]. The quality and content of the water are dependent on local environmental factors and dictate the complexity of the water purification system (e.g., the array of filters before the RO unit) required to produce water suitable for dialysis use [23]. Globally, the dialysis population generates approximately 3675 million litres of wastewater a year [8, 27].

Water Consumption

Water consumption is dependent on the type of home HD machine being used. Broadly, there are two categories of home HD machines, the conventional single-pass system (SPS) and the low-flow system (LFS). The former requires the translation of a hospital-based infrastructure for dialysate water production in the home (including reverse osmosis (RO) unit), is the most used form of home HD globally and supports standard-hours and extended-hours HD [18, 23, 28]. The latter was developed as a miniaturised system for the home, is more prevalent in the United States, does not require an RO unit and supports short daily and nocturnal HD [28–30].

Conventional Single-Pass System (SPS)

The volume of water consumed in a single-pass conventional HD system for 7–8 h of dialysis per treatment for 4–5 nights a week is estimated to be 800 L/treatment and 200,000 L per patient per year [31]. It uses a large volume of dialysate that is poorly saturated with urea to achieve a high clearance rate, particularly of small molecules [18, 32]. Water treatment in this setting is a sequential system of pre-treatment, comprising sediment filters, carbon filters and water softeners to produce water free of particulate matter, followed by RO to remove inorganic solutes, bacteria and endotoxins, to produce high-grade water for dialysis [23, 27, 33]. Two types of water results from each session of dialysis—RO reject water (RW) and the dialysate effluent. The former is water that did not meet the standard after passing through the RO and has not encountered the patient or any component of the patient's blood. The latter is generated through the process of dialysis—it has moved through the dialyser and is generated from the clearance of solutes and toxins from the patient's blood.

Low-Flow System (LFS)

Where SPS uses a dialysate flow to blood flow (Qd:Qb) ratio of 2:1, the LFS reverses this ratio (Qd:Qb of 1:2 or 1:3), maximising urea saturation of the dialysate and allowing for shortened but more frequent treatment time [18, 28]. Clearances with LFS are reduced in efficiency compared to conventional SPS, necessitating increased intensity of prescription, typically an average of 17.5 h a week [28, 32, 34]. Although not widely available or used internationally, the NxStage system is the most frequently used LFS in the United States [18]. The NxStage system's approach is similar to peritoneal dialysis, where low dialysate volumes are used compared with conventional HD, increased dwell time allows greater equilibration across a semi-permeable membrane and dialysate is lactate based [32]. It consists of two primary components: one, the cycler which incorporates the user interface, the electronic and mechanical functionalities required to conduct dialysis and two, a disposable treatment cartridge that is inserted into the cycler and serves to contain the blood and fluid circuits [29]. Dialysate is obtained from the supplier in pre-made bags like in peritoneal dialysis or can be easily prepared from drinking-quality tap water using a disposable water purification system (PureFlow™) that provides 60 L of ultrapure dialysate over 7 h and does away with the need for routine water testing or an RO unit [28, 29]. Dialysate volume is much lower in LFS (15–60 L per short daily treatment, 90–360 L/week) compared to conventional HD (90–200 L per treatment, 270–600 L/week) [28], and only a dialysate effluent is generated at the end of each treatment. Online dialysis fluid generation requires large volumes of water, thus by doing away with this and using lower dialysate flows, less water is consumed in LFS [34].

Reject Water

RW makes up approximately two-thirds of the typical 500–800 L volume of mains water drawn up for each dialysis session [16, 31, 35]. This water is safe for use, meeting World Health Organisation (WHO) criteria as potable water, but is not yet legally acceptable for drinking [36], and is often drained as waste. An analysis of RW collected using a sterile technique from the inflow pipes and outflow ports of the RO (RW) in a satellite HD unit in a regional town in Australia showed the RW was one, comparable to the town's standard potable water reporting limits for bacteriological and biochemical analytes except for conductivity and turbidity and two, even these fell well within the limits of US EPA standards for potable water [37]. A similar analysis performed in Morocco had drew the same conclusions in demonstrating the safety of RW for human consumption [38]. Indeed, the term 'reject water' seems a misnomer when the water quality does in fact exceed that of regular water from the tap.

RW is now being reused in hospitals around the world (Australia, United States (US), Canada, United Kingdom (UK), China, France, Spain and Morocco) for sterilisation of medical equipment (steam generation for sterilising and autoclaving), toilet flushing, floor cleaning and hospital landscape use [36, 39]. An innovative group in Malaysia were the first to report their experience in the creation of an aquaponics system, utilising RW from their in-centre dialysis unit to sustain aquaculture (farming of fish in this case) and hydroponics (farming of vegetables using a water-based medium), distributing their crop amongst staff and patients [40, 41]. On a community level, RW was being given, free-of-charge, to the local Aged Care Centre, sporting clubs and school grounds [37]. The significant socioeconomic impact RW reuse had on sustaining agriculture, food production and job opportunities in a remote, water-scarce community in the Australian outback using a simple system of collection and drainage is an inspiring example of what could be achieved with simple innovation to serve a need [27, 33]. On a legislative level, efforts should be made to mandate the reuse of RW [2, 42].

In the home HD setting, RW can be reused in two ways: tanking and piping for reuse in cleaning, laundry, agriculture and animal care [33, 36, 39] or recycling back through a closed-loop system for representation to the RO which can result in up to 80% of water saving [26]. This can be done in two ways: first, internal recycling of the RW or second, storage of RW in a separate storage tank for representation to the filtration system at a different time [33]. The former has been used in the United Kingdom, Australia and France through retrofitted water-conserving equipment and has shown to be financially viable and potentially profitable [2]. Recycling will cause conductivity at the RO membranes to eventually rise, which is thus monitored by a meter and the water is discarded if the conductivity exceeds safe RO membrane extraction limits. If this happens, water from the mains is subsequently re-engaged to maintain dialysis feed flow, although this is a rare occurrence [33, 39]. Regular water testing for bacterial contamination should be performed [43]. Recycling RW is generally limited to areas where feed water quality is high and conductivity does not exceed 1000 mSm/cm (most urban areas typically have water conductivity <500 mSm/cm) due to the impact this will have on reducing the efficiency and, thus, the lifespan of the RO membrane [26].

Dialysate Effluent Water

Worldwide, dialysis effluent is discarded into the sewerage [36]. This nutrient-rich water is generated in large quantities (500 mL/min per patient in conventional SPS dialysis and 160 mL/min in LFS dialysis for a standard treatment session) in dialysis [32, 39]. A group in Morocco investigated the possibility of dialysate effluent reuse and discovered that the water quality of the spent dialysate effluent, apart from its high conductivity, met WHO and UN Food and Agriculture Organisation criteria for use in agriculture in all other aspects including bacteriology and chemical composition [36]. In fact, the level of bacteria detected in dialysate effluent fell below industry standards and the culture of this water did not detect any coliform species [38]. Despite high conductivity and salinity limiting its use, this water is rich in phosphate, magnesium, potassium and urea, and more effort should be made to finding innovative uses for it. A proof-of-concept trial showed the successful use of dialysis effluent in the aquaculture of seaweed [39, 44], which plays a role in absorbing carbon emissions, regenerating marine ecosystems, being a food source and creating renewable plastics [45]. The group explored the possibility of putting the dialysate effluent through further RO and nanofiltration to reduce its conductivity and achieve water quality that is suitable for irrigation and proposed a potential cost saving compared with desalination of seawater [36]. With technological advances and increasing water scarcity, this may become another viable and cost-effective option for dialysate effluent reuse.

Reduce Water Use

As we seek to find ways to reuse and recycle dialysis wastewater, we should also examine strategies to reduce the overall water consumption in HD. Optimising dialysis prescriptions to allow for maximal clinical benefit whilst minimising waste should become routine practice. The use of dialysis machines and ROs with good efficiency ratings may represent a higher initial cost but prove to be more resource- and cost-effective in the longer term [46]. Where suitable and available, LFS may be a viable treatment option for both the patient and the environment. Finally, sorbent technology continues to be investigated. This is not a new technology, but rather, one that has made a resurgence in the research and development of smaller, portable dialysis machines which relies on battery power and uses less water and does not require complex RO water preparation compared to conventional HD [2, 33].

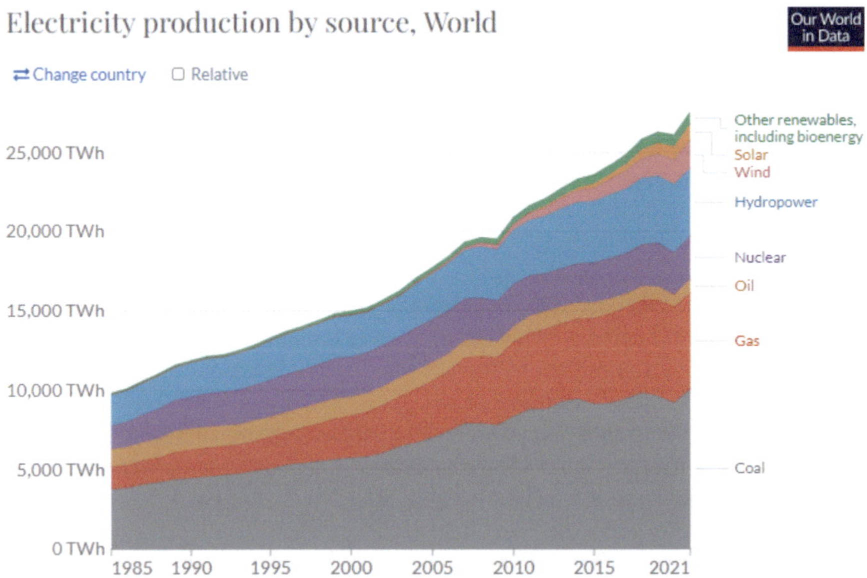

Fig. 17.1 Sources of electricity in the world, [our world in data], 2022. 'Other renewables include biomass and waste, geothermal, wave and tidal [47]

Energy (Electricity)

Energy accounts for the majority of GHG emissions in many countries [8]. Globally, more than one-third (36.7%) of electricity is now produced from renewable sources although coal, followed by gas, remains the largest source of electricity. Of the renewable sources of energy, nuclear and hydropower contain the largest share although solar and wind power are increasingly used. Through climate change policies, many countries are increasing their share of renewable sources of energy for electricity production (Fig. 17.1), for example, the United Kingdom, whose coal use has fallen from 60% in 1980 to 2% by 2021 [47].

Electricity Consumption and Consequence

HD using a Fresenius 4008B machine together with an individual Gambro WRO 10-1 RO unit consumes about 6.2 kWh of electricity per session [2], compared with the average 18 kWh per day of electricity in a 4-person household in Australia in 2014 [2] or 27 kWh per day in the US in 2020 [48]. Electricity is used in HD to start up and prime the machine and RO, warm the dialysate and heat disinfection resulting in a significant amount of electricity use in proportion to the amount of electricity used for regular daily activities.

The cost of energy consumption is passed on to the patient in the home HD setting, which should become an additional point of interest to clinicians: to not only reduce the environmental impact of kidney replacement therapy but to also relieve the social burden this life-saving therapy has on the patient. The cost of renewable energy is declining and may become a cheaper alternative to coal [49]; however, the uptake of nuclear energy remains controversial due to the cost and political complexities it holds on to a world stage, and hydropower would have to take place on a larger scale than what is relevant to the individual on home HD [50]. Many countries have a scheme for subsidising the cost of electricity on the home HD patient through government-funded reimbursement programs [18, 51] and thus, increasing the use of renewable sources of energy is expected to not only provide an environmental benefit but also translate to household and governmental cost savings.

Unsurprisingly, dialysis equipment and prescription also play a role in energy consumption. In the United States, home HD is often performed in short daily sessions (6 × 2–2.5 h) using the NxStage system which uses far less electricity compared with the single-pass machine with an RO system (for 4 × 5–8 h commonly used in other countries [35, 50, 52]. Many of these decisions will depend on patient location and equipment availability.

Renewable Sources

Two main renewable energy sources that have been of interest in the home dialysis setting are solar and wind energy [8, 50, 53]. Factors to consider in selecting an energy source include space availability, population density and availability of the natural resources of the location. Wind power requires reasonable land area, is less predictable compared with solar energy and risks contention from noise and sight pollution [50]. It is thus less feasible for urban households but remains available to the consumer through third-party providers.

Solar Energy

The benefits of solar energy are its accessibility to households in both urban and rural settings, dependability, silence and finally, its longevity. A common misconception is the need for access to bright, direct sunlight to be able to harness sufficient energy, whereas solar exposure can differ significantly from the individual's impression. Solar exposure can be measured either by direct measure of solar radiation or indirectly by solar insolation—the amount of solar radiation incident upon a unit horizontal surface over time [50]. Information on region-specific levels of solar insolation is readily available, with the southwest region having the highest solar insolation in the United States (see Fig. 17.2).

There are two ways solar energy can be sourced and utilised. The first is through array donation and service draw from the national grid with reimbursement from the local electricity provider. The second is through onsite battery storage which is

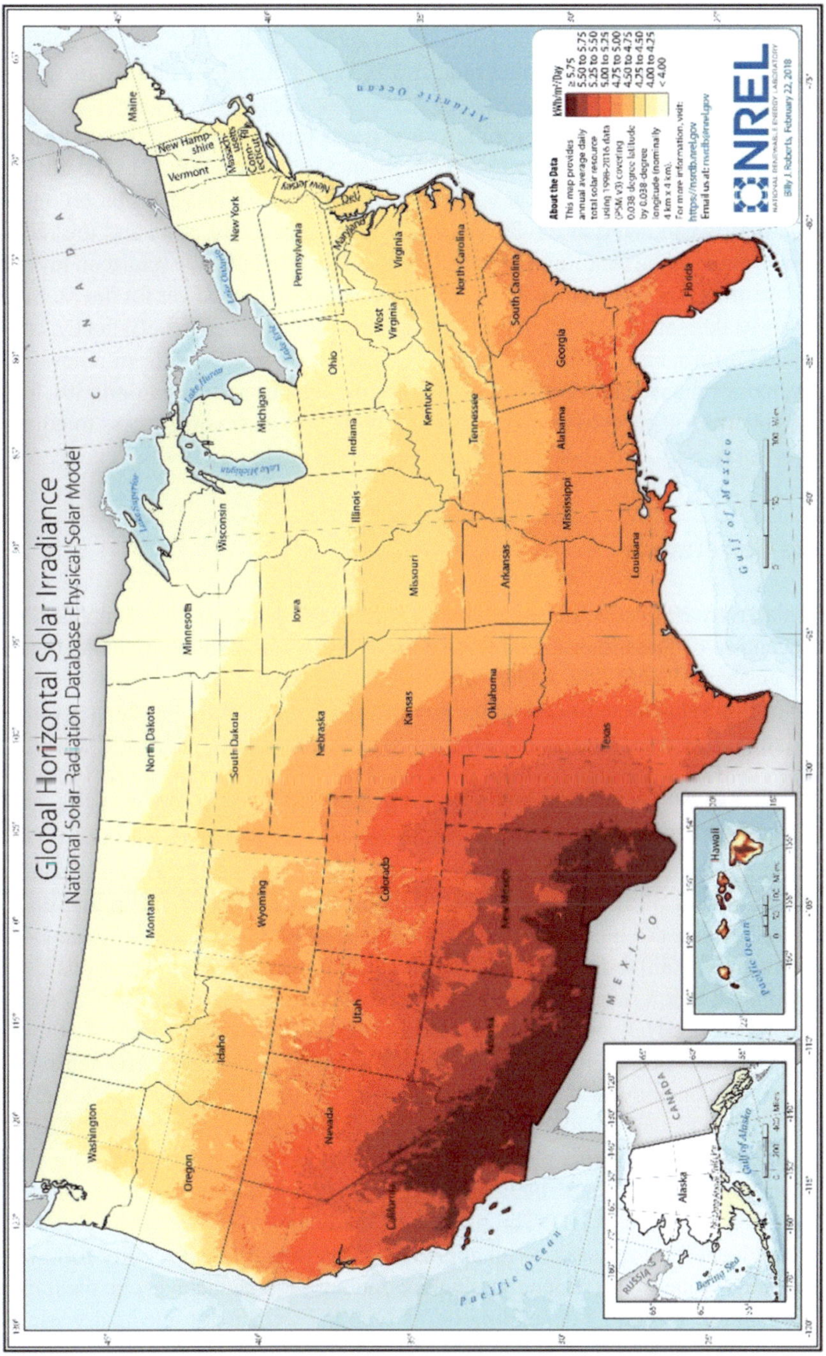

Fig. 17.2 Annual Solar Global Horizontal Irradiance (GHI) in the United States [54]

more commonly used in off-grid settings and has a higher cost. Once solar energy is harnessed, an inverter converts the direct current (DC) electricity to alternate current (AC) which HD and household electricity requires. The solar energy required for a 12-h week of home HD would require 15 kWh of electricity and 4.8 m^2 of the solar array [50].

Solar augmentation of power for dialysis use was found to reduce grid consumption by 91% and electricity costs by 76.5% in an Australian study [2]. The cost of the solar array and its installation varies between countries, however, based on its lifespan that is estimated at 25–30 years and using electricity costs and the reimbursement rates at the time, an Australian group calculated that the return on investment is estimated at 7–8 years with the cost-free generation of power for the lifetime of the array thereafter [2, 39]. With technological advances in the efficiency, reliability and affordability of battery storage of electricity harnessed from renewable energy, more reliance can be placed on this form of electricity generation [39]. The role of government incentives and dialysis providers in increasing access to equipment for solar-assisted dialysis may serve to improve the uptake of solar energy use.

Waste Generation

Human activity results in waste generation. In the healthcare setting, emphasis on the prevention of infectious spread from clinical waste has resulted in the tendency toward ensuring health and safety, with reduced emphasis on the environmental impact of this behaviour. To date in the healthcare sector, priority has been given to achieving good patient outcomes and maintaining staff safety with little time and energy placed on sustainability from both the perspective of the consumer (patients and medical staff) and the industry. Adding to the burden of existing waste loads in healthcare facilities, the Covid-19 pandemic resulted in significant waste contribution from the healthcare sector with approximately 87,000 tonnes of personal protective equipment (PPE) being procured, the majority of these would ending up as waste: 2600 tonnes of non-infectious waste and 731,000 L of chemical waste from test kits, and 144,000 tonnes of additional waste from vaccine administrations [55]. It is estimated that a patient dialysing in an in-centre HD unit generates 2.5 kg of clinical waste per HD session, which adds up to an estimated 390 kg of clinical waste per patient per year and this figure is increased in the home HD setting to 650 kg per person per year just in hazardous waste [8, 16]. This figure reaches about 600,000 tonnes per annum globally [8]. Hazardous, or medical, waste in the dialysis setting includes components that have encountered or contain blood and are thus considered infectious. These include needles, dialysers, infusion and bloodlines, and syringes [56] used in HD. The process of medical waste disposal involves the storage and transport of waste to an approved waste management facility followed by treatment of the waste which may include incineration, autoclave, chemical disinfection and/or shredding depending on its type [57]. Once non-medical waste is placed together with medical waste, it is classed as medical waste, undergoing the same high cost and energy waste management procedures.

Non-hazardous waste comprises general waste and waste that can be recycled [2]. General waste usually ends up in landfill, and toxins from the breakdown of this waste can seep into surrounding soil and groundwater, becoming environmental and health hazards. On top of that, organic waste in landfill emits methane, a GHG, that is 25–28 times more potent than carbon dioxide at warming the earth (contributing to global warming) despite being far lower in concentration and half-life in the atmosphere compared to carbon dioxide. Thus, any reduction in methane emission would potentially have a rapid and significant effect in decreasing the earth's warming potential [58, 59]. The use of bagged dialysis fluid in the NxStage system leads to a much higher amount of non-hazardous plastic waste generated per session (731 g) compared with conventional HD machines (approximately 200 g), a phenomenon also noted in peritoneal dialysis [2, 34].

The management of recyclable waste, comprising mostly of plastic in the HD setting [2], poses a different challenge. First, the rate of recycling of plastic, which is estimated to be recycled 14–18% of the time on a global level, is low compared to industrial metals and paper, whose recycling rates exceed 50%. Most plastic is either incinerated (24%) or enters landfill or nature (58–62%) which has a significantly higher GHG footprint compared to recycling [60]. The breakdown of polyvinyl chloride (PVC), which is abundant in plastic, produces toxic substances [2]. However, plastic recycling rates vary greatly between countries with the highest rate seen in high-income countries in the European Union, and this rate is not accurately known in low-middle-income countries. Second, the combination of its high usage rate and plastics' longevity results in a situation where plastics linger in the environment over hundreds or thousands of years, fragmenting into nanoplastics during this time [60]. Third, the carbon footprint of recycled plastics is significantly less than that of virgin plastics use which should not only encourage the practice of recycling more but is also important when considering product manufacturing and design for both equipment and packaging.

The home HD setting is a good place to start efforts in waste reduction and recycling. At an individual level, education should be provided to patients as part of dialysis training on waste reduction as well as conscientious waste classification and separation. Training to avoid wastage of consumables in HD will reduce waste generation and education in appropriate waste segregation will prevent contamination of recyclables and other non-hazardous waste. A study performed in an HD unit in Italy showed that the process of waste classification and segregation made a significant reduction in financial and ecological cost to the unit and only increased practice time by 1–2 min [56]. Waste clearance demands significant cost in the healthcare setting, where despite making up a smaller proportion of total waste, hazardous waste contributes to a large proportion of cost.

Financial costs aside, the ecological impact of this level of waste generation should not be taken lightly as any method of waste clearance comes at a cost to the environment. On an individual level, waste reduction and appropriate waste segregation should be practised. On an industry level, a collaboration between manufacturers and dialysis care providers focussing on reducing water and energy consumption of dialysis provision and overall carbon footprint of products used in dialysis by examining the entire life cycle of each product: through its development, production, transport, storage, use and waste management [19]. Assessment of entire product life cycles involves examining direct emissions of product use and indirect emissions from upstream (production and transportation) and downstream (waste disposal management) activities. It also provides comprehensive information on overall energy consumption and allows thorough evaluation of the environmental impact of each product which consists of 15 items and is subdivided into 5 main categories (human health preservation, terrestrial conservation, water protection, atmosphere protection and resource conservation) [19, 56, 61]. This may shed light on areas which can be optimised to improve the overall ecological sustainability of dialysis [8, 19]. Rather than considering a product as a finite entity, existing only in a linear fashion from manufacture (cradle) to final use (grave), let us be challenged to adopt a cradle-to-cradle philosophy to each product, where items we use are carefully thought-of by their components and potential to be reused or refashioned to become part of a new generation of products [56]. This is beautifully illustrated by Piccoli et al. in the analogy of the organic components of a dead tree nourishing growth of new plants without losing its biological components [56]. More effort is needed, on an industry and legislative level in improving management of waste in dialysis, particularly plastic waste.

Carbon Emissions

A comprehensive understanding of the impact of carbon emissions requires an understanding of the carbon cycle and is inseparable from local government and global policy and legislation. Calculation estimates like these are difficult to do and vary widely based on hospital practices, product supply chains and a country's, region's and unit's [62] level of information collection, capacity for conservation and access to renewable energy sources. A neutral carbon cycle requires a balance between emissions (from natural sources like decomposition or respiration, or human sources like burning of coal, oil and natural gas) and absorption (the role of forests as a carbon sink). The Kyoto Protocol, signed in 1997 as an international treaty setting mandatory limits on GHG emissions in industrialised nations identifies multiple GHGs with global warming potential (GWP) although only three are commonly reported: carbon dioxide (CO_2), methane (CH_4) and nitrous oxide (N_2O) [53]. Out of these, carbon dioxide is most used as the reference gas, and a unit of GWP is expressed as carbon dioxide equivalent (CO_2-e) [53]. Health care services in general are major contributors to climate change although these proportions vary widely depending on the country [3]. Between 2003 and 2013, the healthcare sector in the US represented 7–10% of the total US carbon dioxide emissions [62], and this number was 7% in 2014–2015 in Australia and 4% in England in 2012 [3]. Dialysis contributes to carbon emissions by water usage, energy consumption, waste generation and pharmaceutical manufacturing and supply. Despite the low proportion of patients on dialysis overall (0.4% of patients in the UK) dialysis contributed to about 65% of healthcare emissions in the UK in 2010 [63]. Further illustrating the 'high cost, low volume' nature of dialysis provision, calculations done in the Australian context show dialysis contributes to 10.2 tonnes carbon dioxide equivalent (CO_2-e) per patient, which is a significant proportion of the estimated emissions per person in general of 18.8 tonnes CO_2-e [8]. The contribution of each component of activity within the dialysis sector on carbon emissions differ by country. Procurement of pharmaceuticals and consumables (which includes emissions generated from manufacturing) made up majority of carbon emissions in Australia and the UK (59.1% and 72%, respectively), with energy consumption and travel included in the top three contributors to emissions [7, 8, 39, 52, 53]. This contrasts with energy consumption (28%) making up the largest proportion of carbon emissions, followed closely by procurement (27%) in Morocco [53]. Home dialysis eliminates the need for patient and staff travel although requires individual waste collection and product delivery.

More data is needed in this area to better understand the impact of dialysis-related trends on carbon emissions to aid us with implementing strategies and policies that will reduce our impact in this area. Monthly data collection on Key Performance Indicators (KPIs) related to ecological matters (electricity consumption, water usage and waste generation) began in 2005 for the French NephroCare group under Fresenius, allowing them to monitor practice trends over the subsequent decade [62] and is a good foundation that will aid in designing action plans to reduce the impact of dialysis on the environment. A thorough understanding of the sources of carbon emissions in dialysis would also pave the way for collaboration with pharmaceutical and equipment industries in product design and manufacturing to reduce the impact on carbon emissions.

Global Initiatives

In 2009 the UK established the Green Nephrology network within the National Health Service (NHS) Sustainable Healthcare Programme, documenting and implementing eco-friendly practices across dialysis units across the country and contributing to significant reduction in cost, water and energy consumption and GHG emissions [2, 8, 39, 64]. The European Renal Association European Dialysis and Transplant Association committed to implementing 'green' policies in the kidney sector in 2018. Recently, the Australia New Zealand Society of Nephrology released a position statement on green nephrology and has developed the existing Green Dialysis website with information for the implementation of 'green' changes in dialysis in their units [2, 64]. These strategies have been aimed largely at reducing the environmental impact of dialysis units but there are many practical recommendations which can be extrapolated and applied in the home HD setting.

Conclusion

HD is a resource-intensive treatment modality which has a significant impact on the environment. As clinicians, we need to acknowledge this burden and contribute to data collection, research, implementation of environmental-conservation policies and education of renal staff and the younger generation of nephrologists. It is also necessary to acknowledge that the clinician cannot function alone, and collaboration with industry experts, patients, dialysis staff and policymakers is key to achieving these goals. Whilst this undertaking may seem daunting with many variables on a large scale, the progress made by this movement, considering its humble beginnings two decades ago lends some encouragement. Despite this, there is still much work remaining in advancing sustainable dialysis practices.

References

1. IPBES. Summary for policymakers of the global assessment report on biodiversity and ecosystem services of the Intergovernmental Science-Policy Platform on Biodiversity and Ecosystem Services. Bonn: IPBES Secretariat; 2019. https://ipbes.net/sites/default/files/inline/files/ipbes_global_assessment_report_summary_for_policymakers.pdf.
2. Barraclough KA, Agar JWM. Green nephrology. Nat Rev Nephrol. 2020;16(5):257–68.
3. Nagai K, Suzuki H, Ueda A, Agar JWM, Itsubo N. Assessment of environmental sustainability in renal healthcare. J Rural Med. 2021;16(3):132–8.
4. Environmentally sustainable health systems: a strategic document. World Health Organization. Regional Office for Europe. 2017. https://apps.who.int/iris/handle/10665/340375.
5. World Health Organization. The Global Health Observatory: public health and environment. Environment and Health (WHO). [cited 2022 Oct 2]. https://www.who.int/data/gho/data/themes/public-health-and-environment.
6. Prüss-Üstün A, Wolf J, Corvalán CF, Bos R, Neira MP. Preventing disease through healthy environments: a global assessment of the burden of disease from environmental risks. Geneva: World Health Organization; 2016. [cited 2022 Oct 2]. 147 p. https://apps.who.int/iris/handle/10665/204585.
7. Tomson C, Connor A. Implications of climate change for nephrology. Nat Rev Nephrol. 2015;11(1):8–9.
8. Dunbar-Reid K, Buikstra E. The environmental impact of healthcare and haemodialysis: the Jekyll and Hyde dilemma. Ren Soc Australas J. 2017;13(2):38–44.
9. Johnson RJ, Wesseling C, Newman LS. Chronic kidney disease of unknown cause in agricultural communities. N Engl J Med. 2019;380(19):1843–52.
10. Sanchez Polo V, Garcia-Trabanino R, Rodriguez G, Madero M. Mesoamerican nephropathy (MeN): what we know so far. Int J Nephrol Renovasc Dis. 2020;13:261–72.
11. Sorensen C, Garcia-Trabanino R. A new era of climate medicine—addressing heat-triggered renal disease. N Engl J Med. 2019;381(8):693–6.
12. Fresenius medical care annual report 2018: care and live. Fresenius Medical Care AG & Co. KGaA; 2019. p. 267. https://www.freseniusmedicalcare.com/fileadmin/data/com/pdf/Media_Center/Publications/Annual_Reports/FME_Annual-Report_2018.pdf.
13. Himmelfarb J, Vanholder R, Mehrotra R, Tonelli M. The current and future landscape of dialysis. Nat Rev Nephrol. 2020;16(10):573–85.
14. World Health Organization. Climate change and health. Washington, DC: World Health Organization; 2021. [cited 2022 Oct 2]. https://www.who.int/news-room/fact-sheets/detail/climate-change-and-health.
15. James R. Dialysis and the environment: comparing home and unit based haemodialysis. J Ren Care. 2007;33(3):119–23.
16. Connor A, Mortimer F, Tomson C. Clinical transformation: the key to green nephrology. Nephron Clin Pract. 2010;116(3):c200–6.
17. Agar JWM, Hawley CM, George CRP, Mathew TH, McDonald SP, Kerr PG. Home haemodialysis in Australia—is the wheel turning full circle? Med J Aust. 2010;192(7):403–6.
18. Agar JW, Perkins A, Heaf JG. Home hemodialysis: infrastructure, water, and machines in the home: Home HD-Setup in the home. Hemodial Int. 2015;19:S93–111.
19. Apel C, Hornig C, Maddux FW, Ketchersid T, Yeung J, Guinsburg A. Informed decision-making in delivery of dialysis: combining clinical outcomes with sustainability. Clin Kidney J. 2021;14(Suppl 4):i98–113.
20. Marshall MR, Chan CT, The Global Forum for Home Hemodialysis. The Global Forum for Home Hemodialysis: a new open-source practical manual: Global Forum for Home Hemodialysis. Hemodial Int. 2015;19:S1–3.

21. UNICEF. Reimagining WASH: water security for all; 2019. p. 24. https://www.unicef.org/reports/reimagining-wash-water-security-for-all.
22. UNESCO, editor. UN world water development report 2019: leaving no one behind. Paris: UNESCO; 2019. 186 p. (The United Nations world water development report). https://unesdoc.unesco.org/ark:/48223/pf0000367306.
23. Damasiewicz MJ, Polkinghorne KR, Kerr PG. Water quality in conventional and home haemodialysis. Nat Rev Nephrol. 2012;8(12):725–34.
24. ACI Renal Network DWG. Water for dialysis: a guide for in-centre, satellite and home haemodialysis in NSW. Australia: Agency for Clinical Innovation; 2018. p. 88. Report no.: V1.5. www.aci.health.nsw.gov.au.
25. Coulliette AD, Arduino MJ. Hemodialysis and water quality. Semin Dial. 2013;26(4):427–38.
26. Dheda S, Van Eps C, Hawley C, Johnson DW. Water treatment for centre and home-based haemodialysis. In: Suzuki H, editor. Updates in hemodialysis. London: IntechOpen; 2015. [cited 2022 Jun 26]. http://www.intechopen.com/books/updates-in-hemodialysis/water-treatment-for-centre-and-home-based-haemodialysis.
27. Agar JWM, Simmonds RE, Knight R, Somerville CA. Using water wisely: new, affordable, and essential water conservation practices for facility and home hemodialysis. Hemodial Int. 2009;13(1):32–7.
28. Lockridge R, Cornelis T, Van Eps C. Prescriptions for home hemodialysis: prescriptions for home HD. Hemodial Int. 2015;19:S112–27.
29. Hoenich NA, Ronco C. Perspectives in home hemodialysis therapy. In: Ronco C, Rosner MH, editors. Contributions to nephrology. Basel: S. Karger AG; 2011. p. 25–9. [cited 2022 Oct 1]. https://www.karger.com/Article/FullText/327339.
30. Ibrahim A, Chan CT. Managing kidney failure with home hemodialysis. Clin J Am Soc Nephrol. 2019;14(8):1268–73.
31. Agar J. Haemodialysis: going green. Home haemodialysis central. 2014. https://homedialysis.org/news-and-research/blog/49-haemodialysis-going-green.
32. Glickman JD, Teitelbaum I, Golper TA. Prescribing home hemodialysis. Adv Chronic Kidney Dis. 2021;28(2):157–63.
33. Agar JWM. Reusing and recycling dialysis reverse osmosis system reject water. Kidney Int. 2015;88(4):653–7.
34. Haroon S, Davenport A. Haemodialysis at home: review of current dialysis machines. Expert Rev Med Devices. 2018;15(5):337–47.
35. Agar JWM. Dialysis and the environment: seeking a more sustainable future. Artif Organs. 2019;43(12):1123–9.
36. Tarrass F, Benjelloun M, Benjelloun O, Bensaha T. Water conservation: an emerging but vital issue in hemodialysis therapy. Blood Purif. 2010;30(3):181–5.
37. Agar JW. Conserving water in and applying solar power to haemodialysis: 'green dialysis' through wiser resource utilization: natural resource conservation in dialysis. Nephrology. 2009;15(4):448–53.
38. Tarrass F, Benjelloun M, Benjelloun O. Recycling wastewater after hemodialysis: an environmental analysis for alternative water sources in arid regions. Am J Kidney Dis. 2008;52(1):154–8.
39. Agar JWM. Green dialysis: the environmental challenges ahead. Semin Dial. 2015;28(2):186–92.
40. Agar JWM, Barraclough KA. A novel way to re-use reverse osmosis reject water. J Nephrol. 2021;34(1):27–8.
41. Chang E, Lim JA, Low CL, Kassim A. Reuse of dialysis reverse osmosis reject water for aquaponics and horticulture. J Nephrol. 2021;34(1):97–104.
42. Ponson L, Arkouche W, Laville M. Toward green dialysis: focus on water savings: toward green dialysis. Hemodial Int. 2014;18(1):7–14.
43. Layman-Amato R, Curtis J, Payne GM. Water treatment for hemodialysis: an update. Nephrol Nurs J. 2013;40(5):383–404, 465 quiz 405.
44. Agar JWM, Barraclough KA. Water use in dialysis: environmental considerations. Nat Rev Nephrol. 2020;16(10):556–7.

45. Godin M. The ocean farmers trying to save the world with seaweed. TIME. 2020. https://time.com/5848994/seaweed-climate-change-solution/.
46. Gauly A, Fleck N, Kircelli F. Advanced hemodialysis equipment for more eco-friendly dialysis. Int Urol Nephrol. 2022;54(5):1059–65.
47. Ritchie H, Roser M. Electricity mix. Our world in data. 2020. https://ourworldindata.org/electricity-mix.
48. What is the average electricity use for a family of four? Green energy efficient homes. 2016. https://green-energy-efficient-homes.com/average-electricity-consumption.html.
49. Masterson V. Renewables were the world's cheapest source of energy in 2020, new report shows. Cologny: World Economic Forum; 2021. https://www.weforum.org/agenda/2021/07/renewables-cheapest-energy-source/.
50. Agar JWM, Perkins A, Tjipto A. Solar-assisted hemodialysis. Clin J Am Soc Nephrol. 2012;7(2):310–4.
51. Damasiewicz MJ, Polkinghorne KR. Global dialysis perspective: Australia. Kidney360. 2020;1(1):48–51.
52. Connor A, Lillywhite R, Cooke MW. The carbon footprints of home and in-center maintenance hemodialysis in the United Kingdom: the carbon footprint of hemodialysis. Hemodial Int. 2011;15(1):39–51.
53. Mtioui N, Zamd M, Ait Taleb A, Bouaalam A, Ramdani B. Carbon footprint of a hemodialysis unit in Morocco. Ther Apher Dial. 2021;25(5):613–20.
54. Sengupta M, Xie Y, Lopez A, Habte A, Maclaurin G, Shelby J. The National Solar Radiation Data Base (NSRDB). Renew Sustain Energy Rev. 2018;89:51–60. https://www.nrel.gov/gis/solar-resource-maps.html.
55. WHO Water, Sanitation, Hygiene and Health Unit. Tonnes of COVID-19 health care waste expose urgent need to improve waste management systems. Washington, DC: World Health Organization; 2022. https://www.who.int/news/item/01-02-2022-tonnes-of-covid-19-health-care-waste-expose-urgent-need-to-improve-waste-management-systems.
56. Piccoli GB, Nazha M, Ferraresi M, Vigotti FN, Pereno A, Barbero S. Eco-dialysis: the financial and ecological costs of dialysis waste products: is a 'cradle-to-cradle' model feasible for planet-friendly haemodialysis waste management? Nephrol Dial Transplant. 2015;30(6):1018–27.
57. IWRG612.1: clinical and related waste—operational guidance. Environment Protection Authority Victoria. 2009. https://www.epa.vic.gov.au/about-epa/publications/iwrg612-1.
58. Importance of methane. United States Environmental Protection Agency. 2022. https://www.epa.gov/gmi/importance-methane.
59. Borunda A. Methane, explained. National Geographic. 2019. https://www.nationalgeographic.com/environment/article/methane.
60. Improving plastics management: trends, policy responses, and the role of international co-operation and trade. Organisation for Economic Co-operation and Development; 2018.
61. Sherman JD, Thiel C, MacNeill A, Eckelman MJ, Dubrow R, Hopf H, et al. The green print: advancement of environmental sustainability in healthcare. Resour Conserv Recycl. 2020;161:104882.
62. Bendine G, Autin F, Fabre B, Bardin O, Rabasco F, Cabanel JM, et al. Haemodialysis therapy and sustainable growth: a corporate experience in France. Nephrol Dial Transplant. 2020;35(12):2154–60.
63. Connor A, Lillywhite R, Cooke MW. The carbon footprint of a renal service in the United Kingdom. QJM. 2010;103(12):965–75.
64. Barraclough KA, Holt SG, Agar JW. Climate change and us: what nephrologists should know: climate change and nephrology. Nephrology. 2015;20(10):760–4.

18 Anemia Management in Home Hemodialysis

Ramy M. Hanna, Rebecca S. Ahdoot, Anjay Rastogi, and Edgar V. Lerma

Introduction

Anemia in chronic kidney disease (CKD) is one of many complications that require a broad spectrum of clinical expertise beyond simple management of serum electrolytes. This highlights the ongoing and evolving understanding of the kidneys' endocrine functions, like parathyroid hormone (PTH) response, 25 hydroxyvitamin D-1 alpha hydroxylation, phosphatonin and Fibroblast growth factor 23 (FGF23) regulation, erythropoietin generation, and iron metabolism [1].

As CKD patients transition into end-stage renal disease (ESRD) two main modalities await them: peritoneal dialysis (PD) or hemodialysis (HD). The PD at-home model is drastically different from the hemodialysis model of in-center care [2]. The home hemodialysis (HHD) model is a hybrid of in-center hemodialysis (ICHD) with different dialyzer clearances, a higher order of medical skills that patients need to be trained on, and a higher risk of a serious mechanical failure (given extracorporeal blood pumping) [3]. The benefits of HHD include superior efficiency versus in-center, as it allows for more frequent HD, which results in superior solute clearance, volume control, blood pressure control, phosphorous control, and lower need for erythropoietin stimulating agent (ESA) use [2].

R. M. Hanna (✉) · R. S. Ahdoot
Division of Nephrology, Department of Medicine, University of California Irvine Medical Center, Orange, CA, USA
e-mail: ramyh1@hs.uci.edu; Ahdoot@uci.edu

A. Rastogi
UCLA Medical Center, Los Angeles, CA, USA
e-mail: rastogiadmin@mednet.ucla.edu; ARastogi@mednet.ucla.edu

E. V. Lerma
Section of Nephrology, University of Illinois at Chicago/Advocate Christ Medical Center, Oak Lawn, IL, USA
e-mail: elerma@uic.edu

A. Shah et al. (eds.), *Applied Home Hemodialysis*,
https://doi.org/10.1007/978-3-031-77244-3_18

The downside of HHD, however, is the requirement for a medically proficient patient, and family to support patients and to help handle medical emergencies [4]. The patients recruited to HHD must be able and comfortable with self-canulation, handling dialysis machine functionality, and being able to understand the balance of ultrafiltration to avoid hypotension, manage weight, and track weight as a marker of volume [4]. HHD patients must be on guard against adverse effects against residual renal function, which declines with hypotension and aggressive ultrafiltration [5].

The management of anemia in HHD is similarly expected to be more independently managed by the patient [6]. ESA use and iron supplementation can be coordinated algorithmically with nursing or medical support [6]. However, instead of intravenous dosing of ESAs (both fast-acting alpha or slow-acting beta erythropoietin agents) are typically administered subcutaneously [6]. The somewhat slow emergence of hypoxia-inducing factor-prolyl hydroxyl inhibitors (HIF-PHIs) also stand to provide an oral agent alternative to the standard subcutaneous injections now used to manage anemia in ESRD, and soon also anemia in CKD [7]. Iron infusions may be handled differently in this case (orally) or by intravenous infusion at the in-center dialysis unit. CKD patients currently have an indication for ferric citrate as a phosphorous binder and to help alleviate anemia in CKD, currently no indication exists for in-center HD or HHD. The dual use of this agent however should be included in discussions of oral iron therapy [8].

This chapter will review anemia in ESRD management from the maximal freedom from in-center services that HHD programs provide [2]. It is believed that the national emphasis on de-emphasizing ICHD and increasing HHD and PD, that future directions of development in HHD will de-emphasize in-center services [9]. In lieu of this, artificial intelligence, algorithms, and remote support will very likely emerge to minimize in-person healthcare burden to systems and provide comparable or improved healthcare outcomes at equivalent or modestly lower costs [10].

Pathophysiology of Anemia of End-Stage Renal Disease

The main problem in ESRD is the reduction of healthy, functional filtering nephron mass to a critically low level [11]. This results in decreased filtration of solute, acid, organic anions, potassium, salt, free water, urea/nitrogenous waste, as well as decreased generation of hormonal mediators [11]. This is reflected in a drop in erythropoietin levels, and dysregulation of iron metabolism due to inflammation leading to an anemia of chronic disease (ACD) clinical picture [6, 12]. HD can also theoretically result in increased and unwanted filtration of water-soluble B vitamins necessary for erythrogenesis [6, 12]. Add to this the risk of blood loss by clotting, bleeding from dialysis access, blood loss, and bleeding caused by the transient heparinization frequently used in dialysis circuits [6, 12]. The use of warfarin, antiplatelet agents, or other novel oral anticoagulants is also needed in certain medically complex ESRD patients [6, 12].

This can increase the risk of bleeding from non-renal access-associated causes: hemolysis, gastrointestinal bleeding, or gynecological bleeding in females. Access de-clotting with tissue plasminogen activator (TPA) or thrombectomies provides another avenue for surgical blood loss in ESRD patients [6, 13].

The result, of course, is the clinically apparent drop in hemoglobin with accompanying increased cardiac risk, cerebrovascular risk, fatigue [6, 12], drop in health-related quality of life (HRQoL) assessments [14], and the need for workups to ascertain the cause of anemia in patients who may not respond as completely to ESAs and iron supplementation [15].

In addition to the loss of erythropoietin production, there is a growing body of evidence that CKD and ESRD are inflammatory processes that affect nutrition, ESA responsiveness, and iron metabolism [6, 12]. This inflammatory state is increasingly thought to be related to middle molecules that aren't well cleared by dialysis modalities in the United States (usually more favorably cleared by hemofiltration than hemodialysis) [6, 12]. In addition, the failure to normalize phosphorous despite PTH and FGF23 activation can result in increasing levels of inflammation that affect hepcidin and the HIF-PHI pathway [1]. In extreme cases, calcium and phosphorous deposition may result in even more extreme inflammation and the clinically grim specter of calciphylaxis [1]. Volume excess is also postulated to not only result in cardiac morbidity and mortality but also may affect endothelial cell homeostasis adversely [12].

In summary, the mechanisms of anemia in ESRD are legion. They include lower bone marrow production of red cells, iron deficiency, iron utilization block by inflammation, nutritional deficiency, dysfunction of red cells from middle molecule uremic toxins, inflammation from other toxins, blood loss from access/dialysis tubing, and endothelial factors that affect red blood cell health and longevity [6, 12, 16, 17]. See Figs. 18.1 and 18.2.

Treatment of Anemia in CKD and ESRD

CKD and ESRD are cardiovascular risk factors from a variety of mechanistic standpoints—calcification, dyslipidemia that often accompanies epidemiological metabolic syndrome, volume overload, and anemia are the most clinically significant ways that CKD and ESRD contribute to worsening cardiovascular risk [6, 12]. The endothelial inflammation caused by inappropriately cleared middle molecules also contributes to an increased risk of thrombosis, coronary, cerebrovascular, and peripheral artery disease as CKD evolves into ESRD [6, 12]. Atherosclerotic cardiovascular disease (ASCVD) is a major mortality concern and, with worsening CKD, cardiovascular mortality risk can be higher than the risk of progression to ESRD [6, 12]. The current hemoglobin target is 10–11.5 g/L. There is a strong target to avoid hemoglobin levels >12 g/dL [18], which paradoxically and unacceptably increases the risk of thrombosis [6, 12, 18]. While quality of life improves with increased hemoglobin levels, the cardiovascular, cerebrovascular, and thromboembolic risk factors far outweigh any benefits symptomatically so as to preclude recommending hemoglobin levels >12 g/dL [12]. While ESRD centers often have advanced

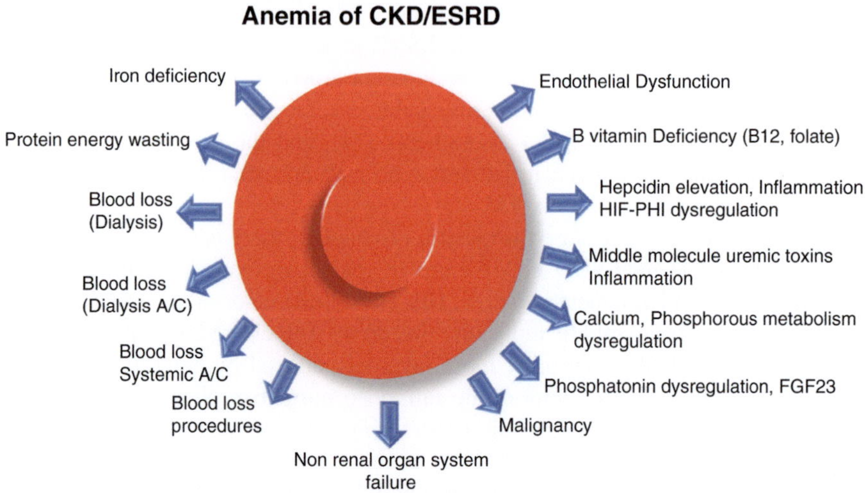

Fig. 18.1 Why do CKD and ESRD cause anemia? ACE, angiotensin converting enzyme; ARB, angiotensin receptor blockers; B12, cyanocobalamin; BM, bone marrow; BUN, blood urea nitrogen; Ca, calcium; CKD, chronic kidney disease; EPO, erythropoietin; ESRD, end-stage renal disease; HD, hemodialysis; HIF, hypoxia-inducing factor; Phos, phosphorus; TDC, tunneled dialysis catheters

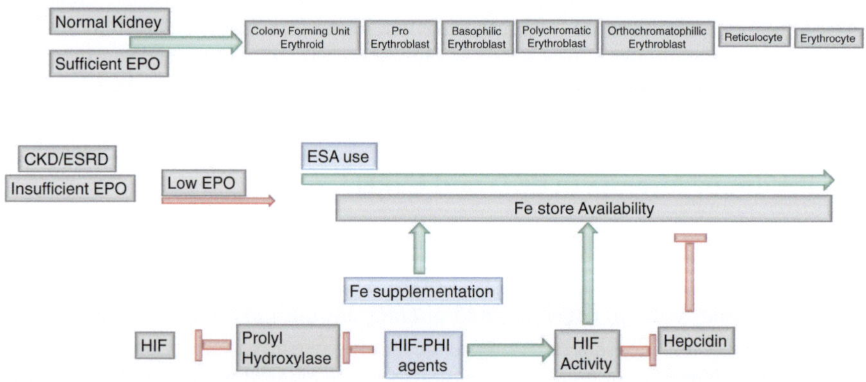

Fig. 18.2 Erythrogenesis and ESA mechanisms of action. EPO, erythropoietin; ESA, erythropoiesis-stimulating agents; Fe, iron; HIF-PHI, hypoxia-inducing factor-prolyl hydroxylase inhibitor; $T_{1/2}$, half-life

algorithms for the treatment of ESRD-related anemia, there are few such programs validated for use in CKD [19].

Novel therapeutic treatment options in CKD, difficulty with insurance coverage or financial cost, and required patient/caregiver training make anemia management in CKD even more challenging. The rationale as outlined is focused on increasing hemoglobin while minimizing the increased risk of ASCVD-related adverse outcomes [12]. Negative cardiac outcomes also include congestive heart failure (CHF) and increased left ventricular hypertrophy in addition to the dramatic coronary events caused by increased work of myocardium required in anemia combined with reduced oxygen carrying capacity (Fig. 18.1) [12].

The main tools available to increase serum hemoglobin today are very different than those used in the past [6]. Previously, anemia management was focused on transfusions and testosterone therapy [6]. Currently, the cornerstone of anemia management is IV iron and ESA [6]. HIF-PHIs are currently expeditiously being developed and the information presented is likely to rapidly change even from the time of writing this chapter to its publications [6]. Below we describe the available evidence for each intervention.

IV Iron

CKD and ESRD patients have reduced red cell counts for a number of reasons, including loss of ESA action from reduced renal mass, comorbid conditions, and the dialysis state itself which can lead to blood loss and inflammation from reduced middle molecule clearance. Additionally, dialysis membrane exposure can produce an inflammatory state increasing hepcidin and reducing iron utilization, contributing to an anemia of chronic disease pattern. Adding to this, the use of ESAs prompts higher iron demands over and above physiologic needs to support red blood cell production [20–25].

Iron therapy in earlier-stage CKD can typically be managed with oral iron administration. While this modality is easier to take and convenient, oral iron can be sub-optimally absorbed and is not always well tolerated [20]. Side effects include constipation and stomach irritation [20]. Alternatively, IV iron has superior bio availability, which has previously been demonstrated [23]. IV iron has been shown to be superior in inducing ESA response with a proactive rather than a reactive study. IV iron also presents a risk of exacerbating systemic infections due to iron being a growth-limiting factor in bacterial replication [21]. Many algorithms are based on data first revealed in the PIVOTAL trial. This trial revealed that proactive IV iron use results in equivalent anemia control with less ESA usage in HD patients (PIVOTAL trial) [24] and is highly likely to be relevant to the home hemodialysis population. Lower ESA usage in the dialysis population has also been linked with improved clinical outcomes as well as improved cost utilization from an organizational point of view [6].

The key measure of ESA effectiveness is the avoidance of blood transfusions with proper IV iron usage in conjunction with ESAs [6]. IV iron is much easier to utilize in ICHD vs. PD or CKD patients [2, 4]. HHD patients have the advantage of having access established while doing dialysis more easily allowing IV administration of medications [2, 4]. However, the risk of a negative allergic transfusion reaction of IV iron remains highlighting the importance of a test dose and ensuring the patient can tolerate the IV infusion. Otherwise, this may necessitate the need for in-center IV iron infusions even in HHD patients [6].

Table 18.1 Iron formulations for home hemodialysis

Agent	Usual schedule	Usual dose	Route	Side effects
Iron sulfate	TID	325 mg	Oral	Constipation, poor bioavailability, and absorption
Iron gluconate	TID to QID	240–320 mg	Oral	Poor bioavailability and absorption Less constipation than iron sulfate
Iron dextran Low molecular weight	2–3 times a week for limited duration	100 mg injection	Intravenous	Anaphylaxis, infection risk, renal oxidative stress risk in CKD
Iron dextran High molecular weight	2–3 times a week for limited duration	100 mg injection	Intravenous	Anaphylaxis, infection risk, renal oxidative stress risk in CKD
Iron sucrose	2–3 times a week for limited duration	100 mg injection	Intravenous	Anaphylaxis, infection risk, renal oxidative stress risk in CKD
Ferumoxytol	Followed by 1 repeat dose 3–8 days after initial dosing	510 mg injection	Intravenous	Will cause enhancement on MRI scanning up to 3 months after
Ferric gluconate	2–3 times a week for limited duration	125 mg injection	Intravenous	Benzyl alcohol reactions
Ferric citrate	2–3 tabs with meals	210 mg	Oral	Constipation

CKD, chronic kidney disease; MRI, magnetic resonance imaging; QID, four times a day; TID, three times a day

Downsides to IV iron use would be to avoid/minimize active infection [23], volume overload, and in sensitized/allergic patients. Though the downsides to blood transfusion certainly also warrant minimizing those procedures given risks of transfusion reactions, elevated immune sensitization (especially problematic for potential transplant recipients) [6], volume and potassium load as well [6]. Table 18.1 lists current readily available oral and IV iron repletion regimens and their most common side effects.

ESAs

Erythropoietin stimulating agents (ESAs) are synthetic recombinant agents that mimic the endogenous hormone erythropoietin [26, 27]. The clinical effect is to stimulate the line of red cell progenitors in the bone marrow, a role typically played by endogenously renally produced erythropoietin (Fig. 18.2) [26, 27]. There are two broad classes differing in potency and half-lives, also they generate different clinical responses given differing rates of onset of action. ESAs can be given both intravenously and subcutaneously. In the setting of HHD patients, either method is possible. It is, however, important to note that subcutaneously administered ESAs tend to have a longer biological half-life [28–37].

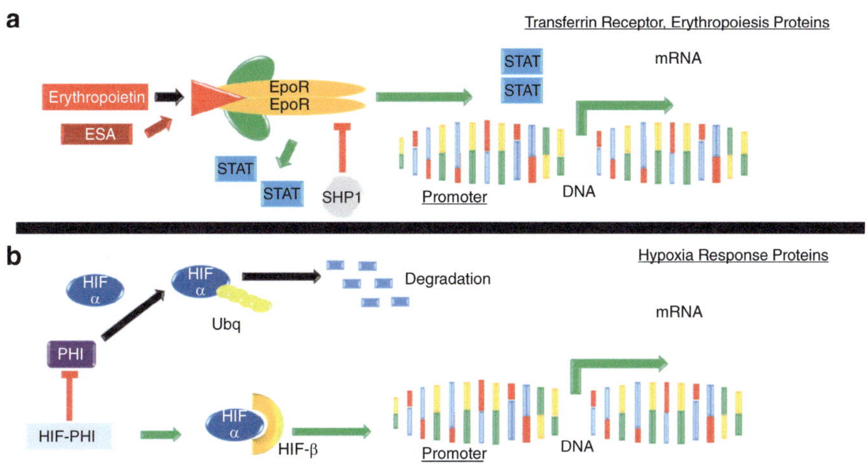

Fig. 18.3 ESA and HIF-HIF-PHI mechanisms of action. (**a**) EpoR, erythropoietin receptor; ESA, erythropoiesis-stimulating agent; mRNA, messenger RNA; HIF-α, hypoxia-inducing factor alpha; (**b**) HIF-β, hypoxia-inducing factor beta; PHI, prolyl hydroxylase inhibitor; SHPI-1; SH2-domain containing protein; STAT, signal transduction and transcription protein; Ubq, ubiquinone. Note ubiquinone tagged proteins are marked for proteasome degradation

Half-life considerations and variation in degradation speed aside, these agents function molecularly by promoting phosphorylation of signal transducer and activation of transcription protein (STAT) protein that then undergoes nuclear translocation and binds the promotor of various erythropoiesis promoting proteins (Fig. 18.3) [33].

The history of these agents is one of the greatest successes in modern nephrology practice. They were first described and used experimentally in the 1980s and 1990s. The three broad categories of ESAs are discussed briefly below [6].

Erythropoietin Alpha

The erythropoietin alpha (ESA-α) category is a shorter-acting variety that has a rapid onset of action similar to biological erythropoietin and similar rapid degradation. These were the first agents to be successfully used in CKD and ESRD population [38]. They are approved for CKD and ESRD populations and their use is a marker of quality CKD care. They are more easily given in the algorithmic form, including some algorithms that are commonly employed by large dialysis organizations (LDOs) that are using artificial intelligence [19]. They typically have the shortest half-lives and require the most frequent redosing [6]. While this may be acceptable for ICHD patients, it is less optimal for home dialysis patients (PD and HHD), who are less frequently present in-center [6]. This can be mitigated in patients who can self-administer and may need to use older generations of ESAs due to formulary limitations (Table 18.2) [6].

Table 18.2 Doses of erythropoietin analogs used in end-stage renal disease

Agent	Usual dose	Usual schedule	Route	Side effects
Erythropoietin alpha-α	300 units/kg 2000–20,000 units	TIW ($T_{1/2}$ = 4–13 h)	IV SQ	High hemoglobin >12 g/L associated with adverse CV and cerebrovascular events Worsening of existing malignancy
Methoxy-polyethylene-glycol-erythropoietin-beta β	0.6 μg/kg 60–360 μg doses	60–180 μg every 2 weeks 120–360 μg every 4 weeks $T_{1/2}$ 119–124 h (HD lower $T_{1/2}$, PD higher $T_{1/2}$)	IV SQ	High hemoglobin >12 g/L associated with adverse CV and cerebrovascular events Worsening of existing malignancy
Darbepoetin-alpha-α	0.45 μg/kg 25–500 μg doses	Every 4 weeks ($T_{1/2}$ = 24–144 h)	IV SQ	High hemoglobin >12 g/L associated with adverse CV and cerebrovascular events Worsening of existing malignancy
Erythropoietin βΔΩ not approved in the United States by the FDA at this time of this writing				

CV, cardiovascular; FDA, US Food and Drug Administration; EU, European Union; HD, hemodialysis; V, intravenous; PD, peritoneal dialysis; SQ, subcutaneous; $T_{1/2}$, half-life; TIW, three times a week

(PEG) Erythropoietin Beta

Methyl-polyethylene glycol (PEG) erythropoietin beta (ESA-β) make up the family of beta ESAs that have a longer half-life and less hemoglobin variation with a slower onset of action and longer duration of action. These agents are more naturally useful in patients who are in the center for fewer visits or see their provider less often, which is the current case with HHD/PD patients (Table 18.2) [6, 38].

Darbepoetin Alpha

Darbepoetin alpha is a chemical modification of the original erythropoietin alpha which allows for extremely long half-lives, they are typically re-dosed at every 4-week intervals. This allows less frequent injections and greater sustainability of patient hemoglobin targets. While algorithmically they need more careful control given a longer duration of action, their effect tends to be slower and the rise and fall of hemoglobin is slower with the longer-acting agents (Table 18.2) [6, 38].

HIF/PHI

Hypoxia-inducing factor (HIF)/prolyl hydroxylase inhibitors (PHI) offer a very interesting frontier in CKD/ESRD anemia therapeutics. The oral route of administration is highly enticing and would likely improve compliance, patient satisfaction, and quality of life over injections. The mechanism of action is unique. Rather than targeting the endogenous erythropoietin pathway, the target is prolyl hydroxylase. PHIs stabilize HIF by inhibiting ubiquitin tagging which leads directly to proteasome degradation (Fig. 18.3), resulting in endogenous Erythropoietin production, in turn, organically raising serum hemoglobin [7, 38–51].

The very first agent to be explored, Roxadustat, is a cautionary tale of the difficulties in drug development. After an initial bid for FDA approval [42], Roxadustat was reevaluated in light of concerns about cardiovascular safety, liver function test elevations, and risk of worsening malignancy [42]. Despite the fact that the same risks exist with ESAs further data is requested by the FDA and it may in fact eventually win approval with more rigorous data. The current risks cited are cardiovascular, liver function test abnormalities, and risk of worsening malignancies [42].

Currently, the approved drugs in the HIF-PHI class include Daprodustat in April 2023 [52]. Vadadustat was close to an approval in the United States [53] but has been held back since March 2022 pending safety trials [54]. It is approved in Japan as of March 2022 [55]. There are several other agents that are being given orally either daily or 3 times a week. The current direction indicates approvals are likely for some (as they are approved in India, the EU, Japan, and other developed nations).

HIF-PHIs stand to greatly impact CKD anemia management and the management of anemia of ESRD due to its oral route. Perhaps, with more safety data algorithmic management can be combined with modern communications to streamline HIF-PHI use at home with artificial intelligence guidance with continued vigilance from physician or advanced practice nursing oversight [43–46]. See Table 18.3 for details.

Final Thoughts on HHD Anemia Management

Currently, it is very important with the 2019 Advancing American Kidney Health Act to recognize that an unstoppable momentum is building for changing the way dialysis is currently organized. While ICHD allows a maximum of patient services being done in facilities, it runs into patient satisfaction, cost, and logistical difficulties. The changing face of dialysis will evolve into a primarily home dialysis modalities (PD and HHD) system rather than in center given the Advancing Kidney Care Act [9, 56].

With a potential approaching explosion in HHD and PD, a great need arises to streamline ESA use at home or to look to new advancements (like HIF-PHI) to fill the gap that will be formed by large dialysis organizations cutting back ICHD in compliance with governmental and payor dictates [6].

Table 18.3 Doses of HIF stabilizers-PHI inhibitors in end-stage renal disease

Agent	Route	Usual dose (mg)	Usual schedule	Side effects
Roxadustat	Oral	50–300	TIW ($T_{1/2}$ = 12 h)	High hemoglobin >12 g/L is not recommended based on findings with ESAs **Still not FDA approved.** Testing ongoing
Daprodustat	Oral	1–24	Daily	Hemoglobin >12 g/L, not recommended **FDA approved 02/2023**
Vadadustat	Oral	150–600	Daily	Hemoglobin >12 g/L, not recommended **Still FDA approval not yet, re-evaluation after safety trials**
Molidustat	Oral	5–200	Daily	Hemoglobin >12 not recommended, **FDA trials pending**
Enarodustat	Oral	2–24	Daily	Hemoglobin >12 not recommended **FDA currently evaluating approval (soon)**
Desidustat	Oral	100–150	TIW	Hemoglobin >12 not recommended, **FDA approval-not yet**

CKD, chronic kidney disease; ESA, erythropoiesis-stimulating agents; FDA, US food and drug administration; HIF-PHI, hypoxia-inducing factor (stabilizers)-prolyl hydroxylase (inhibitors); $T_{1/2}$, half-life; TIW, three times a week

This section serves to remind the reader that patients will be less well monitored conventionally as more artificial intelligence modalities will likely be used and that the nephrologist will increasingly be required to take on aspects of workup and management done by primary care physicians. As such, a reminder of when patients need further workup for anemia is in order. Finding a high MCV >100 (B12 and folate deficiencies, liver disease) and a low MCV <80 (Iron deficiency) would always trigger a more precise inquiry.

Hematologic syndromes such as atypical hemolytic uremic syndrome and paroxysmal nocturnal hemoglobinuria would demonstrate hemolytic anemia (high LDH, schistocytes) and unexplained thrombotic events, and require quick recognition and a high index of suspicion. Bleeding diathesis should launch an inquiry for malignancy, but the opposite (thrombosis) or the need for high-dose ESAs should also elicit a similar concern. High-dose ESA use without response despite iron repletion should elicit an investigation of the bone marrow or hematological referral [6].

References

1. Hanna RM, Ahdoot RS, Kalantar-Zadeh K, Ghobry L, Kurtz I. Calcium transport in the kidney and disease processes. Front Endocrinol (Lausanne). 2021;12:762130.
2. Vinson AJ, Perl J, Tennankore KK. Survival comparisons of home dialysis versus in-center hemodialysis: a narrative review. Can J Kidney Health Dis. 2019;6:2054358119861941.
3. Miller BW, Himmele R, Sawin DA, Kim J, Kossmann RJ. Choosing home hemodialysis: a critical review of patient outcomes. Blood Purif. 2018;45(1–3):224–9.
4. Pauly RP, Eastwood DO, Marshall MR. Patient safety in home hemodialysis: quality assurance and serious adverse events in the home setting. Hemodial Int. 2015;19(Suppl 1):S59–70.

5. Kjaergaard KD, Jensen JD, Peters CD, Jespersen B. Preserving residual renal function in dialysis patients: an update on evidence to assist clinical decision making. NDT Plus. 2011;4(4):225–30.
6. Hanna RM, Streja E, Kalantar-Zadeh K. Burden of anemia in chronic kidney disease: beyond erythropoietin. Adv Ther. 2021;38(1):52–75.
7. Haase VH, Chertow GM, Block GA, et al. Effects of vadadustat on hemoglobin concentrations in patients receiving hemodialysis previously treated with erythropoiesis-stimulating agents. Nephrol Dial Transplant. 2019;34(1):90–9.
8. Ganz T, Bino A, Salusky IB. Mechanism of action and clinical attributes of Auryxia((R)) (ferric citrate). Drugs. 2019;79(9):957–68.
9. Quinn RR, Lam NN, Ravani P, Oliver MJ, Blake PG, Tonelli M. The advancing American kidney health initiative: the challenge of measuring success. J Am Soc Nephrol. 2022;33(6):1060–2.
10. Burlacu A, Iftene A, Jugrin D, et al. Using artificial intelligence resources in dialysis and kidney transplant patients: a literature review. Biomed Res Int. 2020;2020:9867872.
11. Cooper BA, Branley P, Bulfone L, et al. A randomized, controlled trial of early versus late initiation of dialysis. N Engl J Med. 2010;363(7):609–19.
12. Hanna RM, Ferrey A, Rhee CM, Kalantar-Zadeh K. Renal-cerebral pathophysiology: the interplay between chronic kidney disease and cerebrovascular disease. J Stroke Cerebrovasc Dis. 2021;30(9):105461.
13. Hanna RM, Barsoum M, Vandross A, Kurtz I, Burwick R. Atypical hemolytic uremic syndrome and complement blockade: established and emerging uses of complement inhibition. Curr Opin Nephrol Hypertens. 2019;28(3):278–87.
14. Spinowitz B, Pecoits-Filho R, Winkelmayer WC, et al. Economic and quality of life burden of anemia on patients with CKD on dialysis: a systematic review. J Med Econ. 2019;22(6):593–604.
15. Evans M, Bower H, Cockburn E, Jacobson SH, Barany P, Carrero JJ. Contemporary management of anaemia, erythropoietin resistance and cardiovascular risk in patients with advanced chronic kidney disease: a nationwide analysis. Clin Kidney J. 2020;13(5):821–7.
16. Locatelli F, Del Vecchio L. The search for the perfect agent for anemia management in chronic kidney disease. J Am Soc Nephrol. 2022;33(4):662–4
17. Locatelli F, Pisoni RL, Akizawa T, et al. Anemia management for hemodialysis patients: kidney disease outcomes quality initiative (K/DOQI) guidelines and dialysis outcomes and practice patterns study (DOPPS) findings. Am J Kidney Dis. 2004;44(5 Suppl 2):27–33.
18. Wish JB. Perspective: will we ever know the optimal Hgb level in ESRD? J Am Soc Nephrol. 2018;29(10):2454–7.
19. Brier ME, Gaweda AE. Artificial intelligence for optimal anemia management in end-stage renal disease. Kidney Int. 2016;90(2):259–61.
20. Alleyne M, Horne MK, Miller JL. Individualized treatment for iron-deficiency anemia in adults. Am J Med. 2008;121(11):943–8.
21. Brookhart MA, Freburger JK, Ellis AR, Wang L, Winkelmayer WC, Kshirsagar AV. Infection risk with bolus versus maintenance iron supplementation in hemodialysis patients. J Am Soc Nephrol. 2013;24(7):1151–8.
22. Hayat A. Safety issues with intravenous iron products in the management of anemia in chronic kidney disease. Clin Med Res. 2008;6(3–4):93–102.
23. Litton E, Xiao J, Ho KM. Safety and efficacy of intravenous iron therapy in reducing requirement for allogeneic blood transfusion: systematic review and meta-analysis of randomised clinical trials. BMJ. 2013;347:f4822.
24. Macdougall IC, White C, Anker SD, et al. Intravenous iron in patients undergoing maintenance hemodialysis. N Engl J Med. 2019;380(5):447–58.
25. Wish JB. Assessing iron status: beyond serum ferritin and transferrin saturation. Clin J Am Soc Nephrol. 2006;1(Suppl 1):S4–8.
26. Gupta N, Wish JB. Hypoxia-inducible factor prolyl hydroxylase inhibitors: a potential new treatment for anemia in patients with CKD. Am J Kidney Dis. 2017;69(6):815–26.

27. van der Weerd NC, Grooteman MP, Nube MJ, ter Wee PM, Swinkels DW, Gaillard CA. Hepcidin in chronic kidney disease: not an anaemia management tool, but promising as a cardiovascular biomarker. Neth J Med. 2015;73(3):108–18.
28. Akaishi M, Hiroe M, Hada Y, et al. Effect of anemia correction on left ventricular hypertrophy in patients with modestly high hemoglobin level and chronic kidney disease. J Cardiol. 2013;62(4):249–56.
29. Can C, Emre S, Bilge I, Yilmaz A, Sirin A. Comparison of recombinant human erythropoietin and darbepoetin alpha in children. Pediatr Int. 2013;55(3):296–9.
30. Drueke TB, Locatelli F, Clyne N, et al. Normalization of hemoglobin level in patients with chronic kidney disease and anemia. N Engl J Med. 2006;355(20):2071–84.
31. Fishbane S, Nissenson AR. The new FDA label for erythropoietin treatment: how does it affect hemoglobin target? Kidney Int. 2007;72(7):806–13.
32. Fishbane S, Spinowitz B. Update on anemia in ESRD and earlier stages of CKD: core curriculum 2018. Am J Kidney Dis. 2018;71(3):423–35.
33. Jelkmann W. Molecular biology of erythropoietin. Intern Med. 2004;43(8):649–59.
34. Kaushik T, Yaqoob MM. Lessons learned from peginesatide in the treatment of anemia associated with chronic kidney disease in patients on dialysis. Biologics. 2013;7:243–6.
35. Koulouridis I, Alfayez M, Trikalinos TA, Balk EM, Jaber BL. Dose of erythropoiesis-stimulating agents and adverse outcomes in CKD: a metaregression analysis. Am J Kidney Dis. 2013;61(1):44–56.
36. Selby NM, Fonseca SA, Fluck RJ, Taal MW. Hemoglobin variability with epoetin beta and continuous erythropoietin receptor activator in patients on peritoneal dialysis. Perit Dial Int. 2012;32(2):177–82.
37. Tonelli M, Winkelmayer WC, Jindal KK, Owen WF, Manns BJ. The cost-effectiveness of maintaining higher hemoglobin targets with erythropoietin in hemodialysis patients. Kidney Int. 2003;64(1):295–304.
38. Minutolo R, Garofalo C, Chiodini P, et al. Types of erythropoiesis-stimulating agents and risk of end-stage kidney disease and death in patients with non-dialysis chronic kidney disease. Nephrol Dial Transplant. 2021;36(2):267–74.
39. Akizawa T, Nangaku M, Yamaguchi T, et al. A placebo-controlled, randomized trial of enarodustat in patients with chronic kidney disease followed by long-term trial. Am J Nephrol. 2019;49(2):165–74.
40. Besarab A, Chernyavskaya E, Motylev I, et al. Roxadustat (FG-4592): correction of anemia in incident dialysis patients. J Am Soc Nephrol. 2016;27(4):1225–33.
41. Chen N, Hao C, Liu BC, et al. Roxadustat treatment for anemia in patients undergoing long-term dialysis. N Engl J Med. 2019;381(11):1011–22.
42. Dhillon S. Roxadustat: first global approval. Drugs. 2019;79(5):563–72.
43. Haase VH. Pathophysiological consequences of HIF activation: HIF as a modulator of fibrosis. Ann N Y Acad Sci. 2009;1177:57–65.
44. Haase VH. The sweet side of HIF. Kidney Int. 2010;78(1):10–3.
45. Haase VH. HIF-prolyl hydroxylases as therapeutic targets in erythropoiesis and iron metabolism. Hemodial Int. 2017;21(Suppl 1):S110–24.
46. Haase VH. Therapeutic targeting of the HIF oxygen-sensing pathway: lessons learned from clinical studies. Exp Cell Res. 2017;356(2):160–5.
47. Haase VH. Hypoxia-inducible factor-prolyl hydroxylase inhibitors in the treatment of anemia of chronic kidney disease. Kidney Int Suppl (2011). 2021;11(1):8–25.
48. Kaplan JM, Sharma N, Dikdan S. Hypoxia-inducible factor and its role in the management of anemia in chronic kidney disease. Int J Mol Sci. 2018;19(2):389.
49. Meadowcroft AM, Cizman B, Holdstock L, et al. Daprodustat for anemia: a 24-week, open-label, randomized controlled trial in participants on hemodialysis. Clin Kidney J. 2019;12(1):139–48.
50. Parmar DV, Kansagra KA, Patel JC, et al. Outcomes of desidustat treatment in people with anemia and chronic kidney disease: a phase 2 study. Am J Nephrol. 2019;49(6):470–8.

51. Provenzano R, Besarab A, Wright S, et al. Roxadustat (FG-4592) versus epoetin alfa for anemia in patients receiving maintenance hemodialysis: a phase 2, randomized, 6- to 19-week, open-label, active-comparator, dose-ranging, safety and exploratory efficacy study. Am J Kidney Dis. 2016;67(6):912–24.
52. Mullard A. FDA approves first hypoxia-inducible factor prolyl hydroxylase inhibitor. Nat Rev Drug Discov. 2023;22(3):173.
53. Chertow GM, Pergola PE, Farag YMK, et al. Vadadustat in patients with anemia and non-dialysis-dependent CKD. N Engl J Med. 2021;384(17):1589–600.
54. Agarwal R, Anand S, Eckardt KU, et al. Overall adverse event profile of vadadustat versus darbepoetin alfa for the treatment of anemia associated with chronic kidney disease in phase 3 trials. Am J Nephrol. 2022;53(10):701–10.
55. Markham A. Vadadustat: first approval. Drugs. 2020;80(13):1365–71.
56. Hippen BE, Reed AI, Ketchersid T, Maddux FW. Implications of the advancing American Kidney Health Initiative for kidney transplant centers. Am J Transplant. 2019;20:1244.

Home Dialysis: Chronic Kidney Disease and Mineral and Bone Metabolism

19

Gates B. Colbert

Case

You are meeting with your end-stage kidney disease (ESKD) patient for their monthly comprehensive home dialysis appointment today. The patient has been on home hemodialysis for 2 years after a long diagnosis of IgA nephropathy. The patient is a 59-year-old Caucasian woman who is using a left-arm arterio-venous fistula without recent complications. As you go over the monthly blood work you mention the portion of CKD-MBD values: calcium 9.8 mg/dL, phosphorous 6.9 mg/dL, parathyroid hormone 480 pg/mL, and vitamin D 32 ng/mL. The patient is not on any oral phosphorous binders secondary to previous constipation with prescribed use. Per the hemodialysis protocol, the patient is receiving doxercalciferol IV 10 μg with each dialysis session. The patient reports adherence to a kidney diet but does enjoy drinking soda several times a day and consumes fast food three times a week. How should this patient be counseled to improve cardiovascular outcomes and reduce her overall risk?

Discussion

Bone and mineral metabolism in its simplest description is the regulation of calcium and phosphate homeostasis. The hormones that control this balance are parathyroid hormone (PTH), calcitriol or 1,25 (O2)2D_3, calcidiol or 24 (OH)D_3, calcitonin, and FGF-23/Klotho [1]. Together these hormones and minerals modulate the absorption, elimination, and deposition of calcium and phosphate and cooperate to maintain serum levels at normal ranges. The organs and glands that produce these hormones are the parathyroid glands, intestine, and kidney. The intricate and

G. B. Colbert (✉)
Texas A&M College of Medicine, Dallas, TX, USA
e-mail: Gates.Colbert@BSWHealth.org

A. Shah et al. (eds.), *Applied Home Hemodialysis*,
https://doi.org/10.1007/978-3-031-77244-3_19

dynamic kidneys are in many aspects the final effector of conserving or eliminating calcium and phosphorous content.

These minerals participate in important biological processes that maintain homeostasis of health regulation. Calcium is the body's most abundant cation with 99% of it stored in bones while only 1% is measurable in the serum, extracellular fluid, and soft tissues. Calcium participates in important life-sustaining functions of cardiac contractility, bone mineralization, and blood coagulation, and in many mechanisms of activation and secretion of other hormones and enzymes [2]. Phosphate as well is an essential mineral with 85% in the bones and 15% measurable in the serum and other tissues. It is a major component of the phospholipids of membranes, nucleotides, and nucleic acids. The kidney is able to exquisitely regulate the absorption and elimination of phosphorus and is capable of nearly complete filtrate reabsorption when necessary for serum maintenance [3]. Diagram 19.1 displays kidney site regulation of filtered phosphorus reabsorption.

When the kidney glomerular filtration begins to decline, the balance of regulation becomes lost. As the eGFR declines to later stages the normal regulatory capacity becomes almost completely eliminated, which will be discussed below. The main alterations from CKD occur in calcium, phosphate, PTH, FGF-23/Klotho, and vitamin D maintenance. Once the balance is disrupted important changes in bone and vascular metabolism lead to negative clinical consequences, such as decreased bone mass, increased fragility fractures, and increased vascular calcification [4]. Normal glomerular filtration down to around 30 mL/min/m^2 eGFR, the kidney can maintain serum calcium and phosphate values, but below 30 mL/min/m^2 eGFR the compensatory mechanisms are no longer effective. In contrast, calcitriol production begins to decline much earlier with eGFR beginning around 70 mL/min/m^2, and compensatory PTH increases around eGFR 60 mL/min/m^2 [5].

For the majority of our understanding of this balanced system, the disruption that occurs in patients with CKD was described as "renal osteodystrophy." But in 2006, the KDIGO (Kidney Disease Improving Global Outcomes) group began coining these imbalances as "CKD-MBD" which includes biochemical and bone abnormalities with the vascular and valvular calcifications as well [6]. Now well into the 2020s, CKD-MBD is the standard vernacular used as we recognize that the vascular complications are just or even more important for mortality risk than bone and mineralization disorders. Alterations of the regulatory axis of bone and mineral metabolism can have a major impact on bone modeling during pediatric growth and adulthood. Progressive CKD-MBD alterations begin in the early stages of CKD and become most impactful at stages 4 and 5 [7]. Vascular and valvular calcification increase the accelerated aging of both the circulatory and integument system.

The earliest events of CKD-MBD dysregulation begins with an increase in FGF-23 secretion, a decrease in Klotho cofactor expression, and a reduction in the kidney mass. These changes lead to the reduction of 1-alpha-hydroxylase production in the kidney parenchyma, which will result in lower levels of calcitriol, the most natural activator of the vitamin D Receptor (VDR). VDR activation is necessary for calcium absorption in the intestine and leads to the synthesis of PTH release from parathyroid glands. PTH release leads to bone turnover and resorption and will

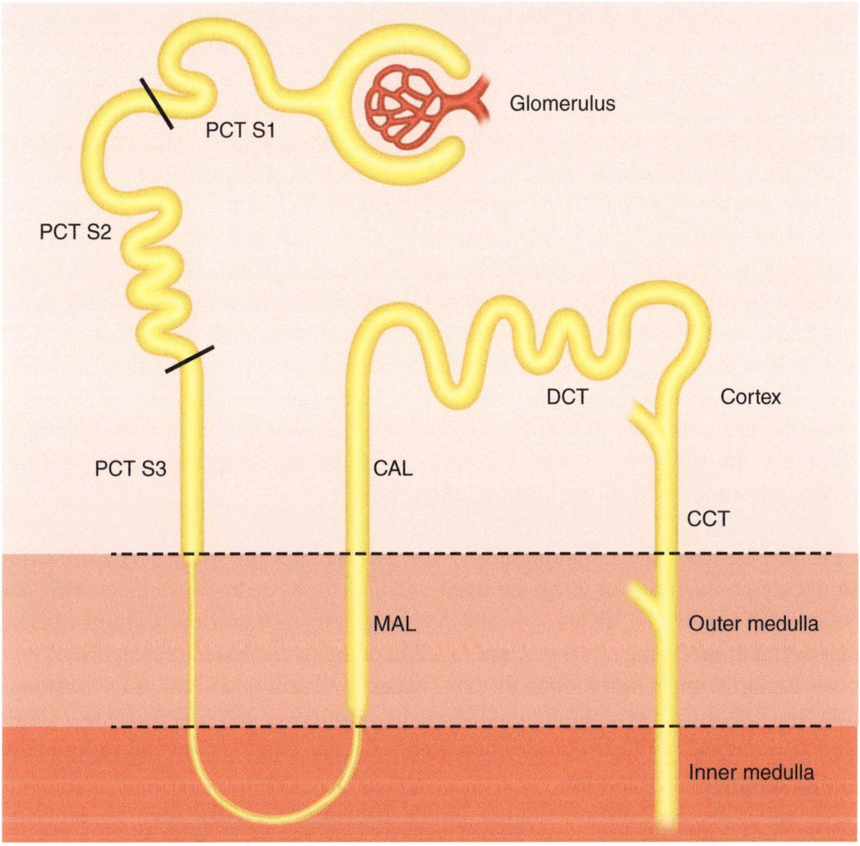

PCT = Proximal Convoluted Tubule
PST = Proximal Straight Tubule
DCT = Distal Convoluted Tubule
MAL = Medullary Ascending Limb
CAL = Cortical Ascending Limb
CCT = Cortical Collecting Limb

Phosphorus reabsorption	
PCT S1+S2	60-70%
PST	15-20%
DCT	5-10%
CAL	0%
MAL	0%

Diagram 19.1 Phosphorus absorption in nephron

go to the kidney to stimulate the production of 1-alpha-hydroxylase to help increase calcium absorption from the intestine via calcitriol. An increase in the FGF-23 and PTH production leads to increased urinary phosphate excretion to maintain normal serum levels. This becomes disrupted by stages 3–4 CKD as the loss of nephron mass develops. PTH will continue to increase over time to accelerate phosphate release from the kidney but will result in negative bone resorption consequences [8].

FGF-23 inhibits 1-alpha-hydroxylase and decreases the synthesis of calcitriol. PTH in opposite effect leads to its stimulation. FGF-23 exerts its tubular effect by binding to a Klotho co-reception whereas PTH has its own specific receptor and is not dependent upon Klotho availability. Both hormones increase phosphorous excretion by reducing the concentration of the sodium cotransporters NaPi2a and NaPi2c [7]. Calcium and calcitriol exert their actions on the parathyroid cells through receptors: calcium-sensing receptor (CaSR) and VDR. The CaSR detects small decreases in extracellular calcium concentrations and can respond within seconds to release stored PTH or halt the unneeded secretion. Unlike calcium and phosphate, calcitriol binds to VDR and exerts its mechanistic effect by reducing the transcription of the PTH synthesis on the parathyroid glands. When CKD stages progress, these complex and tightly interrelated mechanisms begin to break down and fail to control mineral metabolism, despite a compensatory increase in FGF-23 and PTH which leads to a serum phosphate increase and serum calcitriol decrease. With advanced CKD stages, the parathyroid gland is subjected to a permanent proliferative stimulus which leads to a secondary hyperparathyroidism with hyperplasia. Once the gland has mutated in size, it cannot be completely shut off from producing some amount of PTH continuously [9].

Historically patients with CKD had high bone turnover states from unregulated PTH levels. Now the contemporary issue is the opposite with a risk of over-suppressed bone turnover using the many medical tools we have available. This has occurred from several changes in the patient population and our current disease management including advanced age of CKD patients, increased prevalence of diabetes mellitus impacting kidney disease, excess calcium and vitamin D consumption, and historical use of aluminum treatments. Both over and under-turnover states lead to increased bone fragility, increased vascular calcification, and ultimately higher morbidity and mortality.

Bone tissue has several unique biomechanical properties such as fantastic mechanical tension to torsional and tensile stress. These properties allow it to have flexibility and explain why only a small proportion of bone fractures occur despite the many falls and impact traumas patients experience throughout their life. The remodeling units of these bones within a normal response to turnover allows for the building of healthy bone and the removal of old and deteriorated lattice structures. The strength of the bone is determined by its density and quality. Unfortunately, patients with CKD progression have fragile bone with high or low turnover states which leads to increased fracture risk [10]. Frustratingly, the measurement of bone mineral density (BMD) by popular methods such as the bone densitometry (DXA) does not capture bone quality well in patients with CKD. But it still has predictive value for bone fragility fractures. PTH plays a key role in the remodeling process. As PTH increases with progressive CKD, bone turnover will increase at an inappropriately accelerated rate. Osteoid deposition is abnormal and this results in lower strength and greater fragility. Very high PTH levels greater than 450 pg/mL have a reasonably good predictive value for accelerated bone turnover [11]. Low PTH levels, whether from parathyroid removal or over-suppression by medication, are associated with low bone turnover. Generally, a PTH around 120 pg/mL is associated with a low turnover state.

Management of CKD-MBD Abnormalities

Patients with progressive stages of CKD have a worsening inability to excrete excessive phosphate in the serum. The COSMOS study performed on 6790 patients with CKD stage 5 on dialysis showed that a decrease in serum phosphate levels was associated with a significant reduction in mortality [12]. Yet there are many studies that have not shown similar hard outcome improvements with different phosphate therapies. Current recommendations for controlling phosphorus in the normal range include reductions of dietary phosphate intake, appropriate use of oral phosphorous binders with meals, and improved dialysis clearance.

Action by active vitamin D, phosphate content of food, and the bioavailability of ingested phosphorous all impact gastrointestinal absorption. In a typical non-vegetarian Western diet, 60% of phosphorous intake is from protein-rich foods including dairy products, meat, fish, legumes, nuts, and chocolates. Inorganic forms of phosphorous are found in highly processed foods, and these forms have an extremely high bioavailability. This is of great interest to overall public health, as more and more Western diet populations are consuming increasing amounts of processed foods as normal daily diets. Reduction of phosphorus-containing foods is effective in controlling serum phosphorous levels but must be balanced with the risk of malnutrition in some patients.

The use of phosphorus binding agents is the most widely recommended treatment of CKD-MBD phosphorous elevations. Current phosphorous binders are listed in Table 19.1. All available phosphate binders are effective in reducing serum phosphate. There is a linear relationship between high phosphorus binder pill quantity and better phosphorus binding capability. Yet consumption of phosphate binders has many well-known side effects. Calcium-based phosphorous binders have been associated with increased vascular calcifications. Careful evaluation should be

Table 19.1 Phosphorus binders. TID = three times a day

Medication	Pharmacologic factors	Advantages	Starting dose
Calcium carbonate	Calcium based, nonmetal	Effective, inexpensive, good for low calcium states	500 mg tablet TID with meals
Calcium acetate	Calcium based, nonmetal	Effective, less calcium exposure, low cost	667 mg capsule or tablet TID with meals
Lanthanum carbonate	Noncalcium, metal-based	Calcium-free, low pill burden, palatable, safe	500 mg tablet TID with meals
Sevelamer carbonate	Noncalcium, nonmetal	Effective, calcium and aluminum free, not absorbed in GI tract	800 mg tablet or packet sprinkle TID with meals
Aluminum hydroxide	Noncalcium, metal-based	Effective, but not available in the United States	320 mg/5 mL (currently discontinued)
Ferric citrate	Noncalcium, metal-based (iron)	Effective, raises iron levels	1 g tablets, two tablets TID with meals
Sucroferric oxyhydroxide	Noncalcium, metal-based (iron)	Effective, chewable, minimal iron absorption, lower pill burden	500 mg chewable TID with meals

considered if a patient has a trend toward hypercalcemia, vascular calcification, and low bone turnover from low PTH levels. As well, aluminum-based phosphorous binders are associated with aluminum toxicity and are thus not used in the United States currently [4]. Binding agents should not be used as a preventative measure if phosphorus levels are normal or low in patients with CKD.

Hemo- and peritoneal dialysis are excellent removal treatments of phosphorus from the serum. There is no phosphorus content in dialysate and thus with high-quality membranes and fully adhered treatment time, a large quantity of phosphorus can be removed with each treatment. Even though phosphorus is easily dialyzable, the full burden of serum phosphorus is rarely completely removed during standard 3–4 h dialysis treatments as detailed below. Longer and more frequent dialysis has the greatest impact on serum levels, thus making home dialysis treatments ideal for controlling phosphorous levels [13]. Many patients on "prolonged" dialysis will still need phosphorous restriction and oral phosphorous binder intake.

According to various studies, and promoted by a recent KDIGO Home Dialysis report, home dialysis is associated with lowering or even normalizing serum phosphorus levels [14]. Likely this is related to increased frequency and time length of dialysis. Although it should be mentioned, there may be selection bias in that some of the healthiest and most adherent patients are the ones who are capable of doing home dialysis therapy. When looking at phosphorus removal during dialysis, there is usually a surplus of remaining serum phosphorus even after adequate dialysis treatments. Phosphorus behaves like a middle molecule and is negatively charged, leading to reduced dialysis clearance [15]. A typical phosphorus intake in the Western diet may absorb 5000 mg of phosphorus a week. Standard hemodialysis removes 900 mg of phosphorus, amounting to a weekly removal of 2000–2700 mg leaving 2300 mg "toxic" surplus remaining in the body [13]. There is good data from the Frequent Hemodialysis Network Daily and Nocturnal trials [16] on phosphorus removal. In patients receiving nocturnal dialysis six times per week, there was a significant reduction of phosphorus level compared to standard three times per week. Increasing dialysis frequency, which can be done with home treatments or best case scenario prolonged nocturnal dialysis, allows for greater phosphorus removal to match total weekly absorption. Thus, home hemodialysis offers a greater therapeutic advantage for dialytic control of phosphorus levels.

Those patients with CKD stage 3b-4 are suggested to maintain PTH levels in the upper normal range. Worsening stages of CKD 4–5 prior to dialysis, PTH levels can rise to the above normal range limits as this allows for a theoretical maximal phosphaturic loss by the kidney in response to a higher PTH stimulus. In patients with CKD 5 on dialysis, the exact range is more nuanced as medication use can impact values. According to KDIGO guidelines, serum calcidiol should be maintained within the safe and biologically optimal range of (20–40 pg/mL) [17]. This allows for positive effects in all stages of CKD for PTH control, cardiovascular, immune, infectious, and muscular health. The use of calcitriol replacement and other vitamin D analogs is not recommended until CKD stage 4–5 with severe and progressive hyperparathyroidism. Patients on dialysis therapy should use a combination of calcimimetics, calcitriol, or vitamin D analogs in order to reach goal PTH and calcium ranges. In the COSMOS study, the optimal PTH value of 398 pg/mL was associated with the lowest mortality in patients on dialysis [18].

Patients on hemodialysis are suggested to maintain a medication regimen to control PTH excess with calcimimetics and or the use of VDRAs. Although both are effective independently through action on the CaSR and VDR receptors, the combined use together is associated with synergistic effects. A clinician should consider levels of phosphorous and calcium when determining which agent to choose for PTH control. If VDRAs are prescribed, hyperphosphatemia or hypercalcemia will necessitate a lowering of the dose or suspension of its use. Calcimimetics and VDRAs work in concert by limiting hypercalcemia and hyperphosphatemia. If PTH falls below the normal range, both agents should be reduced or discontinued completely as the low bone turnover state is detrimental. Parathyroidectomy is encouraged when patients no longer respond to medical treatment from secondary or tertiary hyperparathyroidism. Currently, there is no exact definition of PTH level that warrants surgical evaluation. The most current practice is if patients have PTH levels above 800 pg/mL for a period longer than 6 months despite adequate medical treatment then surgical removal may be appropriate [19].

Vascular Calcification

Patients with CKD have a high prevalence of vascular calcification, that may be as high as double the population when compared with similar age, sex, and regions [20]. This inappropriate calcification leads to increased cardiovascular disease and increased mortality. One of the highest risk places for vascular calcification is the cardiac valves. Deposition in simple mechanistic terms is a combination of calcium and phosphate precipitation. However, the processes are much more complex and rely on inhibitors and promoters of vascular calcification that become disrupted as CKD progresses [21].

Promoters of calcification are various, but the most important seen in patients with CKD is phosphorus. Phosphorous is able to reach the intracellular space through a specific sodium-dependent channel called Pit1 and exerts important negative actions. When a patient has high phosphorous levels, high intracellular levels result in the activation of osteogenic factors that lead to phenotypic changes [22]. FGF-23 and Klotho are also associated with increased vascular calcification as seen in mice with knockout gene mutations. Inhibitors of vascular calcification that are disrupted in CKD include pyrophosphates and Fetuin A. Pyrophosphates, located in the vascular matrix, preserve smooth muscle phenotypes. Fetuin A is a well-known inhibitor of osteogenesis. Disruption of both of these inhibitors leads to the negative consequences of calcium deposition.

Historically, calcification of vascular tissue was considered a life-threatening complication of CKD with a low chance of improvement. As our understanding of this system has advanced, medical maneuvers and therapies have become available to help patients curb these negative outcomes. Calcification can occur at the vascular intima and media layers of vessels. Intimal calcification is associated with chronic arterial inflammation, hypertension, diabetes, hypercholesterolemia, obesity, and smoking. This progresses throughout life and can result in plaque deposition ultimately resulting in a thrombus [23]. Media calcification occurs in the elastic lamina of arteries. Frequently this is seen in patients with CKD in large-caliber arteries such as the aorta. The deposition in any layer of vascular arteries and veins is associated with a high risk of worsening cardiovascular outcomes.

Currently, there is no consensus on how to diagnose calcification of the vascular system. Advanced calcification can be seen on plain film radiograph images and echocardiograms. Computed tomography (CT) scans can determine calcium locations and have been used to develop a calcium quantification score [24]. The use of scoring and imaging has allowed therapeutic management of CKD and CV risk, but currently do not have hard guidelines [25]. One study in patients on hemodialysis showed that vascular calcifications are located in larger-caliber arteries such as the aorta in 80% of patients, medium-caliber arteries (coronary) in 70%, and small-caliber arteries in 20–30% [20]. Unfortunately, each year of dialysis exposure is associated with an increased risk of developing calcification by 15% [26].

Prevention of calcification deposition is the highest modifiable risk factor to prevent cardiovascular events in patients with CKD. This includes control of disease states known to worsen calcification such as diabetes mellitus, hypertension, and CKD stage progression. Modifiable risk factors such as tobacco avoidance, control of dyslipidemia, and limiting vitamin K inhibitors should be encouraged. Kidney or uremia-related factors should especially be activated by the treating nephrology team. These include appropriate time of dialysis length, control of hyperphosphatemia and hyperparathyroidism, improved nutrition (albumin), and lower use of vitamin D metabolites. Ultimately each patient will have varying responses to these maneuvers, but clinicians should be aggressive in trying to protect the patient's blood vessels that ultimately do not have a true reversible cure once deposition has occurred.

Calcification in some patients leads to a high mortality disease state called calciphylaxis. This affects small cutaneous arteries and is characterized by painful ischemic skin ulcerations that can lead to superimposed infections. Risk factors that have been correlated with calciphylaxis include unregulated PTH, calcium, and phosphate, although they are not always necessary culprits. The use of vitamin K inhibitors has been implicated and should be stopped in patients with calciphylaxis [27]. Management remains a challenge as there is no current cure. Currently, it is recommended to stabilize the three factors above and consider parathyroidectomy in patients with PTH levels above 800 pg/mL. Ulcerated skin lesions should be treated with antibiotics [28]. Anti-inflammatory strategies have been described [29] and the use of sodium thiosulfate is common [30]. However, a recent trial looking at the results of sodium thiosulfate use in patients with calciphylaxis has called into question its utility and effectiveness [31].

Patients with CKD are becoming increasingly older in prevalence. The association between osteoporosis and kidney osteodystrophy is thus compounded in risk in patients with advanced age [4]. Bone fragility and fractures are common and must be evaluated and treated if possible to prevent morbidity. There is increasing evidence that patients with CKD have a higher risk of fractures and associated mortality than the general population [26]. Changes that occur with age-related osteoporosis and renal osteodystrophy can be difficult to separate and thus the term "uremic osteoporosis" is sometimes used [32]. Bone mineral density from DEXA imaging is used in diagnosing osteoporosis and has good predictive utility in fracture risk for patients with CKD. Updates to the KDIGO guidelines in 2017 suggest evaluating patients with BMD in CKD patients who have risk factors [33].

Randomized drug trials of patients with osteoporosis have historically excluded patients with advanced CKD. Yet these patients with Stage 3b-5 are at some of the highest risk for fractures and in most need of treatment. Current recommendations include adequate calcium intake, normalization of calcidiol levels, and use of antiresorptive agents (bisphosphonates or Denosumab) [32]. Denosumab, which decreases the development of osteoclasts, is not eliminated by kidney filtration and should be considered as the best alternative. Hypocalcemia should be monitored closely, similarly to VDRA use in controlling PTH. Teriparatide, an anabolic drug, could be safely used for up to 2 years in parathyroidectomized patients with low bone turnover. Raloxifene, which decreases accelerated bone turnover in postmenopausal women has been used as well but experience is limited. Further studies are still needed and the current debate is ongoing [34].

Home/Nocturnal HD Benefits

Home or nocturnal hemodialysis provides several benefits over traditional three times weekly in-center hemodialysis sessions when accessing CKD-MBD parameters. Home hemodialysis is usually for longer treatment times over 4 h or may be more frequent sessions 4–5× per week. Nocturnal dialysis usually consists of prolonged sessions for 8–10 h at time. This provides increased clearance of phosphorus, uremic solutes, and ultrafiltration volume. Frequently patients on home or nocturnal HD are able to use fewer or no oral phosphorus binders. Some patients may even have hypophosphatemia and will need phosphorus supplementation with diet when pre-dialysis phosphorus levels fall below 1.4 mmol/L. A post-dialysis phosphorus level should be periodically measured in these patients to determine if severe hypophosphatemia has occurred. Chronic hypophosphatemia can lead to CKD-MBD worsening along with muscle pains and weakness. Some patients on nocturnal hemodialysis will require phosphorus added to the dialysate in the form of sodium phosphate enema aqueous solution. This is beneficial as it addresses hypophosphatemia, but avoids GI upset and diarrhea that can occur with increased oral phosphorus supplementation. Additionally, home and nocturnal dialysis patients have been associated with better-controlled PTH and Ca levels [35]. With patients having a tighter range of phosphorus and PTH levels, vascular calcification risk is lowered ultimately leading to less morbidity.

Return to Case

After discussion with the patient and education on why CKD-MBD is important for overall health you determine to start a phosphorus binder. The patient chooses to start ferric citrate as she would like the benefits of possible improvement in iron levels. Previously the patient did not tolerate calcium-based phosphorus binders or sevelamer. As well, education was completed on limiting processed foods such as the fast food that the patient eats several times a week. Counseling was completed on the high phosphorus content of soda, and that this should be limited to special occasions. The home hemodialysis prescription will remain the same given its limited capacity for phosphorus removal. The patient will continue treatments and have labs at the next monthly meeting.

Conclusion

The pathogenesis and management of patients with mineral and bone disorders have been discussed for over 50 years. Recent understanding of the pathogenesis and ways that we can alter the disease states has greatly improved in the last decade. Major guideline organizations such as KDIGO have recognized that CKD patients are at high risk for bone fracture and vascular calcification and must be managed in a more sophisticated manner than previously recognized. Our CKD patients are at the highest risk for bone fracture and cardiovascular disease outcomes, and we should pay close attention to modifying these risk factors. CKD-MBD is much more encompassing and comprehensive than renal osteodystrophy and when looking at both bone and vascular disease under an encompassing umbrella will allow us to care for patients using best practices and the latest guideline-driven treatments.

Key Points

- CKD-MBD is important to prevent cardiovascular outcomes and morbidity for patients with advanced CKD and on dialysis therapy. The main players are calcium, phosphorus, and parathyroid hormone.
- Multiple medical strategies are usually needed to control the CKD-MBD network including controlling phosphorus levels, calcium levels, vitamin D levels, and PTH levels. Diet, dialysis therapy, and medications are used together to control this axis.
- Plant-based phosphorus is much less orally bioavailable as compared with meat and processed foods.
- Diet alone in the Western diet is usually ineffective in controlling phosphorus in advanced CKD. As well, standard dialysis treatments three times per week usually lead to a serum phosphorus surplus.

References

1. Cannata-Andia J, Rodriguez-Garcia M. Metabolismo Calcio-F.sforo y sus alteraciones. In: Avendao H, editor. Nefrologia Clinica. Madrid: L. Editorial Medica Panamericana; 2015. p. 147–60.
2. Favus MJ, Goltzman D. Regulation of calcium and magnesium. In: Rosen CJ, editor. Primer on the metabolic bone diseases and disorders of mineral metabolism. Hoboken: Wiley-Blackwell; 2013. p. 171–9.
3. Vorland CJ, et al. Effects of excessive dietary phosphorus intake on bone health. Curr Osteoporos Rep. 2017;15(5):473–82.
4. Cannata Andia J, et al. Mineral and bone disorders in chronic kidney disease. In: Arici M, editor. Management of chronic kidney disease. Berlin: Springer; 2014. p. 223–39.
5. Levin A, et al. Prevalence of abnormal serum vitamin D, PTH, calcium, and phosphorus in patients with chronic kidney disease: results of the study to evaluate early kidney disease. Kidney Int. 2007;71(1):31–8.
6. Moe S, et al. Definition, evaluation, and classification of renal osteodystrophy: a position statement from kidney disease: improving global outcomes (KDIGO). Kidney Int. 2006;69(11):1945–53.
7. Olgaard K, Salusky I, Silver J. The spectrum of mineral and bone disorders in chronic kidney disease. Oxford: Oxford University Press; 2010.
8. Cannata-Andía JB, Martín-Carro B, Martín-Vírgala J, Rodríguez-Carrio J, Bande-Fernández JJ, Alonso-Montes C, Carrillo-López N. Chronic kidney disease-mineral and bone disorders: pathogenesis and management. Calcif Tissue Int. 2021;108(4):410–22. https://doi.org/10.1007/s00223-020-00777-1. Epub 2020 Nov 15.
9. Tominaga Y, et al. Histopathology, pathophysiology, and indications for surgical treatment of renal hyperparathyroidism. Semin Surg Oncol. 1997;13(2):78–86.
10. Bover J, Ureña-Torres P, Cozzolino M, Rodríguez-García M, Gómez-Alonso C. The non-invasive diagnosis of bone disorders in CKD. Calcif Tissue Int. 2021;108(4):512–27. https://doi.org/10.1007/s00223-020-00781-5. Epub 2021 Jan 4.
11. Sprague SM, et al. Diagnostic accuracy of bone turnover markers and bone histology in patients with CKD treated by dialysis. Am J Kidney Dis. 2016;67(4):559–66.
12. Fernández-Martín JL, Martínez-Camblor P, Dionisi MP, Floege J, Ketteler M, London G, Locatelli F, Gorriz JL, Rutkowski B, Ferreira A, Bos WJ, Covic A, Rodríguez-García M, Sánchez JE, Rodríguez-Puyol D, Cannata-Andia JB, COSMOS Group. Improvement of mineral and bone metabolism markers is associated with better survival in haemodialysis patients: the COSMOS study. Nephrol Dial Transplant. 2015;30(9):1542–51. https://doi.org/10.1093/ndt/gfv099. Epub 2015 Apr 28.
13. Rastogi A, Bhatt N, Rossetti S, Beto J. Management of hyperphosphatemia in end-stage renal disease: a new paradigm. J Ren Nutr. 2021;31(1):21–34. https://doi.org/10.1053/j.jrn.2020.02.003. Epub 2020 May 5.
14. Perl J, Brown EA, Chan CT, Couchoud C, Davies SJ, Kazancioğlu R, Klarenbach S, Liew A, Weiner DE, Cheung M, Jadoul M, Winkelmayer WC, Wilkie ME, for Conference Participants. Home dialysis: conclusions from a Kidney Disease: Improving Global Outcomes (KDIGO) Controversies Conference. Kidney Int. 2023;103(5):842–58. https://doi.org/10.1016/j.kint.2023.01.006. Epub 2023 Jan 31.
15. Bammens B, Evenepoel P, Verbeke K, Vanrenterghem Y. Removal of middle molecules and protein-bound solutes by peritoneal dialysis and relation with uremic symptoms. Kidney Int. 2003;64:2238–43.
16. Rocco MV, Lockridge RS Jr, Beck GJ, Eggers PW, Gassman JJ, Greene T, Larive B, Chan CT, Chertow GM, Copland M, Hoy CD, Lindsay RM, Levin NW, Ornt DB, Pierratos A, Pipkin MF, Rajagopalan S, Stokes JB, Unruh ML, Star RA, Kliger AS, Frequent Hemodialysis Network (FHN) Trial Group, Kliger A, Eggers P, Briggs J, Hostetter T, Narva A, Star R, Augustine B, Mohr P, Beck G, Fu Z, Gassman J, Greene T, Daugirdas J, Hunsicker L, Larive B, Li M,

Mackrell J, Wiggins K, Sherer S, Weiss B, Rajagopalan S, Sanz J, Dellagrottaglie S, Kariisa M, Tran T, West J, Unruh M, Keene R, Schlarb J, Chan C, McGrath-Chong M, Frome R, Higgins H, Ke S, Mandaci O, Owens C, Snell C, Eknoyan G, Appel L, Cheung A, Derse A, Kramer C, Geller N, Grimm R, Henderson L, Prichard S, Roecker E, Rocco M, Miller B, Riley J, Schuessler R, Lockridge R, Pipkin M, Peterson C, Hoy C, Fensterer A, Steigerwald D, Stokes J, Somers D, Hilkin A, Lilli K, Wallace W, Franzwa B, Waterman E, Chan C, McGrath-Chong M, Copland M, Levin A, Sioson L, Cabezon E, Kwan S, Roger D, Lindsay R, Suri R, Champagne J, Bullas R, Garg A, Mazzorato A, Spanner E, Rocco M, Burkart J, Moossavi S, Mauck V, Kaufman T, Pierratos A, Chan W, Regozo K, Kwok S. The effects of frequent nocturnal home hemodialysis: the Frequent Hemodialysis Network Nocturnal Trial. Kidney Int. 2011;80(10):1080–91. https://doi.org/10.1038/ki.2011.213. Epub 2011 Jul 20.
17. Ketteler M, Block GA, Evenepoel P, Fukagawa M, Herzog CA, McCann L, Moe SM, Shroff R, Tonelli MA, Toussaint ND, Vervloet MG, Leonard MB. Executive summary of the 2017 KDIGO chronic kidney disease-mineral and bone disorder (CKD-MBD) guideline update: what's changed and why it matters. Kidney Int. 2017;92(1):26–36. https://doi.org/10.1016/j.kint.2017.04.006. Erratum in: Kidney Int 2017 Dec;92(6):1558.
18. Fernandez-Martin JL, et al. Improvement of mineral and bone metabolism markers is associated with better survival in haemodialysis patients: the COSMOS study. Nephrol Dial Transplant. 2015;30(9):1542–51.
19. Fernandez-Martin JL, et al. COSMOS: the dialysis scenario of CKD-MBD in Europe. Nephrol Dial Transplant. 2013;28(7):1922–35.
20. Rodriguez Garcia M, Naves Diaz M, Cannata Andia JB. Bone metabolism, vascular calcifications and mortality: associations beyond mere coincidence. J Nephrol. 2005;18(4):458–63.
21. Lomashvili K, Garg P, O'Neill WC. Chemical and hormonal determinants of vascular calcification in vitro. Kidney Int. 2006;69(8):1464–70.
22. Montezano AC, et al. Vascular smooth muscle cell differentiation to an osteogenic phenotype involves TRPM7 modulation by magnesium. Hypertension. 2010;56(3):453–62.
23. London GM, et al. Inflammation, arteriosclerosis, and cardiovascular therapy in hemodialysis patients. Kidney Int Suppl. 2003;84:S88–93.
24. Raggi P. Atherosclerosis imaging to refine cardiovascular risk assessment in diabetic patients: computed tomography and positron emission tomography applications. Atherosclerosis. 2018;271:77–83.
25. Ketteler M, Floege J. Clinical management of vascular and soft tissue calcifications in chronic kidney disease patients. In: Olgaard K, Salusky I, Silver J, editors. The spectrum of mineral and bone disorders in chronic kidney disease. Oxford: Oxford University Press; 2010. p. 317–31.
26. Rodriguez-Garcia M, et al. Vascular calcifications, vertebral fractures and mortality in haemodialysis patients. Nephrol Dial Transplant. 2009;24(1):239–46.
27. Fusaro M, Cianciolo G, Evenepoel P, Schurgers L, Plebani M. Vitamin K in CKD bone disorders. Calcif Tissue Int. 2021;108(4):476–85. https://doi.org/10.1007/s00223-020-00792-2. Epub 2021 Jan 6.
28. Torregrosa JV, et al. Successful treatment of calcific uraemic arteriolopathy with bisphosphonates. Nefrologia. 2012;32(3):329–34.
29. Perelló J, et al. Mechanism of action of SNF472, a novel calcification inhibitor to treat vascular calcification and calciphylaxis. Br J Pharmacol. 2020;177(19):4400–15.
30. Singh RP, Derendorf H, Ross EA. Simulation-based sodium thiosulfate dosing strategies for the treatment of calciphylaxis. Clin J Am Soc Nephrol. 2011;6(5):1155–9.
31. Wen W, Portales-Castillo I, Seethapathy R, Durant O, Mengesha B, Krinsky S, Kroshinsky D, Kalim S, Goverman J, Nazarian RM, Chitalia V, Malhotra R, Kramann R, Malhotra CK, Nigwekar SU. Intravenous sodium thiosulphate for calciphylaxis of chronic kidney disease: a systematic review and meta-analysis. JAMA Netw Open. 2023;6(4):e2310068. https://doi.org/10.1001/jamanetworkopen.2023.10068.
32. Bover J, et al. Osteoporosis, bone mineral density and CKD-MBD complex (I): diagnostic considerations. Nefrologia. 2018;38(5):476–90.

33. Kidney Disease: Improving Global Outcomes (KDIGO) CKDMBD Update Work Group. Clinical practice guideline update for the diagnosis, evaluation, prevention, and treatment of chronic kidney disease-mineral and bone disorder (CKD-MBD). Kidney Int Suppl. 2017;7(1):1–59.
34. Evenepoel P, et al. European consensus statement on the diagnosis and management of osteoporosis in chronic kidney disease stages 4 to 5D. Nephrol Dial Transplant. 2019;36(1):42–59. https://doi.org/10.1093/ndt/gfaa192.
35. Nesrallah GE, et al. Canadian Society of Nephrology Guidelines for the management of patients with ESRD treated with intensive hemodialysis. Am J Kidney Disease. 2013;62:187.

Nutrition and Home Hemodialysis

20

Rachel Shi, Kamyar Kalantar-Zadeh, and Shivam Joshi

Hypothetical Case

Ms. Loretta Johnson is a 56-year-old female who presents to your office for follow-up. She is a police officer by day and recently switched to home hemodialysis (HHD) as she was unable to continue her occupation while on in-center dialysis thrice weekly. She is doing well on short daily hemodialysis. She wants to know if she should modify her diet since she has recently switched to HHD. Currently, she consumes a variation of the standard American diet with modifications to limit her sodium, phosphorus, and potassium intake.

Background

Chronic kidney disease (CKD) is known to cause a progressive loss of albumin, muscle, and adipose tissue, with around 30–50% of patients on dialysis developing protein-energy malnutrition [1]. Malnutrition in this vulnerable patient population may be aggravated by poor food intake, insufficient dialysis, chronic inflammation, and reduced physical activity.

R. Shi
University of Central Florida, College of Medicine, Orlando, FL, USA
e-mail: ra102934@ucf.edu

K. Kalantar-Zadeh
The Lundquist Institute at Harbor-UCLA Medical Center, Torrance, CA, USA

Tibor Rubin VA Healthcare System, Long Beach, CA, USA
e-mail: kkalantar@lundquist.org

S. Joshi (✉)
Division of Nephrology, Department of Medicine, Orlando VA Medical Center, Orlando, FL, USA
e-mail: shivam.joshi@va.gov

A. Shah et al. (eds.), *Applied Home Hemodialysis*,
https://doi.org/10.1007/978-3-031-77244-3_20

"Healthy" diet patterns are associated with a lower risk of disease progression and all-cause mortality in patients with CKD [2–4]. In addition, increased fat mass and lean body mass appear to be associated with survival advantage [5–7].

In this chapter, we briefly discuss current guidelines on diet in renal disease, summarize our understanding of electrolytes in hemodialysis (HD), and focus on the current evidence on nutrition and diets for patients on HHD. There is limited information on the nascent field of nutrition and HHD, so much of our understanding is extrapolated from nutrition in conventional hemodialysis.

Evolving Guidelines for the "Renal Diet"

Traditionally, patients on HD were advised to limit intake of fluids, phosphorus, and potassium, which typically excluded fruits, vegetables, nuts, legumes, and whole grains [8, 9]. To prevent malnutrition, the recommended protein intake for patients starting HD treatment is 1–1.2 g/kg body weight per day [6], but this can be incompatible with efforts to reduce phosphate intake [10]. These restrictive and, at times, conflicting dietary guidelines can be cumbersome to follow and deprive the patient of autonomy in one of the basic activities and enjoyments of human life [11]. This in turn may result in disregard of recommendations which can further exacerbate disease progression.

The numerous concerns about the harms of a strict low-potassium, low-phosphorus diet led to suggestions to "liberalize" the diet toward whole foods low in sodium and phosphorus and higher in fiber and antioxidants. In addition, rather than attempt to restrict phosphorus entirely, there was a shift toward reducing inorganic phosphate additives specifically from processed foods which are much more readily absorbed than organic phosphate from plant sources. Prior advice was to also limit potassium-rich foods such as fruits, vegetables, legumes, whole grains, and nuts, but it is unlikely that high-potassium-containing food increases serum potassium levels [12, 13]. For instance, one study reports that the DASH diet (with potassium-rich foods from plant-based sources) was not associated with increased potassium levels in HD patients [14]. Together, these patterns demonstrate how the guidelines for nutrition in CKD have evolved as evidence accumulates (Table 20.1).

Electrolytes

The three major electrolytes relevant to patients with renal disease are sodium, phosphorus, and potassium. Increased sodium intake may increase plasma osmolality resulting in elevated systolic blood pressure, chronic fluid overload, and weight gain [15]. In another study, limiting sodium also reduced inflammatory markers but had no change in blood pressure [16]. However, there are concerns about protein-energy wasting in sodium-restricted diets, so adequate nutritional counseling is necessary to prevent a compromise in energy and protein intake and reduce mortality.

Table 20.1 Renal dietary recommendations for hemodialysis patients. Adapted from Piccoli et al. [10]

Main "enemy" or concern	Risks	Dietary indications	Comments
Potassium	Hyperkalemia and hypokalemia can both increase mortality and arrhythmias	Restrictions on fruits and vegetables (e.g. avocados, bananas, kiwis, and dried fruit)	Can be mitigated by high dialysis efficiency and acidosis control
Phosphate	Vascular calcification, vascular aging	Restrictions on cheese, milk, shellfish	May contrast with the indications of high-protein intake
Malnutrition	Malnourished patients have increased mortality	Increased protein and calorie intake	Difficult to conciliate with previous restrictions

Phosphorus is elevated in end-stage kidney disease (ESKD) and is not removed well by hemodialysis [9]. Hyperphosphatemia contributes to bone density deficits and vascular calcification, but avoiding high-phosphorus foods may be detrimental since they are important sources of protein. This can be mitigated by avoiding processed foods with phosphate additives, boiling foods, and opting for organic sources of phosphorus [13]. Patient education on reading food labels can help decrease serum phosphorus [17], and a thorough nutritional assessment can provide individualized approaches to reducing phosphorus intake for patients without compromising protein and other qualities of their diet.

Hyperkalemia is a rare but potentially deadly complication in dialysis patients, affecting heart function, cellular membrane potential, and skeletal muscle contractility. Conversely, hypokalemia is also associated with increased mortality in dialysis patients [18]. Repeated studies demonstrate no association between dietary potassium intake and serum potassium, and high potassium plant-based diets are not associated with hyperkalemia in dialysis patients, possibly due to alkalinizing effects of plant foods, reduced potassium bioavailability and fiber-dependent potassium absorption [13, 19, 20]. Similar to sodium, guidelines caution about potassium restriction in the face of associated protein-energy wasting and since doing so often concurrently limits dietary fiber. One recommendation is to limit foods with added potassium while liberalizing natural potassium sources (e.g., vegetables and legumes), combined with cooking methods that decrease potassium availability (i.e., boiling and leaching) [21].

Nutrition in Home Hemodialysis

HHD consists of either short daily hemodialysis (6 sessions per week, each lasting 2–3 h) or nocturnal home hemodialysis (NHD; around 5 nights per week, lasting 6–8 h per session). Patients on HHD are maintained on a restriction-free diet and have less disturbance in daytime eating patterns which provides more flexibility, control, and improved quality of life for patients [22]. In addition, because of longer total dialysis time and frequency, HHD is associated with more favorable clinical outcomes compared to in-center HD (standard 3 weekly sessions) [23]. However, its prevalence is only 1.8% in the United States [23] despite known benefits of blood pressure normalization, regression of left ventricular hypertrophy, reduced hyperphosphatemia, and enhanced quality of life [22, 24, 25].

HHD patients tend to be younger and highly motivated to manage their health, so providing careful and comprehensive nutritional assessments and recommendations is crucial to both maintaining quality of life and preventing health complications. In EKRD, there is a distinction between protein-energy wasting from "poor nutrition" versus wasting from clinical conditions such as cardiovascular disease in that the latter tends to be less responsive to nutritional interventions.

Effects of Home Hemodialysis on Nutritional Status

Similar to conventional hemodialysis, HHD patients are encouraged to have high protein intake, and in some studies, NHHD patients may see an increase in appetite, energy, protein intake, dry weight, and lean body mass [23, 26]. One case series reported that NHHD patients developed an increased appetite, body weight, serum calcium and phosphate as well as increased intake of fat, protein, and potassium [27].

In comparing nutritional status on HHD versus standard HD, results are conflicting as some studies report an increased serum albumin and protein intake but no change in BMI or dry body weight in NHHD patients [28, 29], and one case series found that short daily home HD patients had an increase in energy and protein intake, confirmed by an increase in dry weight and lean body mass [26]. On the other hand, meta-analyses report no significant difference in serum albumin and protein intake [23], and analysis of data from the Frequent Hemodialysis Network Trial showed no difference in serum albumin, protein catabolic rate, or total body weight between patients undergoing NHHD versus conventional HD [30]. A cross-sectional study similarly found no difference in protein intake and nutritional status according to the subjective global assessment between HHD and standard HD patients but did find decreased cysteine and homocysteine levels in HHD patients [31]. The discrepancies may be attributed to different patient selection criteria and follow-up times. There is also currently no conclusive evidence of vitamin requirements or deficiencies in HHD patients.

Despite inconclusive and limited data about the impact of NHHD on nutritional parameters, what is more widely understood is that NHHD patients have more frequent dialysis sessions and longer total dialysis hours. This increases phosphate removal, so much that it becomes unnecessary to add phosphate to dialysate [22, 32, 33]. In addition, because of longer duration and more frequent dialysis times facilitating the elimination of waste products, HHD patients might not need to restrict potassium and fluids as much as those on conventional HD [29, 34].

While dietary recommendations for NHHD patients are limited, a recent case series reported that intradialytic total parenteral nutrition (IDTPN) with NHHD can meet daily caloric intake requirements, promote weight gain, and increase serum albumin in patients without liver disease [25], but it is unknown whether IDTPN improves patient outcomes (Table 20.2).

Limited Information on an Ideal Diet for Home Hemodialysis

The majority of Americans follow a Western diet characterized by a higher intake of energy, protein, carbohydrates, fat, phosphorus, and sodium, and lower intake of potassium and sugar compared to a "fruit and vegetable" focused dietary pattern [35]. There have been studies investigating the effects of Western, Mediterranean, "low animal protein," and plant-based diets (defined as having greater than 50% of protein sources coming from plant-based sources) on nutritional status and

Table 20.2 Summary of literature on nutrition and NHD

Topic	Article	Type of study	Main findings
Potassium	Kjellstrand et al. [34]	Multicenter observational study of 262 patients	More effective elimination of potassium and fluids so less dietary restriction of potassium and fluids needed compared to conventional HD
	Ipema et al. [29]	Systematic review with meta-analysis	
	Sikkes et al. [27]	Prospective nonrandomized study of 14 patients	Increased intake of potassium
Nutritional status			Increased appetite, body weight as well as increased intake of fat, protein
	Galland et al. [26]	Prospective nonrandomized study of 8 patients	Increase in appetite, energy, protein intake, dry weight, and lean body mass
	Miller et al. [23]	Literature review	
	Ipema et al. [29]	Systematic review with meta-analysis	Increased serum albumin and protein intake but no change in BMI or dry body weight in NHD patients
	Kaysen et al. [30]	Multicenter, prospective, randomized study using data from the Frequent Hemodialysis Network Trial	No difference in serum albumin, protein catabolic rate, or total body weight
Phosphorus	McPhatter et al. [22]	Prospective study of 12 patients	Increased phosphate removal
	Rocco et al. [33]	Prospective, randomized study of 87 patients	
	Daugirdas et al. 2012 [36]	Multicenter, prospective, randomized study using data from the Frequent Hemodialysis Network Trial	
	Copland et al. [32]	Narrative review	
	Ipema et al. [29]	Systematic review with meta-analysis	
	Sikkes et al. [27]	Prospective nonrandomized study of 14 patients	Increased serum calcium and phosphate

outcomes in hemodialysis patients [37–40]. However, there is little information on the impacts of these diets on HHD patients and if there is any difference.

While the evidence is limited on what constitutes an "ideal" diet for HHD patients, there is a case for a plant-based diet in patients with CKD in general [41, 42]. Plant sources were previously discouraged due to high potassium content in which there were concerns that fluctuations from predialysis hyperkalemia to intradialysis hypokalemia may cause arrhythmias. However, as mentioned previously, consuming high-potassium-containing foods does not always translate to increased serum potassium. In addition, plant-based foods contain higher fiber which is associated with a reduced all-cause mortality in dialysis patients [40], reduced constipation, inflammation, and uremic toxins [38], and increased fecal bulk which can facilitate potassium excretion [13]. A plant-based diet includes "vascular healthy" foods that decrease cholesterol levels [8, 21, 43], and contrary to popular belief, sufficient amounts of protein [39] (Table 20.3).

Challenges to Studying Dietary Intake

There are many explanations for the limited evidence available on nutrition and HHD and reasons to interpret nutritional studies with caution. Most of our knowledge is gleaned from observational studies on self-reported, therefore often underreported or underestimated intake. In addition, many studies on HHD do not distinguish whether effects are from a home versus. center effect or increased dialysis time. There is variable compliance (only 30–50%) with restrictive diets due to the amount of social support, perception of self-efficacy, patient understanding of food labels, cultural factors, changes in salt-taste perception, and taste acuity with increased age, or zinc deficiencies [44, 45].

There are many factors that may confound the exact measurements of electrolyte intake and serum electrolytes. It is difficult to quantify true phosphorus intake since reporting exact quantities in food products is not required by the food industry [46]. Serum potassium depends on other factors related to dialysis (blood and dialysate

Table 20.3 Modern diet for patients on HHD

Topic	Dietary indications for patients on home hemodialysis
Potassium	Fewer restrictions on potassium intake; consider a plant-based diet, especially for cardioprotective effects and to reduce constipation, inflammation, and uremia
Phosphorus	Fewer restrictions on phosphorus intake; may be unnecessary to add phosphate to dialysate
Protein	Limited evidence on this topic in home hemodialysis; recommendation for standard HD patients: 1–1.2 g/kg body weight per day
Fluids	Limited evidence on this topic in home hemodialysis; fewer restrictions on fluid intake may be acceptable
Water-soluble vitamins	Limited evidence on this topic in home hemodialysis; can increase the multivitamin dose without harm [47], but no evidence that this is necessary since deficiencies have not been identified

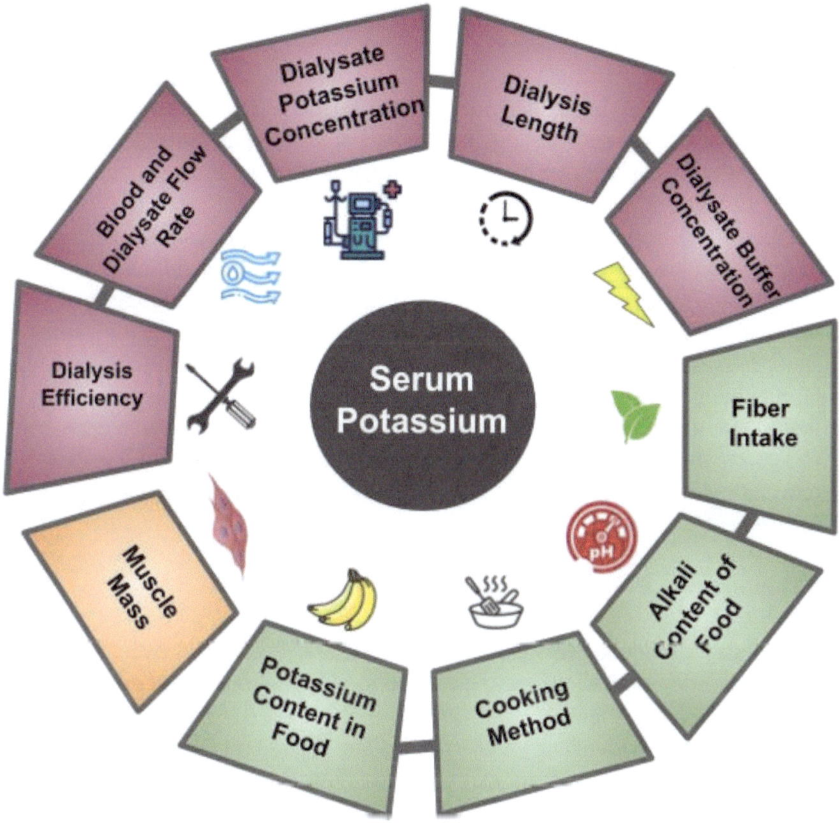

Fig. 20.1 Factors contributing to serum potassium

flow rate, dialysate K^+ and buffer concentrations, dialysis length, and efficiency), diet (fiber, alkali content, cooking methods), and the individual (muscle mass) [35, 48] (See Fig. 20.1). One possibility to overcome some of these challenges and ensure a diet with measurable nutritional qualities is providing home-delivered meals.

Future Directions

Given the proven benefits of patient comfort and improved clinical outcomes of HHD compared to standard hemodialysis, it is startling how little evidence currently exists on nutritional management for patients on HHD. It is unclear how specific diets (Western, Mediterranean, and plant based) affect nutritional status and electrolytes in HHD patients. In addition, research is needed on diet for HHD patients with comorbidities such as diabetes, obesity, and depression, so that optimized dietary recommendations can be made.

Revisiting the Case

– Ms. Loretta Johnson is inquiring about any adjustments to her current modified American diet in light of her transition to HHD. A holistic evaluation of her nutritional needs based on appetite, body weight, dietary intake, and physical examination of muscle mass and body fat would help guide management. Based on the current evidence suggesting more phosphorus removal in HHD, she may not require phosphate binders or strict phosphorus restrictions. She may not have to restrict potassium as much while on HHD and could consider a plant-based, low animal protein, and high-fiber diet for its cardiovascular and anti-inflammatory benefits. Overall, there is limited information on nutrition and short daily hemodialysis, so she will need to be closely monitored through regular biochemical tests for vitamin and electrolyte levels. Caregivers may be solicited to encourage appetite and adequate dietary intake. She may be encouraged to keep a food journal and increase physical activity, which will help reduce mortality and could facilitate her returning to work if she wishes.

Key Points

- The dietary guidelines for patients with ESKD have evolved over the decades from restricting potassium and phosphate to recognizing a protein wasting and malnutrition issue, together which are not feasible for patients to adhere to.
- There is limited evidence from prospective studies and randomized control trials that HHD patients may not need to restrict potassium and phosphate as much because of increased dialysis frequency and total dialysis time.
- No ideal dietary "prescription" for patients on HHD exists, and individualized nutritional assessments with a multidisciplinary team are needed. Improvements in patient quality of life and dietary adherence may be achieved by enhancing patient self-efficacy, education, autonomy, and access to food, as well as addressing other factors related to dietary habits such as attitudes to food, depression, and cognitive function.

References

1. Carrero JJ, Hecking M, Chesnaye NC, Jager KJ. Sex and gender disparities in the epidemiology and outcomes of chronic kidney disease. Nat Rev Nephrol. 2018;14(3):151–64.
2. Kelly JT, Palmer SC, Wai SN, Ruospo M, Carrero J-J, Campbell KL, et al. Healthy dietary patterns and risk of mortality and ESRD in CKD: a meta-analysis of cohort studies. Clin J Am Soc Nephrol. 2017;12(2):272–9.
3. Gutiérrez OM, Muntner P, Rizk DV, McClellan WM, Warnock DG, Newby P, et al. Dietary patterns and risk of death and progression to ESRD in individuals with CKD: a cohort study. Am J Kidney Dis. 2014;64(2):204–13.

4. Hu EA, Coresh J, Anderson CA, Appel LJ, Grams ME, Crews DC, et al. Adherence to healthy dietary patterns and risk of CKD progression and all-cause mortality: findings from the CRIC (chronic renal insufficiency cohort) study. Am J Kidney Dis. 2021;77(2):235–44.
5. Noori N, Kovesdy CP, Dukkipati R, Kim Y, Duong U, Bross R, et al. Survival predictability of lean and fat mass in men and women undergoing maintenance hemodialysis. Am J Clin Nutr. 2010;92(5):1060–70.
6. Ikizler TA, Burrowes JD, Byham-Gray LD, Campbell KL, Carrero J-J, Chan W, et al. KDOQI clinical practice guideline for nutrition in CKD: 2020 update. Am J Kidney Dis. 2020;76(3):S1–S107.
7. Kalantar-Zadeh K, Rhee CM, Chou J, Ahmadi SF, Park J, Chen JL, et al. The obesity paradox in kidney disease: how to reconcile it with obesity management. Kidney Int Rep. 2017;2(2):271–81.
8. Kalantar-Zadeh K, Tortorici AR, Chen JL, Kamgar M, Lau WL, Moradi H, et al., editors. Dietary restrictions in dialysis patients: is there anything left to eat? Seminars in dialysis. Hoboken: Wiley; 2015.
9. Daugirdas JT, Depner TA, Inrig J, Mehrotra R, Rocco MV, Suri RS, et al. KDOQI clinical practice guideline for hemodialysis adequacy: 2015 update. Am J Kidney Dis. 2015;66(5):884–930.
10. Piccoli GB, Moio MR, Fois A, Sofronie A, Gendrot L, Cabiddu G, et al. The diet and haemodialysis dyad: three eras, four open questions and four paradoxes. A narrative review, towards a personalized, patient-centered approach. Nutrients. 2017;9(4):372.
11. Palmer SC, Hanson CS, Craig JC, Strippoli GF, Ruospo M, Campbell K, et al. Dietary and fluid restrictions in CKD: a thematic synthesis of patient views from qualitative studies. Am J Kidney Dis. 2015;65(4):559–73.
12. Clase CM, Carrero J-J, Ellison DH, Grams ME, Hemmelgarn BR, Jardine MJ, et al. Potassium homeostasis and management of dyskalemia in kidney diseases: conclusions from a Kidney Disease: Improving Global Outcomes (KDIGO) Controversies Conference. Kidney Int. 2020;97(1):42–61.
13. St-Jules DE, Goldfarb DS, Sevick MA. Nutrient non-equivalence: does restricting high-potassium plant foods help to prevent hyperkalemia in hemodialysis patients? J Ren Nutr. 2016;26(5):282–7.
14. Garagarza C, Valente A, Caetano C, Ramos I, Sebastião J, Pinto M, et al. Potassium intake—(un) expected non-predictor of higher serum potassium levels in hemodialysis DASH diet consumers. Nutrients. 2022;14(10):2071.
15. DeSimone JA, Beauchamp GK, Drewnowski A, Johnson GH. Sodium in the food supply: challenges and opportunities. Nutr Rev. 2013;71(1):52–9.
16. Rodrigues Telini LS, de Carvalho Beduschi G, Caramori JCT, Castro JH, Martin LC, Barretti P. Effect of dietary sodium restriction on body water, blood pressure, and inflammation in hemodialysis patients: a prospective randomized controlled study. Int Urol Nephrol. 2014;46:91–7.
17. Sullivan C, Sayre SS, Leon JB, Machekano R, Love TE, Porter D, et al. Effect of food additives on hyperphosphatemia among patients with end-stage renal disease: a randomized controlled trial. JAMA. 2009;301(6):629–35.
18. Torlén K, Kalantar-Zadeh K, Molnar MZ, Vashistha T, Mehrotra R. Serum potassium and cause-specific mortality in a large peritoneal dialysis cohort. Clin J Am Soc Nephrol. 2012;7(8):1272–84.
19. Ramos CI, González-Ortiz A, Espinosa-Cuevas A, Avesani CM, Carrero JJ, Cuppari L. Does dietary potassium intake associate with hyperkalemia in patients with chronic kidney disease? Nephrol Dial Transplant. 2021;36(11):2049–57.
20. Babich JS, Kalantar-Zadeh K, Joshi S. Taking the kale out of hyperkalemia: plant foods and serum potassium in patients with kidney disease. J Ren Nutr. 2022;32:641.
21. Biruete A, Jeong JH, Barnes JL, Wilund KR. Modified nutritional recommendations to improve dietary patterns and outcomes in hemodialysis patients. J Ren Nutr. 2017;27(1):62–70.
22. McPhatter LL, Lockridge RS Jr, Albert J, Anderson H, Craft V, Jennings FM, et al. Nightly home hemodialysis: improvement in nutrition and quality of life. Adv Ren Replace Ther. 1999;6(4):358–65.

23. Miller BW, Himmele R, Sawin D-A, Kim J, Kossmann RJ. Choosing home hemodialysis: a critical review of patient outcomes. Blood Purif. 2018;45(1–3):224–9.
24. Trinh E, Chan CT. Intensive home hemodialysis results in regression of left ventricular hypertrophy and better clinical outcomes. Am J Nephrol. 2016;44(4):300–7.
25. Pasricha SV, Allard JP, Alqarni KA, Davis MJ, Chan CT. Case studies of intradialytic total parenteral nutrition in nocturnal home hemodialysis. J Ren Nutr. 2023;33(1):219–22.
26. Galland R, Traeger J, Arkouche W, Cleaud C, Delawari E, Fouque D. Short daily hemodialysis rapidly improves nutritional status in hemodialysis patients. Kidney Int. 2001;60(4):1555–60.
27. Sikkes ME, Kooistra MP, Weijs PJ. Improved nutrition after conversion to nocturnal home hemodialysis. J Ren Nutr. 2009;19(6):494–9.
28. Ipema KJ, van der Schans CP, Vonk N, de Vries JM, Westerhuis R, Duym E, et al. A difference between day and night: protein intake improves after the transition from conventional to frequent nocturnal home hemodialysis. J Ren Nutr. 2012;22(3):365–72.
29. Ipema KJ, Struijk S, van der Velden A, Westerhuis R, van der Schans CP, Gaillard CA, et al. Nutritional status in nocturnal hemodialysis patients—a systematic review with meta-analysis. PLoS One. 2016;11(6):e0157621.
30. Kaysen GA, Greene T, Larive B, Mehta RL, Lindsay RM, Depner TA, et al. The effect of frequent hemodialysis on nutrition and body composition: Frequent Hemodialysis Network Trial. Kidney Int. 2012;82(1):90–9.
31. Kannampuzha J, Donnelly SM, McFarlane PA, Chan CT, House JD, Pencharz PB, et al. Glutathione and riboflavin status in supplemented patients undergoing home nocturnal hemodialysis versus standard hemodialysis. J Ren Nutr. 2010;20(3):199–208.
32. Copland M, Komenda P, Weinhandl ED, McCullough PA, Morfin JA. Intensive hemodialysis, mineral and bone disorder, and phosphate binder use. Am J Kidney Dis. 2016;68(5):S24–32.
33. Rocco MV, Lockridge RS Jr, Beck GJ, Eggers PW, Gassman JJ, Greene T, et al. The effects of frequent nocturnal home hemodialysis: the Frequent Hemodialysis Network Nocturnal Trial. Kidney Int. 2011;80(10):1080–91.
34. Kjellstrand C, Buoncristiani U, Ting G, Traeger J, Piccoli GB, Sibai-Galland R, et al. Survival with short-daily hemodialysis: association of time, site, and dose of dialysis. Hemodial Int. 2010;14(4):464–70.
35. Palmer BF, Clegg DJ. Potassium metabolism in chronic kidney disease. Chronic renal disease. New York: Elsevier; 2020. p. 643–59.
36. John T, Daugirdas GM, Chertow B, Larive A, Pierratos T, Greene JC, Ayus CA, Kendrick SH, James BW, Miller G, Schulman IB, Salusky AS, Kliger. Effects of frequent hemodialysis on measures of CKD mineral and bone disorder. J Am Soc Nephrol. 2012;23(4):727–38. https://doi.org/10.1681/ASN.2011070688
37. Garagarza C, Valente A, Caetano C, Ramos I, Sebastião J, Pinto M, et al. Mediterranean diet: a dietary pattern related to nutritional benefits for hemodialysis patients. J Ren Nutr. 2023;33(3):472–81.
38. Kandouz S, Mohamed AS, Zheng Y, Sandeman S, Davenport A. Reduced protein bound uraemic toxins in vegetarian kidney failure patients treated by haemodiafiltration. Hemodial Int. 2016;20(4):610–7.
39. Joshi S, Shah S, Kalantar-Zadeh K. Adequacy of plant-based proteins in chronic kidney disease. J Ren Nutr. 2019;29(2):112–7.
40. Saglimbene VM, Wong G, Ruospo M, Palmer SC, Garcia-Larsen V, Natale P, et al. Fruit and vegetable intake and mortality in adults undergoing maintenance hemodialysis. Clin J Am Soc Nephrol. 2019;14(2):250–60.
41. Joshi S, McMacken M, Kalantar-Zadeh K. Plant-based diets for kidney disease: a guide for clinicians. Am J Kidney Dis. 2021;77(2):287–96.
42. Dupuis L, Brown-Tortorici A, Kalantar-Zadeh K, Joshi S. A mini review of plant-based diets in hemodialysis. Blood Purif. 2021;50(4–5):672–7.
43. Xie L-M, Ge Y-Y, Huang X, Zhang Y-Q, Li J-X. Effects of fermentable dietary fiber supplementation on oxidative and inflammatory status in hemodialysis patients. Int J Clin Exp Med. 2015;8(1):1363.

44. McMahon EJ, Campbell KL, Bauer JD. Taste perception in kidney disease and relationship to dietary sodium intake. Appetite. 2014;83:236–41.
45. Kim SM, Kim M, Lee EK, Kim SB, Chang JW, Kim HW. The effect of zinc deficiency on salt taste acuity, preference, and dietary sodium intake in hemodialysis patients. Hemodial Int. 2016;20(3):441–6.
46. Curtis PA. OSHA regulations and the food industry. Guide to US food laws and regulations. New York: Wiley; 2013. p. 143–60.
47. Pierratos A, Ouwendyk M, Francoeur R, Vas S, Raj DS, Ecclestone AM, Langos V, Uldall R. Nocturnal hemodialysis. J Am Soc Nephrol. 1998;9(5):859–68. https://doi.org/10.1681/ASN.V95859
48. Sanghavi S, Whiting S, Uribarri J, editors. Potassium balance in dialysis patients. Seminars in dialysis. Hoboken: Wiley; 2013.

Index

A. Shah et al. (eds.), *Applied Home Hemodialysis*,
https://doi.org/10.1007/978-3-031-77244-3

MIX
Papier aus verantwortungsvollen Quellen
Paper from responsible sources
FSC® C105338

If you have any concerns about our products,
you can contact us on
ProductSafety@springernature.com

In case Publisher is established outside the EU,
the EU authorized representative is:
Springer Nature Customer Service Center GmbH
Europaplatz 3, 69115 Heidelberg, Germany

Printed by Libri Plureos GmbH
in Hamburg, Germany